Lower Facial Rejuvenation: A Multispecialty Approach

Editors

SHAI N. ROZEN
LISA E. ISHII

CLINICS IN
PLASTIC SURGERY

www.plasticsurgery.theclinics.com

October 2018 • Volume 45 • Number 4

ELSEVIER

1600 John F. Kennedy Boulevard • Suite 1800 • Philadelphia, Pennsylvania, 19103-2899

http://www.theclinics.com

CLINICS IN PLASTIC SURGERY Volume 45, Number 4
October 2018 ISSN 0094-1298, ISBN-13: 978-0-323-64118-0

Editor: Jessica McCool
Developmental Editor: Meredith Madeira

Clinics in Plastic Surgery (ISSN 0094-1298) is published quarterly by Elsevier Inc., 360 Park Avenue South, New York, NY 10010-1710. Months of issue are January, April, July, and October. Business and Editorial Offices: 1600 John F. Kennedy Blvd., Suite 1800, Philadelphia, PA 19103-2899. Periodicals postage paid at New York, NY and additional mailing offices. Subscription prices are $525.00 per year for US individuals, $882.00 per year for US institutions, $100.00 per year for US students and residents, $595.00 per year for Canadian individuals, $1050.00 per year for Canadian institutions, $636.00 per year for international individuals, $1050.00 per year for international institutions, and $305.00 per year for Canadian and international students/residents. To receive student/resident rate, orders must be accompanied by name of affiliated institution, date of term, and the *signature* of program/residency coordinator on institution letterhead. Orders will be billed at individual rate until proof of status is received. Foreign air speed delivery is included in all *Clinics* subscription prices. All prices are subject to change without notice. **POSTMASTER:** Send address changes to *Clinics in Plastic Surgery*, Elsevier Health Sciences Division, Subscription Customer Service, 3251 Riverport Lane, Maryland Heights, MO 63043. **Customer Service: 1-800-654-2452 (US and Canada). From outside of the United States and Canada, call 314-447-8871. Fax: 314-447-8029. E-mail: JournalsCustomerService-usa@elsevier.com (for print support); JournalsOnlineSupport-usa@ elsevier.com (for online support).**

Reprints. For copies of 100 or more of articles in this publication, please contact the Commercial Reprints Department, Elsevier Inc., 360 Park Avenue South, New York, New York 10010-1710. Tel.: +1-212-633-3874; Fax: +1-212-633-3820; E-mail: reprints@elsevier.com.

Clinics in Plastic Surgery is covered in *Current Contents, EMBASE/Excerpta Medica, Science Citation Index, MEDLINE/ PubMed (Index Medicus), ASCA,* and *ISI/BIOMED.*

Contributors

EDITORS

SHAI N. ROZEN, MD, FACS
Professor of Plastic and Reconstructive
Surgery, Director of the Facial Paralysis
Center and Microsurgery Program at UTSW,
Department of Plastic and Reconstructive
Surgery, The University of Texas Southwestern
Medical Center, Dallas, Texas, USA

LISA E. ISHII, MD, MHS
Associate Professor of Otolaryngology,
Department of Otolaryngology–Head and Neck
Surgery, Johns Hopkins School of Medicine,
Baltimore, Maryland, USA

AUTHORS

ANDRÉ AUERSVALD, MD
Clínica Auersvald de Cirurgia Plástica, Curitiba,
Paraná, Brazil

LUIZ A. AUERSVALD, MD
Clínica Auersvald de Cirurgia Plástica, Curitiba,
Paraná, Brazil

FRANCISCO G. BRAVO, MD, PhD
Clinica Gomez Bravo, Madrid, Spain

LUCAS M. BRYANT, MD
New York Center for Facial Plastic
and Laser Surgery, New York, New York,
USA

KATHERINE H. CARRUTHERS, MD, MS
Resident, Department of Surgery,
Division of Plastic Surgery, West Virginia
University, Morgantown, West Virginia,
USA

DINO ELYASSNIA, MD
Marten Clinic of Plastic Surgery, San
Francisco, California, USA

FRED G. FEDOK, MD, FACS
Facial Plastic and Reconstructive Surgery,
Fedok Plastic Surgery, Foley, Alabama, USA;
Adjunct Professor, Department of Surgery,
University of South Alabama, Mobile, Alabama,
USA

ANDREW JACONO, MD, FACS
Associate Clinical Professor Facial Plastic
Surgery, Department of Otolaryngology/Head
and Neck Surgery, Albert Einstein College of
Medicine, Bronx, New York, USA; New York
Center for Facial Plastic and Laser Surgery,
New York, New York, USA

NATALIE R. JOUMBLAT, BS
Research Associate, Division of Plastic,
Reconstructive, Aesthetic and Transgender
Surgery, LGBTQ Center for Wellness, Gender
and Sexual Health, University of Miami Hospital,
Jackson Memorial Hospital, Miami, Florida, USA

JEFFREY M. KENKEL, MD, FACS
Professor, Chairman, Betty and Warren
Woodward Chair in Plastic and Reconstructive
Surgery, Director, Department of Plastic
Surgery, Clinical Center for Cosmetic Laser
Treatment, Dallas, Texas, USA

TIMOTHY MARTEN, MD
Marten Clinic of Plastic Surgery,
San Francisco, California, USA

AJANI G. NUGENT, MD
Assistant Professor of Surgery, Division of
Plastic, Reconstructive, Aesthetic and
Transgender Surgery, LGBTQ Center for
Wellness, Gender and Sexual Health,
University of Miami Hospital, Jackson
Memorial Hospital, Miami, Florida, USA

T. GERALD O'DANIEL, MD, FACS
Assistant Clinical Professor of Surgery, Department of Plastic Surgery, University of Louisville, Louisville, Kentucky, USA

IRA D. PAPEL, MD
Professor, Division of Facial Plastic and Reconstructive Surgery, Department of Otolaryngology–Head and Neck Surgery, Johns Hopkins School of Medicine, Facial Plastic Surgicenter, Baltimore, Maryland, USA

CHRISTOPHER J. SALGADO, MD
Professor of Surgery, Interim Chief, Division of Plastic, Reconstructive, Aesthetic and Transgender Surgery, Medical Director, LGBTQ Center for Wellness, Gender and Sexual Health, University of Miami Hospital, Jackson Memorial Hospital, Miami, Florida, USA

THOMAS SATTERWAITE, MD
Plastic and Craniofacial Surgeon, Brownstein & Crane Surgical Services, Greenbrae, California, USA

DAVID A. SIEBER, MD
Private Practice, Sieber Plastic Surgery, San Francisco, California, USA

RYAN M. SMITH, MD
Clinical Fellow, Division of Facial Plastic and Reconstructive Surgery, Department of Otolaryngology–Head and Neck Surgery, Johns Hopkins School of Medicine, Baltimore, Maryland, USA

CATHERINE WINSLOW, MD, FACS
Assistant Clinical Professor, Indiana University School of Medicine, Indianapolis, Indiana, USA

Contents

Understanding Deep Neck Anatomy and Its Clinical Relevance 447

T. Gerald O'Daniel

In deep central necklift surgery, the first step to safely and effectively modify all of the relevant components is a thorough understanding of the nuances of the complex anatomic relationships and variations within the confined space of the deep central neck. There are anatomic variations that defy our traditional approaches to create the ideal neck in the aging patient as well as the young patient. This article concentrates on the surgically relevant anatomy of the deep central neck.

Neck Lift: Defining Anatomic Problems and Choosing Appropriate Treatment Strategies 455

Timothy Marten and Dino Elyassnia

Success or failure in treating the neck lies in the diagnosis of underlying problems and the application of a logical surgical plan. Although it is a commonly advocated practice, it is not enough to perform submental liposuction and tighten the skin in most patients, as such an approach ignores a number of anatomic problems present in many patients seeking neck improvement. Removing subcutaneous fat and tightening skin over these problems does not correct them, and the presence or absence of each must be looked for to create and apply an appropriate surgical plan.

Reduction Neck Lift: The Importance of the Deep Structures of the Neck to the Successful Neck Lift 485

Francisco G. Bravo

 Video content accompanies this article at http://www.plasticsurgery.theclinics.com/.

A description of the deep structures of the neck that are responsible for submandibular fullness and a systematic surgical approach to reduce them are presented. The structures susceptible to surgical management include the subplatysmal fat, intersternocleidomastoid origin fat, anterior belly of the digastric muscle, hyoid bone, submandibular gland, and the tail of the parotid gland. A thorough analysis of the key anatomic landmarks of the young and attractive neck is detailed in resting and dynamic positions. A clinical classification of parotid reduction in the face lift/neck lift patient is also presented.

Management of the Submandibular Gland in Neck Lifts: Indications, Techniques, Pearls, and Pitfalls 507

André Auersvald and Luiz A. Auersvald

 Video content accompanies this article at http://www.plasticsurgery.theclinics.com/.

Neck contour deformities are common among patients who present for facial rejuvenation. A thorough physical examination and photographic analysis, including an upward view of the flexed neck, enable the surgeon to determine which structures should be treated. Common causes of neck concerns include hypertrophy of the subplatysmal fat, the anterior belly of the digastric muscle, and/or the submandibular salivary glands. Partial removal of the submandibular salivary glands requires advanced knowledge of subplatysmal anatomy and surgical expertise but can be performed safely and reliably to yield favorable results of neck rejuvenation.

procedure is performed through a submental incision without any removal of skin and relies on modification of deep-layer structures to improve neck contour. "Excess" skin is allowed to redistribute itself over the increased neck surface area created when deep-layer maneuvers are performed, neck contour is improved, and the cervicomental angle deepened. For properly selected patients, the procedure can produce a marked improvement in facial appearance.

CLINICS IN PLASTIC SURGERY

FORTHCOMING ISSUES

January 2019
Plastic Surgery After Weight Loss
Jeffrey A. Gusenoff, *Editor*

April 2019
Pediatric Craniofacial Plastic Surgery: State of the Craft
Edward P. Buchanan, *Editor*

July 2019
Repairing and Reconstructing the Hand and Wrist
Kevin C. Chung, *Editor*

RECENT ISSUES

July 2018
Gender Confirmation Surgery
Loren S. Schechter and Bauback Safa, *Editors*

April 2018
Gluteal Augmentation
Robert F. Centeno and Constantino G. Mendieta, *Editors*

January 2018
Contemporary Indications in Breast Reconstruction
Jian Farhadi, Stefan O.P. Hofer, and Jaume Masia, *Editors*

SERIES OF RELATED INTEREST

Facial Plastic Surgery Clinics
Otolaryngologic Clinics
Advances in Cosmetic Surgery
Dermatologic Clinics

Preface
Lower Facial Rejuvenation

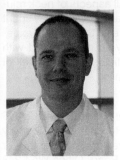 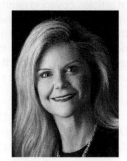

Shai N. Rozen, MD, FACS   Lisa E. Ishii, MD, MHS

Editors

Traditionally, when facial rejuvenation was discussed, the face would receive the majority of the attention. Over the last decade, it has increasingly recognized that, in most cases without excellent concomitant neck rejuvenation, the overall result of a face–neck-lift will be average rather than superb. In fact, some authors would argue that the highest yield in satisfaction is provided by an excellent result in the neck component of the facial rejuvenation. The motifs in neck rejuvenation have also changed over the years, similarly to the face, but lagging by several decades. Initially, during the Skoog days, the emphasis in face-lifts was on skin excision and later evolved into manipulating the deeper layer (the SMAS); analogously, the neck has also undergone a parallel evolution, although at a slower pace and perhaps with more controversy. Before any discussion on surgical technique occurs, an in-depth understanding of anatomy is essential. Dr O'Daniel provides an outstanding and in-depth review of deep neck anatomy and its clinical relevance. Procedures of the deep layers of the neck, including the submandibular gland and digastric muscle reductions, may provide the desired result in a considerable number of patients and can result in superb outcomes that otherwise may not have seemed possible. Yet, gland and muscle reduction are technically demanding, involve a steep learning curve, and are still controversial. Superb and incredibly detailed and thoughtful articles are provided by Drs Marten and Elyassnia, emphasizing how to analyze the neck and provide logical and problem-oriented solutions, followed by technically detailed articles by Dr Bravo and Drs André Auersvald and Luiz Auersvald. As previously noted, most patients will have combined midface and neck rejuvenation as these are often inseparable, and a harmonious result is provided when both are addressed. Drs Jacono and Bryant provide excellent insights on this relationship and necessary steps to blend the midface, jawline, and neck. The platysma is without doubt the one common structure that is invariably addressed in neck rejuvenation, yet there is certainly not one common approach. Drs Marten and Elyassnia provide a very thoughtful and analytical approach to the platysma, avoiding the temptation of a cookie cutter approach but rather providing a very patient, problem-oriented approach. They also address the less common patient group, which may benefit solely from a neck lift without a concomitant midface rejuvenation, providing insights regarding patient selection and technical details on performing short-scar neck-lifts.

As we all know, midface rejuvenation is incomplete without addressing the periorbital region and the skin. Similarly, to attain optimal neck rejuvenation results, the surgeon frequently needs to also address the skin and the perioral area. In fact, with the increasing use of fillers, lasers, IPLs (intense pulsed lights), and other emerging technologies, it is very common that patients will initially ask for these procedures, later committing to surgery. These modalities are necessary in the armamentarium of surgeons interested in facial and neck rejuvenation. Excellent and comprehensive articles are provided by Drs Sieber and Kenkel discussing noninvasive

Clin Plastic Surg 45 (2018) ix–x
https://doi.org/10.1016/j.cps.2018.07.001
0094-1298/18/© 2018 Published by Elsevier Inc.

methods for lower facial rejuvenation and Dr Winslow discussing surgical and nonsurgical perioral and lip rejuvenation beyond solely volume restoration.

This or any issue would not be complete without discussing challenges and unsolved problems. Drs Papel and Smith masterfully discuss this difficult and essential subject. Dealing with complications and more importantly avoiding or minimizing them is probably one of the most difficult and important subjects in any surgical discussion. Most surgeons prefer to discuss these in private or not at all. It is only the experienced and confident surgeon that is willing to tackle such a subject so we may all benefit from their experience. We thank Dr Fedok for sharing his knowledge and willingness to attack this subject with such agility.

Last, but not least, perhaps one of the fastest emerging areas in facial rejuvenation, which truly enables us to learn and develop techniques for all populations, is gender reassignment. This fascinating field provides insights about patient preferences and further expands our surgical horizons into areas that have traditionally not been part of traditional neck rejuvenation discussion. Dr Salgado, one of the leaders in this area, shares his vast experience and superb insights in this emerging field.

We want to thank all of the surgeons who helped create this fantastic and comprehensive collection of articles covering nearly all aspects of neck rejuvenation. It is not only the valuable time they spent that we appreciate, but more so the years of experience and knowledge they so aptly shared with us, further developing the field and helping all of us optimize our patient results.

Shai N. Rozen, MD, FACS
Department of Plastic and Reconstructive Surgery
University of Texas Southwestern Medical Center
1801 Inwood Road, Office WA4.248
Dallas, Texas 75390-9132, USA

Lisa E. Ishii, MD, MHS
Department of Otolaryngology–
Head and Neck Surgery
Johns Hopkins School of Medicine
10751 Falls Road, Suite 406
Lutherville, MD 21093, USA

E-mail addresses:
shai.rozen@utsouthwestern.edu (S.N. Rozen)
learnes2@jhmi.edu (L.E. Ishii)

Understanding Deep Neck Anatomy and Its Clinical Relevance

T. Gerald O'Daniel, MD*

KEYWORDS

• Necklift • Submandibular gland reduction • Subplatysmal fat • Digastric muscle • Platysma muscle

KEY POINTS

- Surgery of the central neck is complex due to the number of anatomic structures encountered in a confined space with limited distant access.
- A thorough understanding of the complex anatomy and the 3-dimensional relationship of these structures is crucial to safely and efficiently perform surgery on the subplatysmal structures.
- Clinical pictures from surgery and anatomy laboratory dissections are used to illustrate the most pertinent structures encountered in subplatysmal surgery.

INTRODUCTION

In aesthetic neck surgery, we are more widely recognizing that all necks are not created equally. There is increasing interest in understanding surgery of the deep central neck that previously has been practiced by few surgeons. There are anatomic variations that defy our traditional approaches to create the ideal neck in the aging patient as well as the young patient. These variations are related to the 3-dimensional relationship of the volume of deep central neck soft tissue structures, deep fat, musculature, fascial attachments, and submandibular glands, to the skeletal confinements of the mandible. When this discrepancy between soft issue volume and the skeletal structure that must contain it occurs, we are often required to give surgical attention to these anatomic characteristics and modify relative deep neck components to create an optimal aesthetically pleasing cervicomental angle (**Figs. 1** and **2**).

In deep central necklift surgery, the first step to safely and effectively modify all of the relevant components is a thorough understanding of the nuances of the complex anatomic relationships and variations within the confined space of the deep central neck. This article concentrates on the surgically relevant anatomy and is presented in the order that the surgeon will encounter each structure.

SUBMENTAL TRIANGLE

The platysma are paired, broad elastic muscles that originate from the deltopectoral fascia and inserts into the base of the mandible and into the modiolus of the lower lip. The labial component of the platysma is referred to as the pars labialis platysma and runs beneath the depressor anguli oris and lateral to the depressor labia inferioris muscles.[1] The cervical branch of the facial nerve innervates the platysma. The platysma acts as a depressor to the lateral lip and injury to the platysma or its innervation can lead to lower lip depressor dysfunction. The platysma muscle and the deep investing fascia form the roof of the submental and submandibular triangles. The paired platysma muscle has varied interdigitations in the

Disclosure Statement: The author has nothing to disclose.
Department of Plastic Surgery, University of Louisville, Louisville, KY, USA
* 132 Chenoweth Lane, Louisville, KY 40207.
E-mail address: jerry.odaniel@gmail.com

Clin Plastic Surg 45 (2018) 447–454
https://doi.org/10.1016/j.cps.2018.06.011

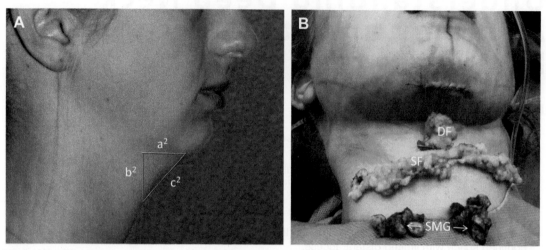

Fig. 1. (*A*) A 20-year-old preoperative. Space within the triangle is occupied by soft tissue in a tight skin envelope. (*B*) Volume is reduced by removal of 6 mL of deep subplatysmal fat (DF), 6 mL of supra-platysma fat (SF), and 8 mL of submandibular glands (SMG) during an isolated necklift. A chin implant was added.

midline, most often (85%) the muscle fibers interlace in the midline ranging from less than 2 cm area of decussation in half and greater than 2 cm in the other half. In 15%, the platysma does not meet in the midline.[2]

The superficial cervical fascia and deep cervical fascia are important in central neck surgery. The superficial cervical fascia is a translucent membrane that covers the superficial surface of the platysma (**Fig. 3**). The fascia fuses with the deep fascia of the pectoralis and deltoid muscles inferiorly and becomes the superficial musculoaponeurotic system above the jawline. Maintaining the integrity of the superficial cervical fascia during

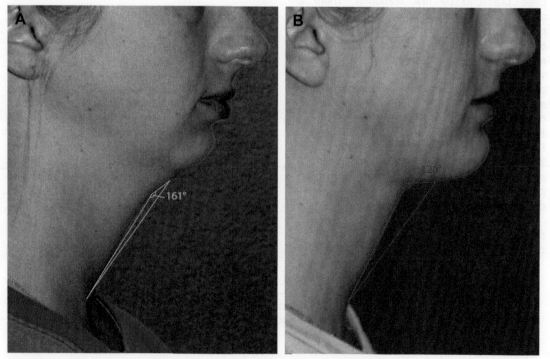

Fig. 2. (*A*) A preoperative cervicomental angle of 161°. (*B*) One-year postoperative cervicomental angle of 120°.

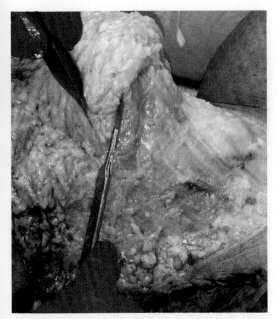

Fig. 3. Superficial cervical fascia covering the platysma muscle.

contouring of the superficial fat is important for optimal strength of the muscle-fascial system when plicating and tightening the platysma.

The deep investing layer, also known as the superficial layer of the deep cervical fascia, wraps the deep neck structures in a connective tissue sleeve. Anteriorly, the deep investing fascia splits to encase the submandibular gland forming the capsule of the submandibular gland. This deep investing fascia has significant implications when partial resection of the submandibular gland is performed and postoperative bleeding occurs. The fascia will contain the bleeding, thereby directing the blood posteriorly potentially leading to airway compression.

Two ligaments, the mandibular cutaneous and submental ligaments, are frequently released in

both isolated necklift and facelift surgeries. The mandibular ligament is an osteocutaneous ligament that arises from the anterior mandible 1 cm above the mandibular border and inserts into the dermis creating the anterior border of the jowl fat. The fibers penetrate the inferior portion of the depressor anguli oris muscle. The fibers are short and tough and the terminal branch of the marginal mandibular nerve will traverse the ligament below the platysma and superficial muscular aponeurotic system.[3] There are typically vessels intimately associated with the ligament, so care must be taken when controlling these vessels with cautery to avoid injury to the terminal branch of the marginal mandibular nerve. The submental ligament creates the submental crease where it holds the skin to the platysma muscle.

The fat in the central neck can greatly impact submental fullness. The fat is distributed in the supraplatysmal and subplatysmal planes. The subplatysmal fat has been described to inhabit 3 different compartments: central, medial, and lateral. The central compartment subplatysmal fat is a more fibrous-type fat when compared with medial and lateral compartments, where the consistency is similar to the buccal fat. The subplatysmal fat is covered by the platysma and the superficial cervical fascia in the midline where the platysma separates. The subplatysmal central compartment covers the mylohyoid muscle centrally and extends over the digastric muscles. The medial compartment continues over the digastric muscle just above the digastric tendon and extends into the lateral neck, becoming the lateral compartment covering the submandibular gland[4] (**Fig. 4**).

The digastric muscles are paired muscles with 2 bellies: anterior and posterior. The anterior bellies of the digastric muscles form the lateral boundary of the submental triangle and originate from the digastric fossa at the midline of the mandible. The

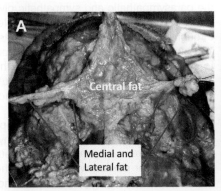

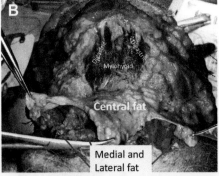

Fig. 4. (*A*) Subplatysmal fat elevated showing pyramidal shape. (*B*) Subplatysmal fat reflected revealing the floor of the submental triangle made by the mylohyoid muscle and the lateral boundaries made up by the digastric muscles.

anterior digastric muscle is joined to the posterior digastric muscle by a tendon at the hyoid where a fascial sling holds the tendon to the body and greater horn of the hyoid. Medially the digastric muscle will frequently fuse with the mylohyoid muscle. The anterior digastric muscle is innervated by a branch of the mylohyoid nerve and the muscle assists in opening the mouth against resistance and elevating the hyoid bone during swallowing. The blood supply is from the submental and mylohyoid artery and submental vein.

The mylohyoid muscle is a paired muscle with the fibers originating from the mylohyoid line on the medial surface of the mandible and runs inferomedially to insert on the hyoid bone. At the midline, each side is fused to the other by a midline raphe. The posterior edge is open and the deep lobe of the submandibular gland is located superior and deep to it. The mylohyoid is innervated by the mylohyoid nerve and elevates the hyoid and floor of the mouth during swallowing. The blood supply is from the submental and mylohyoid artery and submental vein.

The peri-hyoid fascia is a condensation of deep cervical fascia at the hyoid bone. The fascia covers the mylohyoid muscle and extends to join the infrahyoid muscles and extends to each digastric tendon (**Fig. 5**). The thickness of the fascia is highly variable and can sometimes be thick enough to contribute to an obtuse cervicomental angle that requires release by transection or excision (**Fig. 6**).

The submental triangle can have robust vasculature from the submental artery and veins. The size and location of these vessels can be highly variable. The submental veins join the facial vein and as they descend to the hyoid fascia they join the anterior jugular vessels. There is wide variation in location and size of these vessels. There is the occasional communicating branch between the anterior jugular vein and the facial vein that can be quite large and presents itself when approaching the medial capsule of the submandibular gland (**Fig. 7**).

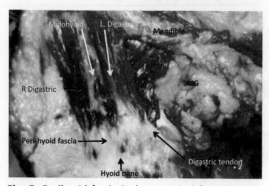

Fig. 5. Perihyoid fascia is deep cervical fascia joining structures at the hyoid bone.

Vigilance and control of these vessels is mandatory with any surgery in the submental triangle.

SUBMANDIBULAR TRIANGLE

The submandibular triangle is bound superiorly by the lower border of the mandible and a line drawn from the angle to the mastoid process. The posterior inferior border is the posterior digastric muscle and the anterior inferior border is the anterior digastric muscle. The roof is the platysma muscle with its underlying deep cervical fascia and the floor is formed by the mylohyoid and hypoglossus muscle. The triangle contains the submandibular gland and a number of important anatomic structures that may be encountered with any surgery of the submandibular gland. These include submandibular lymph nodes, facial artery and vein, and the lingual, hypoglossal, and mylohyoid nerve with the marginal coursing along the roof of the triangle.

For the aesthetic surgeon, the submandibular gland is the most difficult structure to manage; therefore, the anatomy is described as the surgeon would encounter each structure. The submandibular gland is enveloped by the deep cervical fascia and has a thicker capsule anteriorly versus the posterior capsule. The marginal mandibular and facial vein pass just anterior to the anterior capsule. Therefore, staying within the fascia during management is crucial to protecting the nerve and vein.

Submandibular Gland

The submandibular gland is between 7 and 15 g in size and is responsible for 20% to 30% of the 1.0 to 1.5 L of saliva produced per day. The submandibular gland is responsible for most of resting saliva production. The submandibular gland is classified as a mixed gland that predominantly produces serous saliva. The volume of saliva production is high compared to its mass. The production is almost completely controlled extrinsically by both the parasympathetic and sympathetic divisions of the autonomic nervous system. The arterial flow through the glands is high relative to its weight. The high volume of saliva produced is partly due to this high blood flow rate through the gland. This accounts for the highly friable glandular tissue bleeding easily and briskly from its surface during partial resection.[5]

The submandibular gland is c-shaped with most of the gland laying on the mylohyoid and hypoglossus muscle and makes up the superficial lobe. A smaller portion wraps around the posterior edge of the mylohyoid muscle and makes up the deep lobe of the submandibular gland. In aesthetic surgery, it is the superficial gland that is reduced.

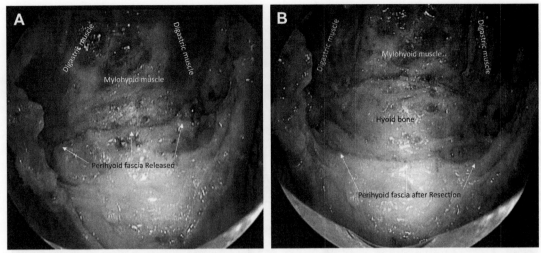

Fig. 6. (*A*) Perihyoid has been transected and released from mylohyoid muscle and digastric tendons. (*B*) The thickened perihyoid fascia has been resected showing the hyoid bone.

Vasculature of Submandibulat Triangle

The submandibular gland derives its arterial supply predominately from the submental and sublingual arteries, which are branches of the facial and lingual arteries. The facial artery is a tortuous branch of the external carotid artery. It travels superiorly beneath the posterior belly of the digastric muscle and immediately loops back over the posterior digastric muscle to enter the capsule of the submandibular glad. The artery travels upward lateral or deep to the tail of the superficial lobe of

the gland. Here the facial artery supplies the gland through a variable number of very short 2-mm to 4-mm arterial branches. These branches are easily torn and can be difficult to control during resection of the tail of the superficial gland (**Fig. 8**). The superior course of the facial artery can be variable, sometimes running deep to the superficial lobe and sometimes running through the tail of the gland (**Fig. 9**). Before the facial artery exits the capsule, it gives off the submental artery approximately 0.5 cm below the mandibular border. It then exits the capsule and continues across the mandible in the facial groove to ascend the face.

The submental artery runs under the border of the mandible superficial to the mylohyoid muscle. Over its course, it has branches to the superficial lobe of the submandibular gland, the platysma, mylohyoid, and anterior digastric muscles. The medial most of the branches to the superficial submandibular gland are frequently encountered while removing a portion of the superficial lobe, and care must be exercised to control them as they are short and easily torn.

The lingual artery branches inferior and posterior to or with the facial artery off the external carotid artery. It runs deep to the posterior digastric muscle and capsule on the lateral surface of the middle constrictors to pass anterior and medial to the hypoglossus muscle. Along the course, accompanying veins coalesce to form the lingual vein. Frequently there is a branch of the lingual artery that penetrates the capsule to enter the deep lobe of the submandibular gland and continue into the posterior third of the superficial lobe of the submandibular gland. This artery is frequently encountered during resection (**Fig. 10**).

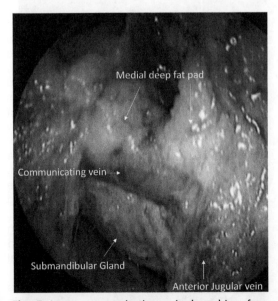

Fig. 7. Large communicating vein branching from anterior jugular vein, passing on the anterior surface of the submandibular gland.

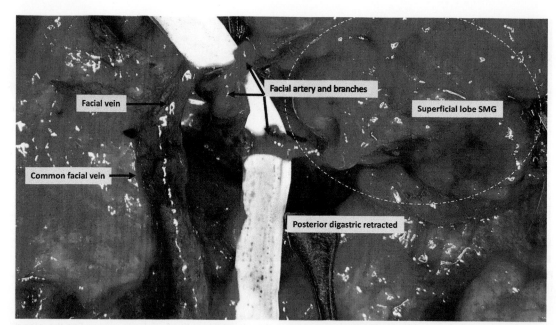

Fig. 8. The facial artery running lateral to the superficial lobe of the submandibular gland with 2 small branches supplying the tail of the gland.

The submandibular gland is mainly drained by the anterior facial vein and the superficial lobe is emptied by small venules that drain into the submental veins. The facial vein enters the capsule just below the mandibular border where it is joined by the submental vessels medially, and on the lateral side it is joined by the anterior branch of the retromandibular vein to form the common facial vein. The common facial vein courses over the middle or lateral third of the superficial lobe

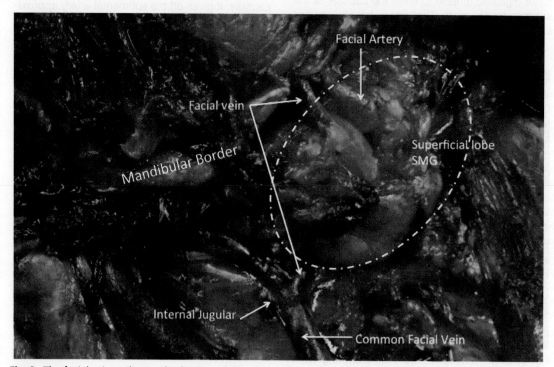

Fig. 9. The facial vein and artery both entered the lateral gland and exit the submandibular gland at the mandibular border.

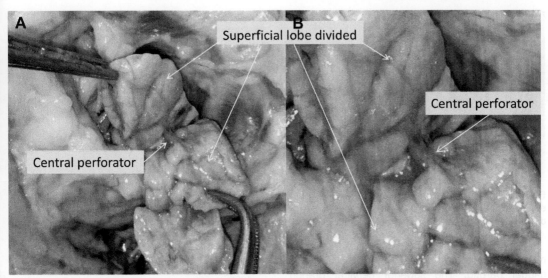

Fig. 10. (*A*) The central perforating artery passes through the posterolateral aspect of the superficial lobe of the submandibular gland. (*B*) The same view zoomed in to show the central perforating artery.

of the submandibular gland. The facial vein enters the internal jugular vein at the greater horn of the hyoid bone.

Nerves in Submandibulat Triangle

The marginal mandibular and cervical branches of the facial nerve are the nerves of most importance. Most investigators, including this one, experience a temporary weakness in the depressor function of the lower lip in as many as 9.6% of patients undergoing subplatysmal surgery.[6] Therefore, a thorough understanding of the course and variation of the marginal mandibular and cervical nerve in relationship to the subplatysmal elements is needed.

The marginal mandibular nerve is a branch of the inferior cervicofacial branch of the facial nerve that innervates the depressors of the lower lip, including the depressor anguli oris, depressor labii inferioris, and occasionally the pars labialis platysma. In addition, it innervates the mentalis muscle, which pulls the chin upward and elevates and protrudes the lower lip. The nerve exits the anterior border of the parotid gland approximately 0.5 to 1.5 cm anterior to the posterior border of the mandible. It runs on the posterior surface of the platysma. There can be 1 to 4 branches of the nerve that can course above or below the mandibular border. The branches can be as high as 2 cm above the border to 3 cm below the border.[7] The marginal mandibular nerve runs anterior to the facial vein and vein and capsule of the submandibular gland (**Fig. 11**). Singer and Sullivan[8] identified the marginal mandibular nerve to lie approximately, on average, 3.7 cm cephalad to the inferior extent of the submandibular

gland. As the marginal mandibular nerve crosses the submandibular gland it runs anterior to the capsule of the gland. Care must be taken when retracting or cauterizing within the capsule to avoid injury to the nerve.

The cervical branch of the facial nerve innervates all 3 platysmal components: par modiolaris platysma, par labialis platysma, and par mandibularis platysma. All components insert into the lower lip and act as depressors of the lower lip to varying degrees. Ellenbogen[9] first described the platysma as a depressor of the lower lip and that injury to the innervation can happen during facelift platysma surgery. The cervical branch descends within the parotid gland and splits from the marginal

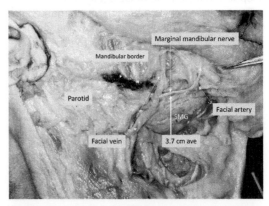

Fig. 11. The marginal mandibular nerve runs anterior to the facial vein and vein and capsule of the SMG. The marginal mandibular nerve lies approximately, on average, 3.7 cm cephalad to the inferior extent of the submandibular gland.

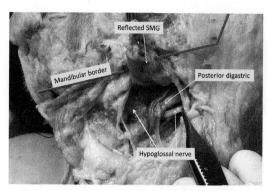

Reflected SMG

Mandibular border

Posterior digastric

Hypoglossal nerve

Fig. 12. The hypoglossal nerve travels from inferolateral to superior-medial passing beneath the posterior digastric muscle. The SMG is reflected superiorly.

mandibular nerve before exiting through the caudal parotid. The superior cervical branch quickly becomes more superficial just below the platysma and runs parallel to the mandibular border. The inferior branch runs a similar pattern inferior to the superior branch, parallel to the mandibular border lower neck. Both the superior and inferior branches penetrate the platysma in the lateral aspect of the platysma such that it is less susceptible to injury during central neck surgery.

The hypoglossal nerve supplies motor function to the extrinsic and intrinsic muscles of the tongue. The hypoglossal nerve emerges from beneath the occipital branch of the external carotid artery to travel beneath the posterior belly and common tendon of the digastric muscle. It then passes through the submandibular triangle deep to the thin posterior capsule of the submandibular gland to pass posterior to the anterior digastric muscle. It then ascends anterior to the lingual nerve and deep to the mylohyoid muscle (**Fig. 12**).

The lingual nerve is a branch of the mandibular division of the mandibular branch of the trigeminal

nerve that supplies general sensation and taste to the anterior two-thirds of the tongue. The nerve courses laterally between the medial pterygoid muscle and ramus of the mandible and enters the oral cavity and travels across the hypoglossus muscle along the floor of the mouth.

The mylohyoid nerve supplies motor innervation to the anterior digastric muscle and mylohyoid muscle. The nerve runs on the inner surface of the mandible until it enters the posterior edge of the mylohyoid muscle. The submental artery runs superficial to it.

REFERENCES

1. Salmons S. Section 7: muscle. In: Williams PL, Bannister LH, Berry MM, et al, editors. Grays anatomy. 38th edition. New York: Churchill Livingston; 1995. p. 789.
2. Cardoso de Castro C. The anatomy of the platysma muscle. Plast Reconstr Surg 1980;66:680–3.
3. Furnas DW. The retaining ligaments of the cheek. Plast Reconstr Surg 1989;83:11–6.
4. Rohrich RJ, Pessa JE. The subplatysmal supramylohyoid fat. Plast Reconstr Surg 2010;126:589–95.
5. Varga G. Physiology of the salivary glands. Surgery 2012;30(11):578.
6. Feldman JJ. Neck lift my way: an update. Plast Reconstr Surg 2014;134:1173–83.
7. Savary V, Robert R, Rogez JM, et al. The mandibular marginal ramus of the facial nerve: an anatomic and clinical study. Surg Radiol Anat 1997;19:69–72.
8. Singer DP, Sullivan PK. Submandibular gland 1: an anatomic evaluation and surgical approach to submandibular gland resection for facial rejuvenation. Plast Reconstr Surg 2003;15:1150–4.
9. Ellenbogen R. Psuedoparalysis of the mandibular branch of the facial nerve after platysmal face-lift operation. Plast Reconstr Surg 1979;63:364–8.

Neck Lift
Defining Anatomic Problems and Choosing Appropriate Treatment Strategies

Timothy Marten, MD*, Dino Elyassnia, MD

KEYWORDS

- Neck lift • Short scar neck lift • Extended neck lift • Submental liposuction • Double chin
- Witch's chin • Submandibular gland reduction • Partial digastic myectomy

KEY POINTS

- Success or failure in treating the neck lies in the diagnosis of underlying problems and the application of a logical surgical plan.
- Although it is a commonly advocated practice, it is not enough to perform submental liposuction and tighten the skin in most patients as such an approach ignores a number of anatomic problems present in many patients seeking neck improvement.
- Removing subcutaneous fat and tightening skin over deep layer neck problems does not correct them, and the presence or absence of each must be looked for to create and apply an appropriate surgical plan.

INTRODUCTION

Why perform a neck lift? Why not just lift the cheeks and jawline or perform other procedures that rejuvenate the eyes or upper face? The simple answer is that a well-contoured neck is an artistic imperative to an attractive and appealing appearance. A good neckline conveys a sense of youth, health, fitness, confidence, and vitality, and lends an appearance of decisiveness, sensuality, and beauty (**Fig. 1**). Neck improvement is of high priority to almost every patient seeking facial rejuvenation, and the results of "face lift" procedures are judged largely by the outcome obtained in the neck. If the neck is not sufficiently improved, our patients will feel we have failed them.

It is unlikely there will ever be a consensus on how a neck lift should be performed and it is a fact that no one procedure will be best for all patients. The technique used cannot be arbitrary, will depend on the problems present, and will necessarily vary from patient to patient. Success or failure in treating the neck, like the nose, breast, and body, lies in the diagnosis of underlying problems and the application of a logical surgical plan, and any surgeon capable of identifying the anatomic basis of patient problems and forming a sound plan for their correction can achieve excellent outcomes.

So how should one perform a neck lift? Perhaps it is easiest to start by recognizing what not to do. Although it is a commonly advocated practice, it is not enough to perform submental liposuction and tighten the skin in most patients, as such an approach ignores a number of anatomic problems present in many patients seeking neck improvement, including platysmal laxity, platysma bands,

Disclosure: The authors have nothing to disclose.
Marten Clinic of Plastic Surgery, 450 Sutter Street Suite 2222, San Francisco, CA 94108, USA
* Corresponding author.
E-mail address: tmarten@martenclinic.com

Clin Plastic Surg 45 (2018) 455–484
https://doi.org/10.1016/j.cps.2018.06.002

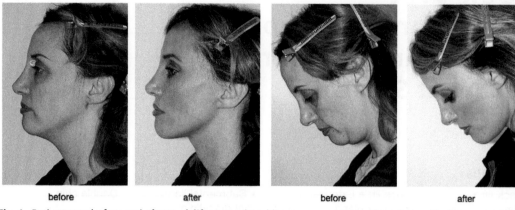

before　　　　　after　　　　　before　　　　　after

Fig. 1. Patient seen before and after neck lift. A good neckline conveys a sense of youth, health, fitness, confidence, vitality, decisiveness, sensuality, and beauty. (The patient is seen before and 1 year and 3 months after facelift, temple lift, lower eyelid surgery, and facial fat injections). Surgical procedure performed by Timothy J. Marten, MD, FACS. (*Courtesy of* Timothy J. Marten, MD, FACS, Marten Clinic of Plastic Surgery, San Francisco, CA.)

excess subplatysmal fat, large submandibular glands, digastric muscle hypertrophy, and developmental factors, such as the size and shape of the bony jaw and chin. Removing subcutaneous fat and tightening skin over these problems does not correct them, and the presence or absence of each must be looked for to create and apply an appropriate surgical plan (**Fig. 2**).

STRATEGIES FOR NECK LIFT

Patients seeking neck improvement have a range of options available to them depending on the problems present, the degree of improvement they seek, and the time, trouble, and expense they are willing to undergo to obtain the improvement they desire. And although it is essential to discuss these options and the advantages and disadvantages of each, patients are also seeking our guidance as to

what is possible, what is practical, and what is really best. It is not enough to steer patients to procedures we are comfortable with. We are professionally bound and ethically obliged to refer patients for the care they need and desire if we are not able to provide it ourselves.

Submental Liposuction

Submental liposuction (and arguably "noninvasive" treatments including cryolipolysis, deoxycholic acid injections, and radiofrequency and ultrasound "skin shrinking" treatments) is the simplest and likely the most commonly performed surgical procedure to improve neck contour in the range of options available to patients. It does not constitute a true neck lift, however, and only occasionally produces optimal outcomes. Patients and surgeons are predictably

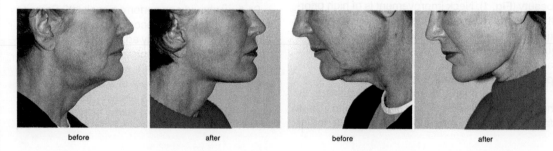

before　　　　　after　　　　　before　　　　　after

Fig. 2. Patient seen before and after neck lift. It is not enough to perform submental liposuction and tighten the skin in most patients. Such an approach ignores anatomic problems present in many patients seeking neck improvement. A careful evaluation shows patient preoperatively (*before*) to be troubled by platysmal laxity, platysma bands, excess subplatysmal fat, large submandibular glands, and digastric muscle hypertrophy. Removing subcutaneous fat and tightening skin over these problems does not correct them, and cannot produce the type of improvement shown (*after*). Surgical procedure performed by Timothy J. Marten, MD, FACS. (*Courtesy of* Timothy J. Marten, MD, FACS, Marten Clinic of Plastic Surgery, San Francisco, CA.)

drawn into a sense of denial of this, however, by the fact that subliposuction will occasionally produce worthwhile improvement in select cases, and it is these atypical outcomes that are predictably displayed in offices, placed in advertisements, shown on TV and Web sites, published in the beauty press, and even included in presentations at plastic surgery symposia. Adding to the deception is that these photographs have usually been taken in the early postoperative period when swelling is still present that obscures irregularities and underlying but untreated deep layer problems.

In reality, submental liposuction (and noninvasive procedures that target subcutaneous neck fat) is an incomplete solution to neck problems for most patients. As a standalone treatment, it suffers the significant drawback that it falsely assumes poor neck contour to be solely the result of the accumulation of subcutaneous fat, and it is conceptually flawed in that it does not address platysma laxity and other deep layer problems, which together typically play a much larger and more important role in the aging neck and neck contour deformities. As such, most patients undergoing this procedure achieve arguably marginal improvement, but not comprehensive correction of their neck problems, and ultimately relying on this technique as the only method to obtain improved neck contour will seldom be successful (**Fig. 3**).

Submental liposuction is also a frequent cause of many vexing patient problems and complications, as it often leads to unintended but inappropriate removal of subcutaneous fat essential to a natural and youthful appearance, and this can, in turn, expose underlying problems of deep layer origin. Misapplied and overused, or when aggressive "ultrasonic" and "laser" techniques or other "power tools" are overenthusiastically applied, submental liposuction all too commonly also can result in overresection of precious subcutaneous fat and unnatural and objectionable appearances. These problems are typically not evident in the operating room or in the early postoperative period when cervicosubmental tissues are swollen, however, but appear later, and once present, are very difficult to correct (**Fig. 4**).

Liposuction, in combination with ill-conceived overtightening of neck skin, can add the additional objectionable problems of hairline displacement and wide postauricular scars, and compound the overall deformity (**Fig. 5**).

Despite its many drawbacks and propensity to precipitate troublesome and difficult to correct problems, the conceptual and comparative technical simplicity of submental liposuction is nonetheless appealing to less experienced surgeons and nonsurgeons seeking to improve the neck. Indeed, these aspects of the technique almost guarantee that, appropriate or not, it will continue to be overused and misapplied to patients who are not good candidates for the procedure.

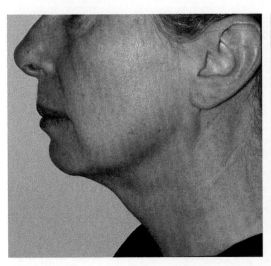 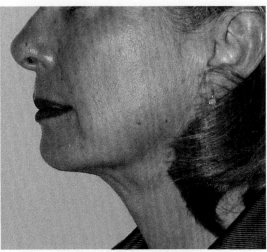

before   after

Fig. 3. Typical outcome seen with submental liposuction. Submental liposuction is an incomplete solution to neck problems for most patients, as it falsely assumes that poor neck contour is solely the result of the accumulation of subcutaneous fat, and it does *not* address platysma laxity and other deep layer problems that usually play a much larger role in the aging neck. Note that the large submandibular salivary gland is still present, platysma laxity has not been corrected, and aggressive subcutaneous fat removal has made platysma bands more obvious. (*Courtesy of* Marten Clinic of Plastic Surgery, San Francisco, CA.)

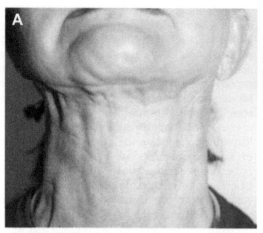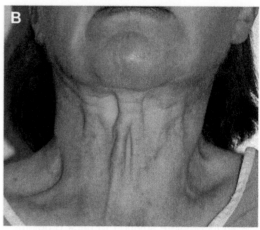

Fig. 4. Overexcision of subcutaneous fat with liposuction. (*A*) The patient (*left*) has had aggressive "small cannula micro-liposculpture" by an unknown surgeon, which resulted in too much fat being removed. The neck and submental region are irregular, unnatural, and unattractive. (*B*) A different patient (*right*) has had "laser liposuction" performed by an unknown surgeon. Inappropriate overresection of fat has resulted in harsh and unnatural contours along with unattractive exposure of platysmal bands. Procedures performed by unknown surgeons. (*Courtesy of* Marten Clinic of Plastic Surgery, San Francisco, CA.)

"Short Scar" Neck Lift (Neck Lift with Submental Incision Only)

Although submental liposuction alone will rarely produce optimal neck improvement, a neck lift performed through a submental incision without any removal of skin can create attractive cervical contour in many patients (**Fig. 6** and see also Timothy Marten and Dino Elyassnia's, "Short Scar Neck Lift: Neck Lift Using a Submental Incision Only," in this issue).

This is because, unlike liposuction, a neck lift performed through a submental incision allows deep layer problems (subplatysmal fat excess and submandibular gland enlargement) and platysmal laxity typically present in most patients

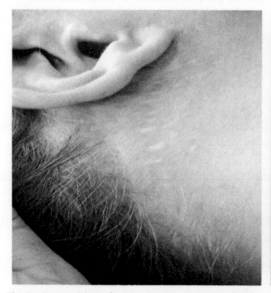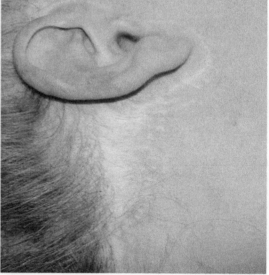

Fig. 5. Overexcision of postauricular skin. It is a common error to attempt to lift the neck by tightening neck skin. It is not possible, however, to create a sustained improvement in neck contour in this manner and ill-conceived overtightening of neck skin will result in wide postauricular scars (and if the incision is planned poorly, hairline displacement). Neck contour is properly created by modification of deep layer structures and only skin that is truly redundant should be removed. In some cases, no skin at all needs be removed (see **Fig. 6** and Timothy Marten and Dino Elyassnia's, "Short Scar Neck Lift: Neck Lift Using a Submental Incision Only," in this issue). Procedures performed by unknown surgeons. (*Courtesy of* Marten Clinic of Plastic Surgery, San Francisco, CA)

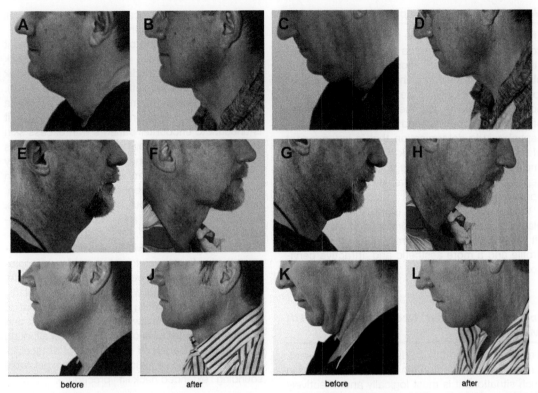

before   after   before   after

Fig. 6. Neck lift with a submental incision only. Although submental liposuction alone will rarely produce optimal neck improvement, a neck lift performed through a submental incision without any removal of skin can create attractive cervical contour in many patients. These patients had their procedures performed through a submental incision only. No incisions were made in the peri-auricular areas and there are no peri-auricular scars. (*A–D*) Surgical procedure performed by Dino Elyassnia, MD, FACS. (*E–H*) Surgical procedure performed by Timothy J. Marten, MD, FACS. (*I–L*) Surgical procedure performed by Dino Elyassnia, MD, FACS. (*Courtesy of* [*A–D*] Dino Elyassnia, MD, FACS, Marten Clinic of Plastic Surgery, San Francisco, CA; and [*E–H*] Timothy J. Marten, MD, FACS, Marten Clinic of Plastic Surgery, San Francisco, CA; and [*I–L*] Dino Elyassnia, MD, FACS, Marten Clinic of Plastic Surgery, San Francisco, CA.)

seeking neck improvement to be addressed. This, however, begs the question, "how can good neck contour be created without removing and tightening the skin, and what happens to the 'excess' skin if only the deeper-layer treatment is made and no skin is excised?" The answer to these question is twofold: First, is the simple yet difficult to accept concept that in a properly performed neck lift, contour is created by modification of deep layers of the neck, *not* by tightening the skin. Skin is intended to be a covering layer and serves a covering function. It was meant to stretch and give as we move and express ourselves. It was not intended to be a structural supporting layer, or to hold up sagging muscle and fat or lift hypertrophied structures lying beneath it. The second part of the answer lies in the increase in neck surface area that occurs when neck contour is improved. Improving neck contour by excising redundant subplatysmal fat and performing other deep layer maneuvers as indicated, followed by

reducing horizontal platysma laxity will result in a deepened cervicomental angle, a longer curvilinear distance from the mentum to the sternal notch, and a more concave and geometrically larger and longer neck surface. When neck skin is re-draped and redistributed over the deeper, more concave surface, "excess" skin is absorbed and none need be removed. These simple but not necessarily intuitive or immediately obvious facts underlie the reason that skin excision need not be performed in patients with good skin quality and mild to moderate apparent skin excess to obtain a good result.

There is a limit to the amount of neck skin that can be absorbed and managed in this manner, however, and an isolated neck lift performed through a submental incision only is typically best for male patients and younger women with mild to moderate skin excess, good skin elasticity, and minimal or modest aging in the mid-face, cheek, and jowl.

Neck Lift with a Chin Implant

The difference between the presence of poor neck contour and microgenia is frequently misunderstood, and it is a common misconception that placement of a chin implant improves neck contour. A chin implant is a treatment for small chin, not a poor neckline, and the presence or absence of microgenia and the need for a chin implant is a cephalometric determination that is independent of the condition of the neck. Placement of a chin implant when microgenia is not present is a conceptual and artistic error that will create unnatural appearances.

When true microgenia is present, however, placing a chin implant in combination with a neck lift will produce a more harmonious and balanced profile and a more aesthetic and attractive cervicofacial profile (**Fig. 7**).

Long Scar "Extended" Neck Lift, and Neck Lift with Facelift

If a significant amount of redundant skin is present, it must be excised to obtain the best result, and in such situations it is most logically and effectively excised in the postauricular areas using periauricular skin incisions. Skin excision from the submental incision is conceptually flawed and will actually degrade neck contour rather than improve it, and skin excision using large midline Z-plasties will result in a poorly concealed odd-appearing geometric scar, and bizarre changes in beard hair inclination in men.

Skin excision can be combined with treatment of the submental neck and subplatysmal neck problems as an "extended" or "long scar" neck lift, or as part of a face lift procedure (**Figs. 8–10**).

Practically speaking, most patients in need of a neck lift with skin excision also need a facelift, as it is unusual to encounter patients with excess skin in the neck but not elsewhere on the face. This is particularly true in women and it is aesthetically inappropriate to perform an isolated neck lift in most women who present for facial rejuvenation. Lifting only the neck but not the cheeks, jowls, and jawline can create an unnatural and unfeminine appearance.

Combining a facelift with a neck lift is almost always the best approach to obtain a balanced, natural, and harmonious rejuvenation of the female face, although not all patients will recognize or accept this (see **Fig. 10**). Performing a facelift in combination with a neck lift also allows for more complete and comprehensive removal of neck skin. And although many men will be put off by the idea of a "facelift," they will readily agree to undergo the more palatable sounding "extended neck lift" procedure.

SURGICAL PLANNING IN NECK LIFT
Planning the Submental Incision

Whether performing a neck lift alone or in combination with a facelift, optimal improvement in

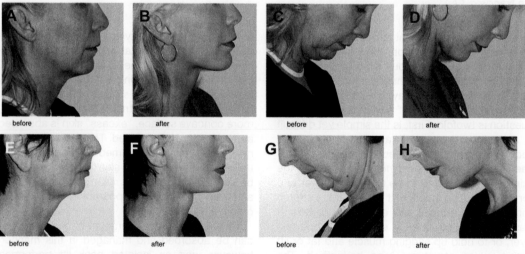

before   after   before   after

before   after   before   after

Fig. 7. Neck lift with a chin implant. The difference between the presence of poor neck contour and microgenia is commonly misunderstood, and it is a common misconception that placement of a chin implant improves neck contour. When true microgenia is present, however, placing a chin implant in combination with a neck lift will produce a more harmonious and balanced profile and a more aesthetic and attractive cervicofacial profile (*Case 1 A-D, Case 2 E-H*). Surgical procedures performed by Timothy J. Marten, MD, FACS. (*Courtesy of* Timothy J. Marten, MD, FACS, Marten Clinic of Plastic Surgery, San Francisco, CA.)

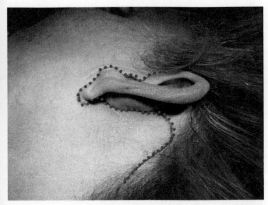

Fig. 8. Incision plan for a long scar or "extended" neck lift. If a significant amount of redundant skin is present on the neck, it must be excised to obtain the best result, and in such situations it is most logically and effectively excised in the postauricular areas using a peri-auricular skin incision rather than one under the chin. This incision plan avoids a temporal incision that is of concern to some patients but provides for significant skin removal from the neck. (*Courtesy of* Marten Clinic of Plastic Surgery, San Francisco, CA.)

neck contour can generally not be obtained in most patients unless a submental incision is made despite the long list of historical but conceptually flawed and failed attempts to avoid doing so. Traditionally, this incision is placed directly in and along the submental crease in a well-intended but counterproductive attempt to conceal the resulting scar (**Fig. 11**).

This incision plan should be avoided, however, as it will surgically reinforce the crease and accentuate a "double chin" or "witch's chin" deformity. Exposure of the submental region will also be compromised, and difficulty will be encountered when suturing or dissecting low in the neck. A more posterior placement of this incision will preclude these problems, but still result in an inconspicuous and better concealed scar (**Fig. 12**).

The submental incision should be placed well within the mandibular shadow and well posterior but parallel to the submental crease at a point lying roughly one-half the distance between the mentum and hyoid. This usually corresponds to a site situated 1.0 to 1.5 cm posterior to the crease (**Fig. 13**).

The submental incision should be approximately 3.0 to 3.5 cm in length, but may be made longer as long as neither end will be advanced up upon a visible portion of the face when skin flaps are shifted. Healing will be best, and the scar will be best concealed, if it is made as a straight, and not as a curved line (**Fig. 14**).

ASSESSING ANATOMIC BASIS OF NECK PROBLEMS
Planning the Modification of the Submental Region

Traditional neck lift techniques do not adequately address many aspects of aging in the submental region, and *it is not enough in most situations to limit treatment of the neck to pre-platysmal lipectomy alone or with postauricular skin excision.* For many patients, subplatysmal fat accumulation,

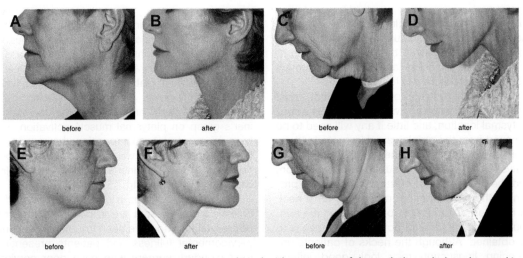

Fig. 9. Extended neck lift. Skin excision can be combined with treatment of the neck through the submental incision as an "extended" or "long scar" neck lift, or as part of a facelift procedure. Both of these patients had skin excised as part of their procedures, and an incision was made in the peri-auricular area *(Case 1 A-D, Case 2 E-H)*. Surgical procedures performed by Timothy J. Marten, MD, FACS. (*Courtesy of* Timothy J. Marten, MD, FACS, Marten Clinic of Plastic Surgery, San Francisco, CA.)

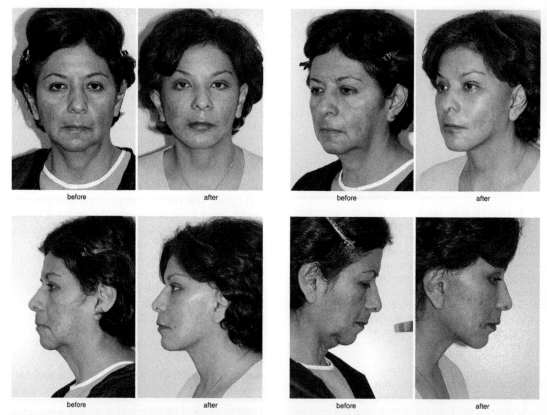

before   after   before   after

before   after   before   after

Fig. 10. Comprehensive rejuvenation of the face. Combining a neck lift with a facelift and related procedures is almost always the best approach to obtain a balanced, natural, and harmonious rejuvenation of the female face, although not all patients will recognize or accept this. This 55-year-old woman underwent facelift, neck lift, limited incision forehead lift, upper and lower blepharoplasties, chin augmentation, and fat transfer to the lips and cheeks. Addressing all regions of the face has produced a natural balanced outcome, and a far better result than neck lift alone (see also **Fig. 1**). Surgical procedure performed by Timothy J. Marten, MD, FACS. (*Courtesy of* Timothy J. Marten, MD, FACS, Marten Clinic of Plastic Surgery, San Francisco, CA.)

submandibular salivary gland "ptosis" (enlargement), and digastric muscle hypertrophy will contribute significantly to the neck contour problems present and necessitate additional treatment if optimal improvement is to be obtained.

In all but the unusual or young patient, most cervical fat accumulation will be present in a *subplatysmal* location, and little if any will need to be removed from the preplatysmal layer. Indeed, as patients age, fat stores generally shift from a preplatysmal location to a subplatysmal location, and the small amount of subcutaneous fat present in the typical patient presenting for a neck lift is necessary and must be preserved if a soft, youthful, natural, and attractive appearance is to be obtained. Although the necks of patients undergoing liposuction may look good initially when swelling is present, once it resolves, they typically display an unnatural and unaesthetic "overresected" appearance. Once one acknowledges this fact and recognizes this occurrence,

the futility and undesirability of cervicosubmental liposuction in most patients becomes obvious.

Abnormal collections of subplatysmal fat can be identified by preoperative palpation of the neck with and without platysmal activation. Fat lying predominantly in a preplatysmal position will generally feel "soft" and will remain in the examiner's grasp on platysmal muscle activation. Fat lying in a subplatysmal position, however, will have a firmer feel, and will tend to be pulled superiorly out of the examiner's grasp when the platysma is contracted (**Fig. 15**).

Two typical scenarios in which subplatysmal fat is likely to be present are in patients with firm, obtuse necks who have been troubled by lifelong cervicomental fullness and patients presenting for secondary surgery who have poor cervical contour (**Fig. 16**). In these individuals, subplatysmal lipectomy will likely be required. Not all fat should be arbitrarily removed from the deep neck, however, and deep cervical fat

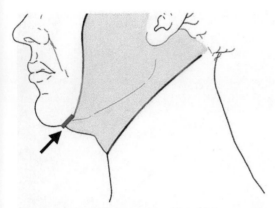

Fig. 11. Traditional, but *incorrect* plan for the submental incision (*red line*). The incision should not be placed directly along the submental crease (*arrow*), as this will reinforce the submental retaining ligaments and accentuate the "double-chin" appearance. Note that typical plan of skin undermining (*yellow area*) also promotes a double-chin appearance because the crease is not undermined, retaining ligaments are not released, and the fat of the chin and the neck cannot be readily blended to create a smooth transition between them. (*Courtesy of* Marten Clinic of Plastic Surgery, San Francisco, CA.)

(interdigastric fat) should not be removed. When deep cervical interdigastric fat is erroneously excised, an objectionable depression in the submental region will result, often referred to as the

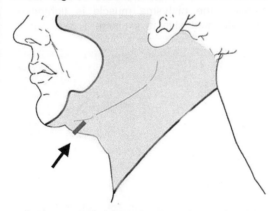

Fig. 12. Correct location for the submental incision (*red line*). Placing the submental incision 1.5 cm *posterior* to the (*arrow* showing incision location [*red line*]) submental crease (see also **Fig. 13**) prevents accentuation of the "double chin" and witch's chin deformities and provides for easier dissection and suturing in the anterior neck (compare with **Fig. 10**). Note that this incision plan allows the submental crease to be undermined and submental retaining ligaments to be released, and the fat of the chin pad and submental neck to be blended to create a smooth and aesthetically pleasing transition between them (see **Figs. 1, 6, 7, 9, 10, 22, 31, 32,** and **33**). Yellow shading shows area of subcutaneous undermining. (*Courtesy of* Marten Clinic of Plastic Surgery, San Francisco, CA.)

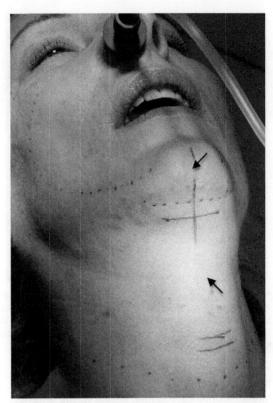

Fig. 13. Plan for the submental incision. The submental portion of the facelift incision (*solid line*) should be placed posterior to the submental crease (*dotted line*), approximately one-half the distance between the mentum and hyoid (*arrows*). Usually this corresponds to a point approximately 1.5 cm posterior to the submental crease. (*Courtesy of* Marten Clinic of Plastic Surgery, San Francisco, CA.)

"dug-out neck" deformity (**Fig. 17**). Typically, this depression is more evident when the neck is flexed somewhat or when the patient swallows.

Planning Treatment of the Prominent Submandibular Gland

Preoperative assessment of the submandibular glands must be made in patients seeking improvement in neck contour, as they often contribute to the appearance of a full, "obtuse," and "lumpy" neck. Large submandibular glands are most easily seen in the upper lateral neck in the patient with secondary facelift who has had prior aggressive cervicosubmental lipectomy (**Fig. 18**). However, large glands are frequently hidden by submental fat or lax platysma muscle in the patient with a full neck presenting for a primary procedure, and a plan that does not recognize this fact will lead to disappointing and unexpected bulges in the lateral submental regions postoperatively.

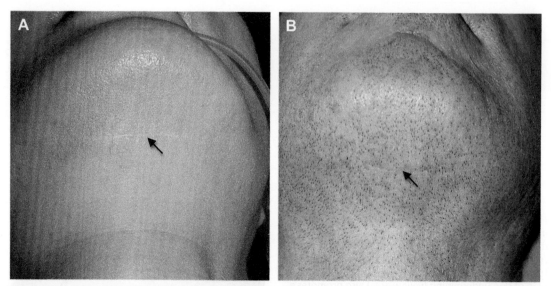

Fig. 14. Healed submental incisions. (*A [woman], B [man]*) Placement of the submental incision posterior to the submental crease will still result in an inconspicuous, well-concealed scar and simultaneously provide better access and exposure when working in the deep layers of the neck (*arrows* show location of healed submental incision). Surgical procedure performed by Timothy J. Marten, MD, FACS. (*Courtesy of* Timothy J. Marten, MD, FACS, Marten Clinic of Plastic Surgery, San Francisco, CA)

Submandibular glands are usually palpable as firm, smooth, discrete, mobile masses in the lateral submental triangle, lateral to the anterior belly of the digastric muscle and medial to the inner aspect of the ipsilateral mandibular border. Submandibular glands lying superior to the plane tangent to the inferior border of the mandible and the ipsilateral anterior belly of the digastric muscle do *not* disrupt neck contour and will usually *not* require treatment. Glands protruding *inferior* to this plane are likely to be problematic, however, if excess cervical fat is removed, the platysma muscle is tightened, and redundant skin is excised. These glands

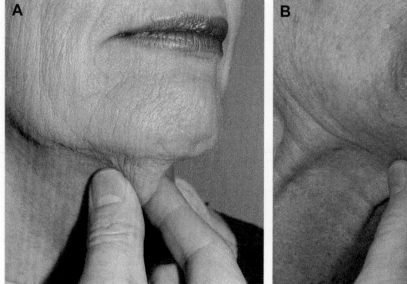
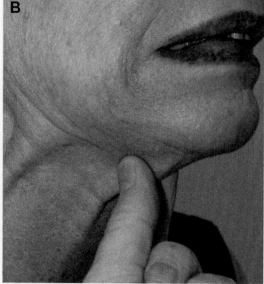

Fig. 15. Assessing the location of cervicosubmental fat. (*A*) Submental "wattle" is grasped with the face and neck in repose. (*B*) The patient is then asked to activate the platysma muscle. In this example fat is pulled superiorly from the examiner's grasp indicating a predominantly *sub*platysmal position. Fat lying predominantly in a subcutaneous, preplatysmal position would tend to remain within the examiner's grasp when the platysma is activated. (*Courtesy of* Marten Clinic of Plastic Surgery, San Francisco, CA.)

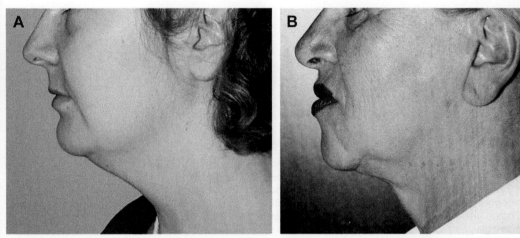

Fig. 16. Patients likely to have subplatysmal fat accumulation. (*A*) Young patient with firm, obtuse neck who has been troubled by lifelong cervicomental fullness. These patients typically have large collections of subplatysmal fat and are suboptimal candidates for submental liposuction. (*B*) Patient presenting for secondary surgery who has poor cervical contour. It can be seen that superficial subcutaneous fat has been stripped out at the primary procedure and the remaining fat is almost completely in a subplatysmal location. (*Courtesy of* Marten Clinic of Plastic Surgery, San Francisco, CA.)

demand treatment if optimal improvement in neck contour is to be obtained.

Despite various claims to the contrary, experience has shown that prominent submandibular glands are actually large, *not* ptotic, and that the platysma contributes little to their position or support. Attempts at tightening the platysma when a prominent gland is present usually results in modest improvement that is short lived. The same is true with the various conceptually flawed suture suspension methods that have been historically proposed and now largely abandoned. Careful

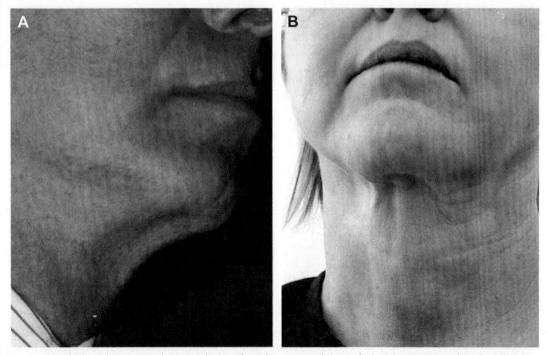

Fig. 17. (*A*, *B*) The "dug-out neck" irregularity. The "dug-out neck irregularity" is a term used to describe situations in which too much subplatysmal and/or deep cervical fat has been erroneously overexcised resulting in an objectionable depression in the submental region. Procedures performed by unknown surgeons. (*Courtesy of* Marten Clinic of Plastic Surgery, San Francisco, CA.)

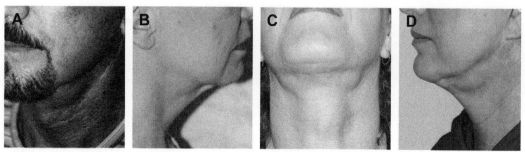

Fig. 18. Prominent submandibular glands. Large submandibular glands are usually evident as protruding masses in the lateral submental triangle, lateral to the anterior belly of the ipsilateral digastric muscle and medial to the mandibular border. (*A*) Patient with residual prominent submandibular gland after facelift and submental liposuction. His prior procedure has made the prominent glands more obvious. (*B*) Patient with residual prominent submandibular gland after "week-end neck lift." Aggressive resection of subcutaneous fat has exposed the prominent gland, which was not treated. (*C*) Patient with residual submandibular glands after "platysma plication." (*D*) Patient with residual submandibular glands after "corset platysmaplasty." Procedures performed by unknown surgeons. (*Courtesy of* Marten Clinic of Plastic Surgery, San Francisco, CA.)

preservation and sculpting of the peri-glandular fat will sometimes allow "small" prominent glands to remain disguised, but large, prominent glands will require that the *protruding portion* be resected if optimal improvement is to be obtained (**Fig. 19**).

The decision to perform submandibular gland reduction should be made in conjunction with the patient after appropriate discussion of the advantages and disadvantages of the procedure have been made. Patients should know that the procedure may prolong submental induration and edema, and carries a small risk of resulting in bleeding, sialoma, salivary fistula, and dry mouth symptoms.

Patients also should be aware, however, that such problems are uncommon, and they should understand that the protruding portion of the gland only is excised, and that most of the gland is left in place and is not removed.

Planning Treatment of Prominent Anterior Belly of the Digastric Muscle

A subgroup of patients will present with large, bulky anterior bellies of their digastric muscles that are evident as *linear paramedian submental fullness* (**Fig. 20**).

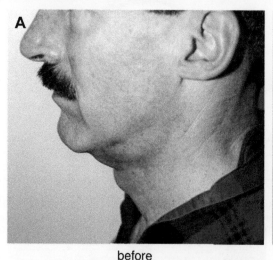
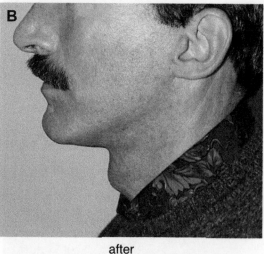

before   after

Fig. 19. Prominent submandibular glands. Despite claims to the contrary, experience has shown that prominent submandibular glands are actually large and not "ptotic" and will require that the protruding portion be resected if optimal improvement is to be obtained. (*A*) Patient with prominent submandibular gland that contributes significantly to poor neck contour. (*B*) Same patient seen after neck lift that included submandibular gland reduction. Surgical procedure performed by Timothy J. Marten, MD, FACS. (*Courtesy of* Timothy J. Marten, MD, FACS, Marten Clinic of Plastic Surgery, San Francisco, CA.)

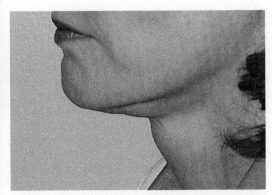

Fig. 20. Prominent anterior belly of the digastric muscle. The anterior belly of the digastric muscle can be seen as objectionable linear paramedian fullness in the submental region. Prominent digastric muscles often go unnoticed at the time of the primary procedure because they are frequently hidden by cervical fat and lax platysma muscle. (*Courtesy of* Marten Clinic of Plastic Surgery, San Francisco, CA.)

Large anterior bellies of the digastric muscles are most easily seen in the patient with secondary face-lift who has had prior aggressive cervicosubmental lipectomy. However, large muscles are frequently hidden by excess submental fat, large submandibular glands, or lax platysma muscle in the patient presenting for primary procedures, and failure to identify them will result in unexpected and objectionable submental bulges postoperatively. When large, prominent digastric muscles are identified, subtotal *superficial digastric myectomy* (excising the protruding portion of the muscle) should be considered. In unclear cases, the final decision as to whether partial digastric myectomy should be performed is often best deferred until the day of surgery and the improvement produced by other modifications of the submental region (subplatysmal fat excision and submandibular gland reduction) can be assessed.

SURGICAL TECHNIQUE
Anesthesia

Properly and comprehensively performed neck lift techniques can be time-consuming, technically demanding, and can test the patience and composure of almost any surgeon. It is highly recommended that any surgeon new to these techniques enlist the services of an anesthesiologist or competent registered nurse anesthetist. This is particularly important when the procedure is to be performed on a patient who is apprehensive, or has a history of anesthetic difficulties, hypertension, sleep apnea, or other significant medical problems.

Most of our and neck lifts are now performed under deep sedation administered by an anesthesiologist using a laryngeal mask airway ("LMA"). The use of a laryngeal mask allows the patient to be heavily sedated without compromise of their airway, but she or he need not receive muscle relaxants and can be allowed to breath spontaneously. An LMA is also less likely to become dislodged during the procedure than an endotracheal tube, and will not trigger coughing and bucking when the patient emerges from the anesthetic. The *flexible* LMA (LMA device with a flexible shaft) is a particularly useful in neck surgery (**Fig. 21**). When this device is used and the breathing circuit is separately draped, the breathing circuit can be moved from side to side as needed to obtain unobstructed access the cervicosubmental region. Most surgeons when initially considering using an LMA airway are understandably fearful that the bladder on the device when inflated will distort the cervical region and interfere with neck assessment and treatment. Fortunately, experience has shown this not to be true and not to be a valid concern.

Preoperative Preparations and Care

Each patient receives a full surgical scrub of the entire scalp, face, ears, nose, neck, shoulders,

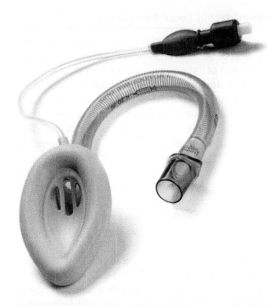

Fig. 21. Flexible LMA. The use of a laryngeal mask airway allows the patient to be heavily sedated without compromise of their airway, but she or he need not receive muscle relaxants and can be allowed to breath spontaneously. An LMA with a *flexible shaft* is particularly useful in neck surgery as it allows the breathing circuit to be easily moved when working in the submental area.

and upper chest with full-strength (1:750) benzal-konium chloride (BAK or Zephran) solution after anesthesia is begun, and bland ophthalmic oint-ment is instilled into each eye. The patient's head is then placed through the opening of a "split sheet" or a split adhesive–backed disposable transverse laparotomy sheet leaving the entire head and neck region unobscured from the clavi-cles up. No "turban" or "head drape" is used. This allows unimpaired examination of the cervico-facial profile in its entirety throughout the proced-ure and provides complete and unobstructed access to the peri-auricular areas when required.

The breathing circuit is draped separately from the patient by wrapping it with a sterile paper drape secured with Steri-Strips (sterile adhesive wound tapes) or other sterile fastener or choice. This allows it to move during the procedure as the patient's head is turned from side to side. When drapes are applied in this manner it is not necessary to secure the LMA with tape or by other means as long as its position is watched by the anesthesiologist and/or other members of the operating room team present. If an endo-tracheal tube is used, it can be conveniently and effectively secured to the peri-oral skin with a TegaDerm or similar sterile adhesive–backed plastic dressing.

Administering Local Anesthesia

Local anesthetic is administered even if deep sedation or general anesthesia is used. This limits stimulation of the patient and the overall amount of narcotics and anesthetics needed. A significant and helpful hemostatic effect is also obtained when epinephrine-containing solutions are used.

Sensory nerve blocks are performed using 0.25% bupivacaine (Marcaine) with epinephrine 1:200,000. This allows the neck or face to be sub-sequently injected subcutaneously with a reduced degree of stimulation. Skin marked for incisions is then infiltrated with the same solution. Areas of subcutaneous dissection are generously infiltrated with 0.1% lidocaine (Xylocaine) with epinephrine 1:1,000,000 solution.

Infiltration of the preauricular cheek and postaur-icular areas are carried out using a 22-gauge spinal needle if an "extended" neck lift or a facelift is being performed. Infiltration of the neck and submental region is carried out with a 1.6-mm multihole blunt-tipped infiltration cannula. No direct infiltra-tion beneath the superficial muscular aponeurotic system (SMAS) or platysma is necessary if the over-lying subcutaneous tissues are infiltrated gener-ously at the beginning of the procedure, as described previously.

Skin Flap Elevation

The submental incision should be made 1.5 cm or more posterior to the submental crease approxi-mately half way between the mentum and hyoid. Making the incision in this location helps conceal it in the shadow of the mandible, avoids surgical reinforcement of the crease and accentuation of the "double chin" and witch's chin deformities, and provides better exposure of the deep neck (see **Figs. 11–14**; **Fig. 22**).

Once the submental incision has been made, the surgeon should stand at the head of the table during dissection of the submental region, while the assistant retracts the edges of the incision with a pair of 10-mm double-pronged skin hooks. Having one's assistant retract frees up the sur-geon's nondominant hand to apply countertrac-tion to the skin being elevated and to assess flap thickness, and provides for optimal teamwork. Skin undermining should be made using a medium curved Metzenbaum scissors and the dissection should be made subcutaneously, leaving most the subcutaneous/preplatysmal fat on the pla-tysma surface. This makes fat excision and sculpt-ing easier later in the procedure if required, and precludes the need for more tedious and demanding excision of fat from the undersurface of the cervical skin flap. Unlike the dissection of the facelift skin flap in which a conscious effort must be made to prevent the flap from becoming too thick and the SMAS for being compromised, a slightly deeper dissection should be made in the neck to preserve a slightly thicker layer of sub-cutaneous fat. Preservation of a thicker layer of fat helps avoid a hard or overresected appearance in the cervicosubmental area, and objectionable overexposure of underlying neck anatomy postop-eratively. In many necks of patients undergoing facelifts, only subplatysmal fat will be removed, and little if any subcutaneous fat will be excised.

Submental dissection is continued inferiorly and laterally. If an "extended (long scar) neck lift" or concomitant facelift is being performed, this dissection will join the upper lateral neck dissec-tion made previously through postauricular and peri-lobular incisions (**Fig. 23**).

On completion of subcutaneous undermining of the anterior neck and submental regions, a retro-grade dissection should be made subcutaneously up onto the inferior chin. This will ensure the sub-mental restraining ligaments have been divided and that the submental crease has been released from its bony attachments, and provides for sub-sequent blending of chin and submental fat after other neck maneuvers have been completed to obtain a visually smooth and optimally seamless,

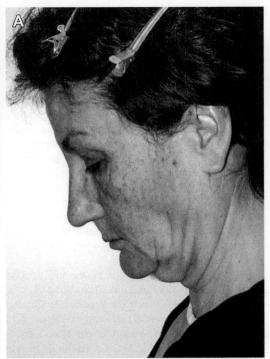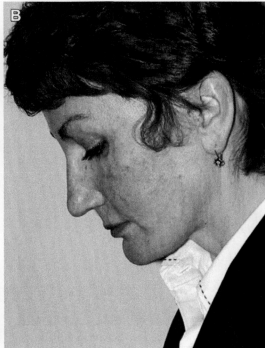

Fig. 22. Correction of the "double-chin" deformity. (*A*) Patient with "double chin" seen preoperatively. (*B*) Same patient seen after face and neck lift. The submental incision was made posterior to the submental crease to allow undermining and release on the submental retaining ligaments and blending of chin and neck fat to create a smooth and aesthetically pleasing transition between them. Surgical procedure performed by Timothy J, Marten, MD, FACS. (*Courtesy of* Timothy J. Marten, MD, FACS, Marten Clinic of Plastic Surgery, San Francisco, CA.)

aesthetic transition for chin to submental region. Some bleeding is usually encountered from perforating vessels that accompany ligaments in this region during this maneuver, but this should not prevent one from carrying out this important step.

If a facelift or "extended" neck lift is being performed, and the upper lateral neck is being approached from a postauricular incision, care must be taken to avoid injury to the great auricular nerve. This nerve provides sensation to the lower two-thirds of the ear and travels superficially superiorly in the upper lateral neck over the sternocleidomastoid muscle fascia. The most superficial portion of the nerve is anatomically constant and lies approximately 6.5 cm inferior to the auditory meatus midway between the anterior and posterior borders of the sternocleidomastoid muscle and it is helpful to mark this spot preoperatively on the neck skin surface to guide one during dissection. If the dissection is performed in the correct plane, however, the nerve will lie deep to the plane of skin flap elevation and will be covered by a thin layer of subcutaneous fat. It is prudent however, that all dissection made over the great auricular nerve is made under direct vision and not blindly.

Patients with thin faces, or those undergoing secondary facelifts, will not uncommonly have little subcutaneous fat between the superficially situated portion of the great auricular nerve and the skin, however. For this reason, extra caution must be taken in these patients if elevating the skin flap in this area, and a clear knowledge of nerve anatomy is required.

Cervical Lipectomy

The key to obtaining good outcomes in the neck is in understanding the distribution of fat in the cervicosubmental region and choosing a treatment plan accordingly. Cervical fat is present in 3 distinct anatomic layers: preplatysmal (subcutaneous), subplatysmal, and deep cervico-submuscular ("interdigastric").

Although our traditional focus has misguidedly and mistakenly been on the preplatysmal layer (submental liposuction and related surgical and nonsurgical procedures that reduce subcutaneous fat), most patients presenting with poor neck contour will be troubled instead by fat excess predominantly in the subplatysmal layer. Understanding and accepting this anatomic reality, and learning

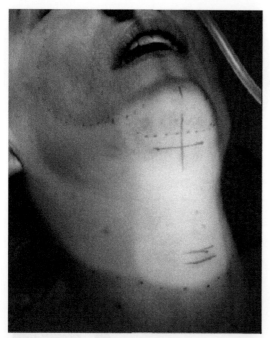

Fig. 23. Subcutaneous skin undermining in neck lift. Orange-shaded area shows subcutaneous skin undermining that is performed through the peri-auricular incisions when a neck lift is performed with a facelift (or during an extended neck lift procedure). Submental skin undermining (*yellow shaded area*) is then completed through the submental incision (*solid line in submental area*). (*Courtesy of* Marten Clinic of Plastic Surgery, San Francisco, CA.)

to appropriately treat subplatysmal fat, is the key to obtaining consistently good outcomes in neck lift procedures.

Cervical lipectomy is a technically demanding maneuver that requires patience, perseverance, and artistic sensitivity, and it should be the aim of the surgeon to produce an attractive neck, and not simply one devoid of fat. Contrary to what is traditionally practiced, if a facelift is being performed in conjunction with the neck lift, subcutaneous lipectomy (including liposuction) should be performed *after* deep neck maneuvers and shifting and suturing of the SMAS and platysma, and not at the beginning of the procedure. If subcutaneous submental liposuction and/or lipectomy is performed at the beginning of the procedure fat will be mistakenly excised from regions of the neck that will be raised onto the face when SMAS flaps are advanced and suspended, and the can result in inadvertent creation of a harsh or irregular mandibular contours (**Fig. 24**). In almost all cases it is best to leave the subcutaneous fat layer untouched until all other maneuvers are completed and improvements obtained with them assessed. Only then should fat be removed from the

subcutaneous layer. Typically what appeared to be excess fat initially will be seen to not be so after deep layer maneuvers have been completed.

Exploration of the subplatysmal space is indicated if preoperative assessment suggests a significant collection of subplatysmal fat is present, large digastric muscles are detected, large submandibular glands are identified, or if uncertainty exists as to any aspect of the subplatysmal condition. Significant accumulations of subplatysmal fat can be demonstrated intraoperatively by placing gentle superior traction on the cheek flaps (if face lift) or cheeks (if isolated neck lift) and flexing the neck. If the neck appears full on this maneuver, consideration should be given to exploration of the subplatysmal space and the removal of redundant subplatysmal fat and/or protruding portions of other enlarged structures.

Subplatysmal exploration is performed through the submental skin incision. The subplatysmal space is entered by incising the superficially situated fascia between the medial platysma muscle borders using a Metzenbaum scissors or electrocautery. A combination of blunt and sharp scissors technique is used to isolate and elevate the medial muscle edge, and it is then grasped and retracted by the assistant using a 10-mm double-prong skin hook or an Allis forceps. The dissection is subsequently carried laterally, over the anterior belly of the digastric muscle hugging the underside of the platysma. If this dissection is carefully made, a well-defined and relatively avascular plane can usually be identified. Small communicating vessels are not infrequently encountered. however, especially near the medial muscle borders. These should be carefully fulgurated and divided as required. Subplatysmal fat should be left on the deep surface of the neck and *not* raised with the platysma flap. This will facilitate subplatysmal fat pad removal, as it is technically more difficult to resect fat from the undersurface of the muscle.

The plane tangent to the anterior bellies of the digastric muscles with the neck in neutral or slightly flexed position should be used as the landmark for subplatysmal fat removal. All fat present in the subplatysmal space lying superficial to this plane theoretically should be removed if optimal contour is to be obtained.

As a practical matter, overall neck contour must be considered, as it is the curvilinear plane across the submental region tangent to the borders of the mandible and the anterior bellies of the digastric muscles that ultimately determines attractive neck contour (**Fig. 25**). If large submandibular glands and/or anterior bellies of the digastric muscles are present and it is elected that they not be treated, subplatysmal fat removal should be more conservative if accentuation of these problems is

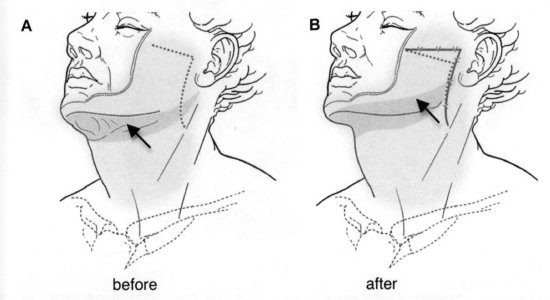

before   after

Fig. 24. Sequencing excision of preplatysmal fat when simultaneous facelift and neck lift are performed. If submental liposuction is performed *before* the SMAS is elevated and sutured, denuded areas will be subsequently advanced onto the lower face. This can result in a harsh mandibular contour. To avoid this problem, preplatysmal fat should be removed, if indicated, *after* the SMAS flap has been raised. (*A*) *Incorrect* plan for preplatysmal fat excision (*gray shaded area*). Submental liposuction is performed at the beginning of the procedure before SMAS flap is raised. (*B*) After SMAS elevation, areas stripped of fat (*gray shaded area*) are moved up onto the lower face. (*Courtesy of* Marten Clinic of Plastic Surgery, San Francisco, CA.)

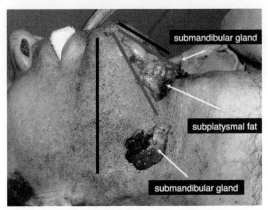

Fig. 25. Anatomy of optimal neck contour. The curvilinear plane across the submental region tangent to the border of the mandible (*near black line*) to the ipsilateral anterior belly of the digastric muscle (*near red line*) to the contralateral digastric (*far red line*), to the contralateral mandibular border (*far black line*) ultimately defines attractive neck contour. Between the border of the mandible and the digastric muscle, poor contour is due to protruding submandibular glands. Between the digastric muscle bellies, the problem is the subplatysmal fat. Additional improvement can be obtained by reducing the anterior digastric muscle bellies themselves. Surgical procedure performed by Timothy J. Marten, MD, FACS. (*Courtesy of* Timothy J. Marten, MD, FACS, Marten Clinic of Plastic Surgery, San Francisco, CA.)

to be avoided. Fibrous fat in the prehyoid region also should not be arbitrarily removed, especially in women, as accentuation and masculinization of the larynx can occur. If prominent submandibular glands and digastric muscles are appropriately treated, however, more aggressive resection of subplatysmal fat can typically be made.

Subplatysmal fat will be evident as a centrally situated triangular shaped fat pad with its base lying at the hyoid and tip near the mentum (**Fig. 26**). It should be removed as appropriate, and as determined by the position and size of the digastric muscles and the size of the submandibular glands. Fat removal should not be arbitrary, and close attention must be paid to the new contours created. Subplatysmal fat excision often results in division of tributaries of small pretracheal vessels and a long-shielded cautery forceps and good suction should be available to obtain adequate hemostasis when required.

Fat situated deep to the plane tangent to anterior bellies of the digastric muscles and beneath the deep cervical fascia (deep cervical or "interdigastric" fat) should not be removed and the overwhelming temptation to "clean out" the deep cervical space resisted. Platysmaplasty, invaginating platysma in a "corset" fashion, suturing the anterior bellies of the digastric muscles together, and other like maneuvers cannot compensate for

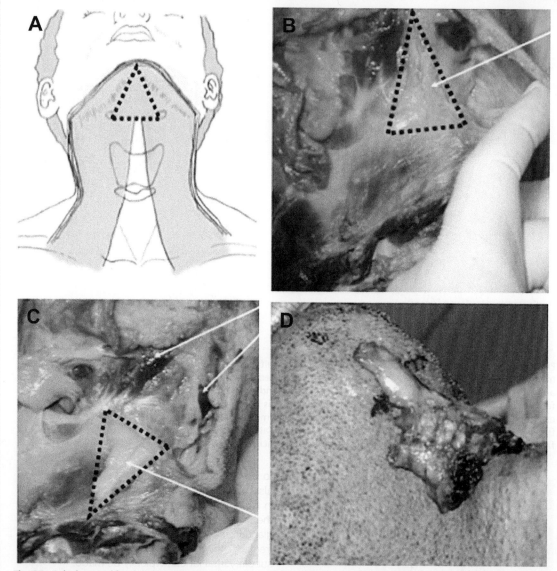

Fig. 26. Subplatysmal fat. (*A*) Illustration showing the position of the triangular-shaped subplatysmal fat pad located in the submental space with its tip near the mentum and base at the hyoid bone. (*B*) Cadaver view of the submental region and subplatysmal fat similar to that shown in illustration in (*A*), but closer-up. The arrow is pointing to the subplatysmal fat that has been outlined with a dashed line. The right and left borders of the platysma have been elevated, showing the contents of the submental space. The subplatysmal fat pad can be seen overlying the digastric muscles to the upper right and left of the triangle. The hyoid bone is at the base of the triangle. (*C*) Cadaver demonstration of subplatysmal fat. The head is slightly turned to the viewer's right and the chin is at the upper right-hand corner of the photo. The two upper arrows point to the anterior bellies of the right and left digastric muscles and the lower arrow to the subplatysmal fat pad. In this photo, the fat pad has been reflected inferiorly but is still attached at its base. The hyoid is now visible along with the interdigastric space. There is a small amount of deep cervical fat visible between the two upper arrows that has been reflected to the right. (*D*). Intraoperative demonstration of the subplatysmal fat specimen lying over the submental space from which it was removed. The patient's chin is pointing superiorly and is in the upper left corner of the photo. The neck is in the lower right corner of the photo. (*Courtesy of* Timothy J. Marten, MD, FACS, Marten Clinic of Plastic Surgery, San Francisco, CA.)

overzealous excision of deep fat and, in time, an objectionable submental depression will appear in the necks of patients so treated (see **Fig. 17**).

Operative Sequence for Subplatysmal Fat Excision

Once the platysma muscles have been raised and the prominent submandibular glands have been identified (see discussion that follows) the subplatysmal fat pad is most easily isolated by identifying each anterior belly of the digastric muscle near its insertion at the chin by making a small incision with scissors in the overlying fat and fascia. Once the muscle is identified in that location, the dissection is carried down inferiorly and laterally on its anterior (inferior) surface to its insertion at the lateral hyoid. If the submandibular glands have been previously mobilized inside their capsules, the dissection along the surface of each digastric muscle can be taken into the submandibular capsule. This dissection along the anterior surface of each digastric muscle defines the lateral border of the subplatysmal fat pad. Overlaying fat is typically divided with electrocautery due to the predictable presence of a branch vein. Once the lateral borders of the fat pad have been dissected, the right and left inferior corners are dissected up off the underlying muscle fascia toward the midline. The plane tangent to each digastric muscle anterior belly is then imagined and all fat lying inferior (superficial) to that plane is removed using electro cautery, leaving the interdigastric fat between the digastric muscles intact and in place. Typically, a vein will be encountered and require cautery in the prehyoid region.

Submandibular Gland Reduction

If large submandibular glands are present, they usually can be seen and palpated lateral to the ipsilateral belly of the anterior digastric muscle on each side within its respective submandibular triangle protruding inferiorly to a plane tangent to the digastric belly and the mandibular border. The protruding portion can be resected through the submental incision before submental platysmaplasty is performed to improve neck contour, if indicated (**Fig. 27**).

Prominent submandibular glands will be encountered as subplatysmal dissection is carried over the anterior belly of the ipsilateral digastric muscle. The prominent gland will appear as a smooth pink to tan-colored mass covered by a smooth capsule. Reduction is begun by incising the capsule overlying the gland inferomedially just lateral to the anterior belly of the digastric muscle. The submandibular gland will be evident once exposed in this manner due to its distinctive lobulated appearance. Its inferior portion can be grasped and easily separated from its capsule using a gentle blunt scissors spreading technique. Although all vital structures are outside the glandular capsule, care should be taken when mobilizing the gland superior-laterally as both the retromandibular vein and the marginal mandibular branch of the facial nerve are in proximity in that area.

An examination of the gland once mobilized inside its capsule will show it to be large, and not merely "ptotic," and this observation forms the basis of the recommendation that partial resection of the protruding portion be performed. Examination of the exposed gland will also clearly demonstrate that attempts to reposition it more superiorly by suture suspension, or by tightening overlying platysma muscle will ultimately be fruitless.

A key step in the safe performance of the procedure is adequate mobilization of the gland, and a modest overmobilization will make both gland resection and the control of any intraglandular bleeding that might be encountered much easier.

Once adequately mobilized inside its capsule, the inferior portion of the gland is grasped, and pulled gently inferiorly and medially out of its fossa and away from adjacent structures. The redundant portion is subsequently excised under direct vision in a medial to lateral direction along the planned line of resection with coagulating current cautery. Excision of the excess part of the gland should be performed in such a manner that the portion protruding inferior to the plane tangent to the ipsilateral anterior belly of the digastric muscle and the ipsilateral mandibular border will be resected. It is usually best that initial resection is conservative and that the gland is incrementally reduced thereafter as required. Never is it necessary or appropriate to remove an entire gland. This could result in a depression or other contour abnormality, and could precipitate an objectionable depression or "dry mouth" condition.

Excision of the redundant and protruding portion of the submandibular gland should be performed using an extended flat-tipped cautery and a long, high-quality pair of atraumatic (DeBakey or similar) forceps. A flat-tipped, extended cautery is superior for controlling bleeding of an intraglandular vessel should it be encountered than is a needlepoint cautery tip. A pair of long, high-quality, insulated coagulation forceps is also required.

As in all surgery of the neck and submental region, a fiberoptic headlight or retractor is mandatory, as is a competent assistant and a second scrubbed team member to pass instruments and sutures as needed. One person cannot effectively perform both these roles. A suction cannula or smoke-evacuating retractor also should be placed, and the position of the cautery tip relative to vital adjacent structures must be known at all times during the resection. If a smoke-evacuating retractor is used, a second suction setup for a Yankauer suction should be available in the event that bleeding is encountered during the resection and suction is needed to obtain hemostasis.

Algorithm for Management of Bleeding Encountered During Submandibular Gland Reduction

Submandibular gland reduction must not be performed without good light, proper instruments, requisite exposure, adequate suction, sufficient personnel, and considered caution, as intraglandular vessels may be encountered. These vessels are

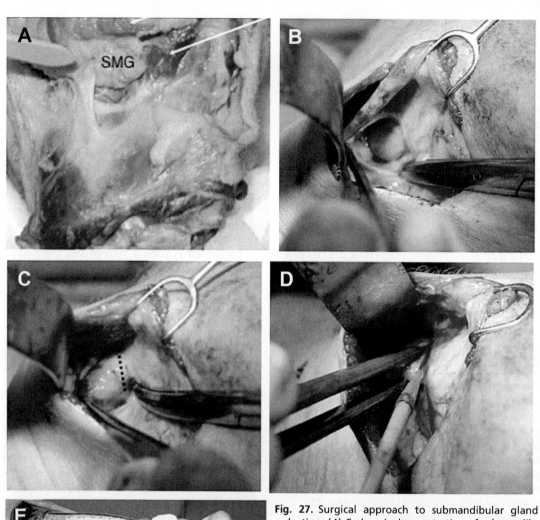

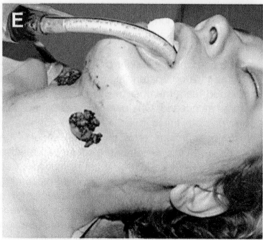

Fig. 27. Surgical approach to submandibular gland reduction. (*A*) Cadaveric demonstration of submandibular triangle. Chin is in the upper right corner of the photo. The excessive portion of the submandibular gland (SMG) is found protruding inferiorly to a plane tangent to the digastric (*small white arrow*) and the mandibular border (*scalpel handle in upper left hand corner of photo*). (*B*) Intraoperative photo demonstrating exposure of the submandibular gland. A submental incision has been made approximately 1 cm posterior to the submental crease and the neck subcutaneously undermined. The right platysma muscle has been elevated and is retracted with a double-pronged skin hook and a malleable retractor. The gland can be seen as a distinct bulge just lateral to the ipsilateral anterior belly of the digastric (scissors tips rest on digastric). The capsule has been incised inferomedially and the submandibular gland isolated using blunt dissection. (*C*). Intraoperative photo before resection of the excess portion of the gland. The gland has been mobilized and gently pulled inferiorly. The dotted line represents the level at which the inferior portion of the gland will be excised. (*D*) Intraoperative photo just before excision of the protruding part of the gland. This should be performed incrementally with electrocautery in such a manner that the portion protruding inferior to the plane tangent to the ipsilateral anterior belly of the digastric muscle and the ipsilateral mandibular border will be resected. (*E*) Patient seen immediately after neck lift that included partial submandibular gland reduction but no skin resection. The photo shows the excellent contour created without skin tightening. The excised portions of the submandibular glands are also demonstrated on both the right and left sides (subplatysmal fat was also excised and the anterior bellies of the digastric muscles reduced). (*Courtesy of* Timothy J. Marten, MD, FACS, Marten Clinic of Plastic Surgery, San Francisco, CA.)

more commonly encountered when larger resections are necessary and are most easily managed by immediate and thorough fulguration before further dissection is made. Typically, bleeding will occur from both the gland and the specimen side and this is usually best controlled by quickly moving the cautery back and forth between each end of the cut vessel. If only the gland side is cauterized, bleeding will often continue from the specimen side, obscuring the surgical field.

If bleeding cannot be readily controlled by direct cauterization of each side of the cut vessel, suction should be applied and an insulated forceps used to directly grasp the bleeding point and the point subsequently cauterized by application of coagulating cautery current to the instrument. If bleeding is brisk and not easily controlled by cauterization as described previously, the gland should be pulled inferiorly and the entire cut edge of it should be compressed proximally with a second pair of forceps. Once bleeding is controlled in this manner, the wound can be irrigated and suctioned to clear the field and the vessel then carefully identified. It can then be grasped with a second instrument and cautery applied.

In the unlikely event that bleeding cannot be controlled by the preceding maneuvers, the submandibular fossae should be packed with a gauze sponge and digital pressure firmly applied for several minutes, pressing the gland against the inner aspect of the mandible and the floor of the mouth. In most cases, when the gauze is carefully removed, the bleeding will be seen to have stopped, the subplatysmal space can be irrigated and suctioned to clear the operative field of any blood, and a search for the bleeding point can be made and any suspicious areas cauterized.

Anatomy of the Submandibular Gland Blood Supply

The submandibular artery enters the submandibular gland superolaterally and will not be directly and specifically encountered when performing conservative resections typically made for aesthetic purposes, and only its terminal branches extending into the gland itself will be encountered. Dissection always should be made carefully in this area, however, and as one becomes more practiced in the procedure and more comprehensive resections as a result are made, this vessel will often be seen as a discrete branch of the much larger submental artery. In many cases, if care is exercised, resection of the most superolateral portion of the protruding portion of the gland can be made without injuring it and it can be isolated and grasped with a hemostatic (Schnitz or tonsil) forceps and ligated.

Once excision of the protruding portion of the gland is complete, the submental region is irrigated and a check for hemostasis along the gland's cut edge is made. It is not necessary or productive to attempt to oversew the cut edge of the gland, or close the glandular capsule. These maneuvers are not only technically difficult, but could result in injury to nearby neurovascular structures. It is also not necessary or productive to overcauterize the cut edge of the gland in an attempt to shrink or seal it. This typically results in more pain and swelling, and prolonged submental induration. Subtotal submandibular gland excision to date has not resulted in any cases of hematoma, airway compromise, salivary fistula, or gustatory sweating in our practices.

Submandibular gland reduction, although important in the rejuvenation of many necks, will not in and of itself result in attractive neck contour. Other problems must be identified and addressed if optimal results are to be obtained.

Submandibular reduction should be regarded as an advanced technique. It should be undertaken by surgeons well versed in cervical anatomy and experienced in more basic maneuvers used to rejuvenate the neck, and the operating surgeon must at all times have the specific algorithm for managing bleeding clearly in mind. It is highly recommended that any surgeon uncertain of the anatomy of the submental triangle or the exact relationships of important structures in this area review them carefully before undertaking this dissection.

Partial Digastric Myectomy

After subplatysmal lipectomy and submandibular gland reduction have been performed, assessment should be made of the anterior bellies of the digastric muscles and whether partial digastric myectomy would produce further improvement in neck contour. In most cases, additional improvement in neck contour can be obtained by performing this procedure.

Typically, large digastric muscles will appear as a linear paramedian fullness lying medial to the rounder and more laterally situated submandibular gland fullness and the difference in appearance of the two problems is a reflection of their differing anatomic origins: the anterior belly of the digastric muscle is a linear paramedian structure and the submandibular gland is a rounder more laterally situated structure (**Fig. 28**).

Usually digastric muscle excess is most evident after subplatysmal lipectomy, and submandibular gland reduction has been performed, but in some cases it may be evident preoperatively in patients seeking secondary, and less commonly, primary surgery. In these situations, additional improvement in neck contour may be obtained

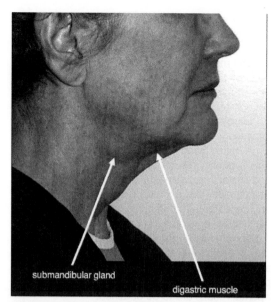

Fig. 28. Surface expression of large digastric muscle. Typically, large digastric muscles will appear as a linear paramedian fullness lying medial to the rounder and more laterally situated submandibular gland fullness and the difference in appearance of the two problems is a reflection of their differing anatomic origins. In some cases, the diagnosis of both problems can be made by simply looking at the patient's neck, as in this one (see also **Figs. 2** and **29**A). (*Courtesy of* Timothy J. Marten, MD, FACS, Marten Clinic of Plastic Surgery, San Francisco, CA.)

by performing superficial, subtotal anterior *digastric myectomy* (excising the protruding portion of the muscle).

Superficial, subtotal anterior digastric myectomy is performed under direct vision, through the submental incision after the subplatysmal space has been opened, the platysma muscle mobilized, and subplatysmal fat and protruding portions of the submandibular gland resected, if indicated. The redundant portion of muscle can be excised by either a tangential strip excision technique or by a partial division and excision technique. Although both are reliable and effective, in most cases tangential strip excision provides the simplest and most intuitive and straightforward means of removing the protruding portion of the muscle belly.

Tangential strip excision is performed by visually gauging the muscle redundancy, grasping the redundant portion with a DeBakey or similar forceps, and tangentially excising a strip of muscle longitudinally from the muscle belly with a Metzenbaum scissors or more commonly with electrocautery using coagulating current. Typically, tangential excision will result in modest bleeding from the excised area that is easily controlled with cautery once muscle reduction is complete if Metzenbaum scissors are used.

Excision is begun near the muscle origin at the mentum and continuing to the muscle belly insertion at the lateral hyoid. The muscle is then reassessed and the action repeated until the protruding portion is fully removed and optimal contour has been established. Approximately 50% of the muscle is removed in the typical case with the most muscle removed near the hyoid and the least near the chin (**Fig. 29**).

In the partial division and excision technique of digastric muscle reduction, the excess muscle present is gauged and isolated on a tonsil forceps by pushing the tips of the instrument through the mid-muscle belly at the level of optimal contour

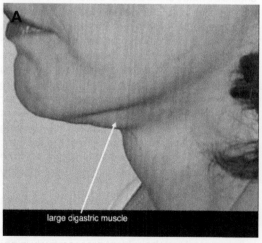

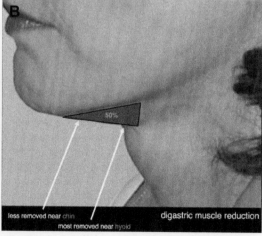

Fig. 29. Digastric muscle reduction strategy. (*A*) Typical appearance of a large anterior belly of the digastric muscle. (*B*) Digastric muscle fullness is treated in a manner that optimizes submental contour. Approximately 50% of the muscle is removed in the typical case, with more muscle removed near the hyoid and less near the chin (*shaded gray area*). (*Courtesy of* Timothy J. Marten, MD, FACS, Marten Clinic of Plastic Surgery, San Francisco, CA.)

and spreading to split the muscle along the length of its fibers. The isolated muscle segment resting on the instrument consisting of the superficial, protruding portion of it is then excised with scissors or cautery by dividing it near the mandible and the hyoid (**Fig. 30**). The neck is reexamined and the maneuver repeated again if necessary until an improved contour is obtained. Usually this entails the excision of the superficial-most half or less of each muscle, with more muscle excised near the hyoid and less near the chin, as is the case when the tangential excision technique is used.

It should be noted that the myectomy, regardless of how it is performed, is a partial and subtotal reduction of the protruding portion of the digastric muscle only, and not an arbitrary exenteration of the entire muscle belly. It also should be understood that optimal contour is achieved when more muscle is resected near the hyoid and less near the chin. In addition, partial, superficial digastric myectomy, although an important maneuver in the rejuvenation of many necks, will not in and of itself result in attractive neck contour. Other problems must be identified and treated if optimal results are to be obtained. Finally, it should be noted that partial, superficial digastric myectomy, although straightforward and conceptually simple, should be regarded as an advanced technique. It should be undertaken by surgeons familiar with cervical anatomy and experienced in more basic maneuvers used to rejuvenate the neck.

Management of the Platysma

Once subplatysmal fat excision, submandibular gland reduction, and partial digastric myectomy have been performed as indicated, and treatment of the subplatysmal space is complete, anterior platysmaplasty is performed. Anterior platysmaplasty is the procedure in which the medial borders of the platysma muscle are sutured together to help consolidate the neck, reduce horizontal platysma laxity, and improve neck appearance when patients flex their neck and look down. It is *not* however, adequate or effective treatment of excess subplatysmal fat, prominent submandibular glands, protruding anterior bellies of the digastric muscles, or the treatment of "hard" dynamic platysma bands. Treatment of these problems will require that other maneuvers be performed. Management of the platysma in neck lift is discussed in detail in the article by Timothy Marten and Dino Elyassnia, "Management of the Platysma in Neck Lift," in this issue.

Final Contouring of Cervicofacial Fat

Once correction of deep layer neck problems has been made and platysmaplasty, platysma myotomy, and suspension of postauricular transposition flaps have been performed as indicated, final contouring of subcutaneous superficial cervicofacial fat should be performed. This can be done under direct vision using Metzenbaum scissors or a small suction cannula. Final fat sculpting should be continued until all contours are smooth and regular, but *it is essential that not all fat be removed if an attractive appearance is to be obtained.* In addition, if a "double chin" or "witch's chin" is present, an extended dissection of the perimental area and chin pad should be made, and fat contributing to these problems sculpted and excised and the two regions seamlessly blended

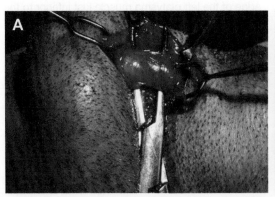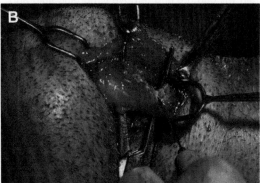

Fig. 30. Partial division and excision technique of digastric muscle reduction. (*A*) Excess muscle present is gauged and isolated on a tonsil forceps by pushing the tips of the instrument through the mid-muscle belly at the level of optimal contour and spreading to split the muscle along the length of its fibers (view from patient's right of left digastric muscle through submental incision; patient's chin is at the left upper corner of the photo and the neck is on right). (*B*) The isolated muscle segment resting on the instrument consisting of the superficial, protruding portion of it is then excised with scissors or cautery by dividing it near the mandible and the hyoid. The neck is reexamined and the maneuver repeated again if necessary until an improved contour is obtained. (*Courtesy of* Marten Clinic of Plastic Surgery, San Francisco, CA.)

to ensure a smooth transition for the chin to the submental area. In full necks, preplatysmal lipectomy can be performed with a suction cannula using an "open" liposuction technique by placing the cannula hole down under the skin flap and holding the skin flap down as resection is made. In thin necks, and in most of our cases, excision is made using a scissors technique.

Drain Placement

Experience has shown that when subplatysmal fat excision and submandibular gland reduction is performed, it is prudent to place a drain in both the subcutaneous and the subplatysmal space for at least several days after the procedure to reduce edema and induration in the submental area to reduce the chance of a fluid collection (lymphatic fluid leakage from the division of lymphatic vessels during subplatysmal fat excision, and saliva leakage from the cut edge of the submandibular gland) and to speed the patient's overall recovery. A 10-F round multiperforated Jackson-Pratt (or similar)-type drain is routinely placed in both the subcutaneous and subplatysmal space and it is safest to perform the platysmaplasty (suturing of the medial platysmal borders together; see Timothy Marten and Dino Elyassnia's, "Management of the Platysma in Neck Lift," in this issue) before subplatysmal drain placement, and then to thread the subplatysmal drain into position afterward. If the subplatysmal drain is placed before platysmaplasty is performed there is a chance that the drain could be caught in one of the platysmaplasty sutures, making its removal problematic.

The vacuum force applied by the subplatysmal drain will capture and remove lymphatic fluid and saliva, close down the subplatysmal space, and pull the underside of the platysmal muscle against the cut edge of each gland. It is convenient to place the exit site of the subcutaneous drain on the opposite side of the neck (opposite the exit site of the subplatysmal drain) so that it is clear which drain is which and output from each can readily be monitored. In a male face, or in a large female face, two subcutaneous drains may be required to adequately drain the subcutaneous space. The vacuum force applied by the subcutaneous drain captures and removes fluid from the subcutaneous space.

Subplatysmal drain placement during deep neck lift should be performed after platysmaplasty is completed (see Timothy Marten and Dino Elyassnia's, "Management of the Platysma in Neck Lift," in this issue) as follows: once platysmaplasty is complete, a stab incision should be made 1 to 2 cm posterior to the occipital facelift incision on the occipital

scalp on right side and the proximal (reservoir) side of the drain pulled retrograde through the incision into position and anchored at its exit site of the scalp with a 4 to 0 nylon suture. The distal part of the drain distal to its point of anchoring is then placed in the subcutaneous space and the tip brought out the submental incision. If a short scar neck lift is being performed and a postauricular incision is not present, a stab incision is made in the right postlobular skin or scalp and a 2.4 or 3.0-mm liposuction cannula is used to tunnel under the lateral neck skin and into the subcutaneous space that has been dissected more anteriorly. The tip of the cannula is brought out the submental incision, the proximal (reservoir) side of the drain is placed firmly over the tip of the cannula, and the cannula is used to drag the drain into position. The drain is then anchored as previously described.

Working through the submental incision, the surgeon then locates the inferior-most platysmaplasty suture and the platysma muscle on the right side just inferior to the inferior-most suture is grasped and the tip of a long "right-angle" (Mixter)-type hemostatic forceps is placed under the muscle edge, then the forceps advanced under the platysma muscle in the subplatysmal space superiorly and laterally up to the approximate location of the right submandibular gland. The tip of the instrument is then pushed through the muscle into the subcutaneous space and the tip of drain grasped and placed over one of the jaws of the forceps. The forceps are then closed and the drain then pulled into the subplatysmal space and back below the inferior-most platysmaplasty suture and out into the subcutaneous space at the midline. The tip of the right-angle forceps is then placed under the medial edge of the left platysma muscle just inferior to the inferior-most platysmaplasty suture and the forceps used to retract the muscle outward to hold open the subplatysmal space on the left. The tip of the drain, now situated subcutaneously in the midline, is then grasped and stuffed into the subplatysmal space on the left side and up to the approximate location of the left submandibular gland. On completion of these maneuvers, most of the drain will be in the subplatysmal space, with a smaller section in the upper lateral right neck in the subcutaneous space.

Skin Closure

If a "short scar" neck lift has been performed, a submental incision only will be present, and this can be conveniently closed in two layers. Before closure, it is important to confirm that the wound edge thickness and amount of subcutaneous fat present on each side of the incision is similar. Typically, the wound edge of the cervical side will be thinner and have less subcutaneous fat due to contact with instruments and retractors during preceding steps in the procedure and the mental, superior side of it will be thicker and have more fat. If a discrepancy is present, as it often will be, fat is carefully removed from the thicker superior side. The first layer of closure consists of several subcutaneous sutures of 5 to 0 Monocryl (or other suture of choice) to ensure that an equal and adequate amount of fat is present behind each edge of the closed wound and so that a depressed or irregular scar is avoided. Final approximation is then made with simple interrupted sutures of 6 to 0 nylon (or other suture of choice).

If an "extended" neck lift is performed, or a face-lift is undertaken in conjunction with a neck lift procedure, skin will be excised from the postauricular area. The postauricular flap is shifted posteriorly and somewhat superiorly, roughly parallel to transverse neck creases and the mandibular border, in such a manner that skin is suspended under minimal or no tension and that *little or no skin need be trimmed from the anterior (postauricular) flap border*. Excessive trimming of skin from the anterior border of the postauricular skin flap will require the flap to be shifted along an incorrect, superiorly directed vector, and this will produce a compromised result. The first point of suspension is located in the postauricular area at the anterior-superior aspect of the occipitomastoid incision. The flap is secured at this point with a simple interrupted suture of 4 to 0 nylon. No incision into the flap is necessary and no deep suture is used.

Once this suspension suture has been placed, the flap overlying the inferior portion of the ear should be carefully divided and the lobule exteriorized. *This is a key step in the procedure that must be performed incrementally and with great care if a visible scar, lobular malposition, and objectionable "pixy earlobe" is to be avoided.* If the incision to exteriorize the lobule is properly made, the apex of the incision should rest snugly against the inferior-most portion of the conchal cartilage. If the incision into the cheek flap is made too far anteriorly or inferiorly, however, artistically appropriate resetting of the lobule will not be possible, and the outcome of the overall procedure significantly compromised.

Postauricular closure along the auriculomastoid sulcus is performed next, and should be completed before trimming and closure of the occipital portion of the incision and resetting of the lobule. It is begun by conservatively trimming the anterior border of the postauricular skin flap into a soft curve to match the curve of the incision made in the auriculomastoid sulcus. The incision is then closed with several interrupted sutures of 4 to 0 nylon. No deep suture is necessary or used.

It is a significant error and conceptually flawed concept to excise any skin over (superior to) the apex of the occipitomastoid incision and to shorten the postauricular flap along the long axis of the sternoclei-domastoid muscle as commonly practiced and shown in many plastic surgery textbooks. Despite an apparent redundancy in this area when the patient is supine on the operating table, there is never any true skin excess at this location. *This pseudo-excess of skin is present only because of the patient's high shoulder position in the supine position. It will vanish when she or he sits up and the shoulders drop to a normal position. Skin along the axis of the sternocleidomastoid muscle is also needed for side-to-side head tilt. Inappropriate excision of skin over the apex of the occipitomastoid defect is the ultimate underlying cause of hypertrophic healing in the postauricular region, and of a wide postauricular scar.*

Trimming and closure of the occipital portion of the incision should be performed after closure of the postauricular area and suspension without trimming along the transmastoid portion of the postauricular incision. A facelift marker should be used to gauge skin flap redundancy along the occipital incision, and all points along the flap should be intentionally trimmed with 2 to 3 mm of redundancy. It must be remembered that the goal of skin excision is to remove redundancy, and not to tighten the cervical skin flap. If trimming is performed correctly, wound edges should abut one another, and no gaps should be present, *before* sutures are placed. The incision is then closed in one layer, with multiple half-buried vertical mattress sutures of 4 to 0 nylon with the knots tied on the scalp side and simple interrupted sutures of 6 to 0 nylon. No deep sutures are required and staples should not be used. This plan will provide precise wound edge alignment and prevent cross-hatched scars (suture marks). In addition, if the incision is closed under no tension as described, an inconspicuous scar will be obtained.

Dressings

After all planned procedures have been completed and all incisions have been closed, the patient's hair is washed with shampoo and conditioner and if long it is placed in a soft braid. The hair is then allowed to dry or is blown dry in the recovery room. A final inspection of sutured incisions is made. If poor alignment is found in any area, it is locally reprepped and sutures are removed and replaced as required.

No dressing is required or applied. Patients are typically discharged with a hat, scarf, and sunglasses following the procedure. The traditional facelift and neck lift dressings consisting of tightly applied mineral oil–soaked cotton and rolled gauze are unnecessary if closed suction drains are used, and a strong argument can be made that they are counterproductive and of potential harm to the patient. These dressings place unnecessary and potentially harmful pressure on thin skin flaps in a critical stage of their healing and can compromise already tenuous circulation in them. In addition, they preclude inspection and monitoring of the operative site and can disguise and delay the diagnosis of serious problems, such as hematoma, flap ischemia, and pressure necrosis. Finally, patients typically find the traditional face and neck lift dressing cumbersome, confining, unhygienic, and claustrophobic, and their family members are often frightened by them.

POSTOPERATIVE CARE

Performance of the procedure itself only fulfills part of our obligation to the patient and the care the patient receives postoperatively is arguably as important as the surgery itself. Diligent postoperative care will also ensure the best result and limit the likelihood that problems and complications will occur.

Patients are discharged with specific written instructions as to how they are to care for themselves, and the surgeon should always be available to answer questions and see any patient, if needed.

Sleeping and Head Position

All patients are instructed to sleep flat on their backs without a pillow. A small cylindrical neck roll is permitted if the patient requests or requires it. This posture ensures a "chin-up" open cervicomental angle and averts dangerous folding of the neck skin flap and obstruction of regional cervical lymphatics that inevitably occurs if the patient is allowed to "elevate the head on pillows" as is commonly recommended after head and neck surgery. If patients are allowed to elevate their heads on pillows, their necks will inevitably end up flexed and their skin bunched and folded. In addition, a flat-in-bed position encourages swelling to drain posteriorly to the back of the head where it is not harmful, less noticeable, and more rapidly transmitted away from the head and neck area when the patient sits upright rather than inferiorly to the anterior neck and along the jawline, as it does when the patient is more upright. This is particularly helpful if a facelift has been performed as part of the procedure.

Patients are shown an "elbows on knees" position that ensures an open cervicomental angle while sitting. This posture places the patient's book, magazine, paperwork, notebook computer, or meal in a position that allows reading, writing, eating, and TV watching to be performed comfortably and safely with the chin up and the neck skin smoothly and uniformly distributed over the neck. If patients are allowed to sit upright during these activities, their neck will inevitably end up flexed and their skin bunched and folded.

Cool Compresses

Patients are asked to rest quietly and apply cool compresses to their face and neck for 15 to 20 minutes of every hour they are awake for the first 3 days after surgery. For most patients, edema peaks at about this time. It is not necessary or productive to apply cool compresses continually throughout the day or at night. Ice and "ice packs" should never be applied directly to the skin.

Medications

All patients are provided oral (usually non-narcotic) analgesics, sleeping pills, oral dissolving anti-emetic tablets, and related and other needed supplies with instructions for their use.

After Surgery Diet

Patients undergoing neck lift are placed on a "salivary rest" diet consisting of soft, wet, easy-to-swallow foods and are encouraged to avoid sweet, salty, sour, dry, and difficult to chew foods and citrus for several weeks. It is particularly important to avoid these sorts of foods that stimulate salivation for 7 to 10 days if submandibular gland reduction has been performed if fluid collections and neck induration is to be avoided. Patients are asked to abstain from the intake of alcohol for 2 weeks after surgery.

Wound Care

Patients are instructed to begin a daily routine of showering and shampooing no later than 3 days after surgery. Patients are allowed to shower even if their drains are still in place. This helps remove crusting about the suture lines, keeps incisions clean, and usually improves the patient's general outlook and well-being. Patients are also informed that they need not be as thorough as usual when washing their hair and assured that shower water, shampoo, and conditioners are not harmful and will not interfere with healing or cause infection.

Drain Removal

Drains are usually left in the neck until the patient's first clinic visit for suture removal 5 days after their surgery. This is because drain output often quickly falls on the first or second day after surgery during the time the patient is mostly supine and resting, but then typically picks up again when the patient begins to spend more time upright, starts to move his or her head about more, and begins to eat more. Leaving the neck drains in longer, for 5 to 7 days, will reduce the likelihood that small collections will form and it will speed the overall resolution of edema, ecchymosis, and induration in the neck area. Their first suture removal visit 5 days after surgery, the progress and drain output are accessed. If healing is progressing well, drain output is minimal, and no fluid collections are present, and if it appears that the patient is following dietary and other instructions, drains are removed at that time. It is prudent to release suction before drain removal and to have the patient or an assistant hold pressure over the anterior neck as the drain is removed for several minutes to avoid inducing the formation of a hematoma.

If a patient's neck appears congested at the fifth postoperative day, if drain output is still significant, or if the patient appears to not be following dietary and other instructions, drains are not removed and are left in place until the patient's second suture removal visit 7 days after surgery. In almost all cases, drains, if still present, are removed at that time.

It is important to carefully monitor the patient's neck for blood and fluid collections at each visit and if found they should be addressed. Often small collections resulting from poor drain function can be removed by "milking" the exteriorized portion of the drain tube to restart drain flow. Loculated collections that have accumulated subcutaneously in an area away from the drain can often be stroked and massaged toward and to it. Collections that cannot be evacuated in these ways should be transcutaneously aspirated with a hypodermic needle. Collections of these sorts may require several serial aspirations performed over a period of several days. It is prudent to see the patient and continue aspiration until the collection no longer reforms. Collections allowed to congeal and consolidate will result in firm, irregular areas that can take many months to resorb and can result in permanent contour irregularities.

Suture Removal

When sutures are removed will vary depending on the type of procedure performed. If a "short scar" neck lift has been performed, a submental incision only will be present and sutures are removed on the fourth or fifth day. If an "extended" neck lift or facelift and neck lift have been performed, 6-0 nylon sutures are removed on the fourth or fifth day. If these sutures are left in longer, telltale and objectionable "suture marks" are likely to occur. Half-buried vertical mattress sutures of 4-0 nylon with the knots tied on the scalp side are removed on the seventh to ninth day.

Return to Work after Surgery

When patients return to work and their social lives will depend on their tolerance for surgery, their capacity for healing, the type of work they do, the activities they enjoy, and how they feel overall about their appearance. Patients are asked to set aside 7 to 10 days to recover depending on the extent of their surgery, and additional time off is recommended if a facelift and related procedures are simultaneously performed. If the patient is doing well and not experiencing problems, she or he is allowed to return to light office work and casual social activities at that time. It is often wise that they begin with a limited workday at first and to adjust their schedules thereafter. If a patient's job entails more strenuous activity or physical labor, a longer period of convalescence may be required. Patients are advised not to drive for the first 10 days after surgery and until they are feeling well, their vision is clear, and they are off pain medications.

After Surgery Activity

Patients are advised to avoid all strenuous activity during the first 2 weeks after surgery. Two weeks after surgery, patients are allowed to begin light exercise and gradually work up to their presurgical level of activity. Four to 6 weeks after surgery, they are allowed to engage in more vigorous activities, including most sports, as tolerated.

CASE EXAMPLES
Patient Example 1

Fig. 31 shows before and after surgery views of a woman, age 65, who has had prior upper and lower eyelifts by an unknown surgeon. Note lax skin, obtuse cervicosubmental contour, paucity of subcutaneous neck fat, and "double-chin" appearance when the patient looks down in before views. A large submandibular salivary gland is clearly visible in the lateral submental triangle in the lateral view, and the patient appears to have a "low hyoid."

Fig. 31 also shows the same patient 13 months after facelift, neck lift, forehead lift, upper and lower eyelifts, peri-oral dermabrasion, and fat transfer to cheeks and lips. The neck lift procedure included excision of excess subplatysmal fat, submandibular salivary gland reduction, superficial digastric myectomy, anterior platysmaplasty and full-width platysma myotomy. Note well-defined

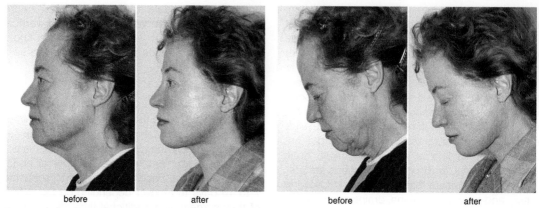

before   after   before   after

Fig. 31. Before and after surgery views of a woman, age 65 who has had prior upper and lower eyelifts by an unknown surgeon. Surgical procedure performed by Timothy J. Marten, MD, FACS. (*Courtesy of* Timothy J. Marten, MD, FACS, Marten Clinic of Plastic Surgery, San Francisco, CA.)

jaw line and attractive, youthful-appearing neckline even when the patient looks down. Comprehensive neck surgery has corrected problems that are commonly misinterpreted as a low hyoid position.

Patient Example 2

Fig. 32 shows before and after surgery views of a woman, age 46, who has had no prior surgery. Note full neck, obtuse cervicosubmental contour, and "double-chin" appearance when the patient looks down in before views. Palpation of the lateral submental triangle revealed a firm mobile mass consistent with an enlarged submandibular salivary gland. Her preoperative appearance suggests the presence of a "low hyoid."

Fig. 32 also shows the same patient 11 months after facelift, neck lift, forehead lift, lower eyelifts, and facial fat injections. The neck lift procedure included excision of subplatysmal fat, submandibular salivary gland reduction, superficial

digastric myectomy, anterior platysmaplasty, and full-width platysmal myotomy. Note attractive, youthful-appearing neckline even when the patient looks down. Comprehensive neck surgery has corrected problems that are commonly misinterpreted as a low hyoid position. The double-chin deformity has also been corrected.

Patient Example 3

Fig. 33 shows before and after surgery views of a woman age 55 who has had prior eyelifts and a peri-oral chemical peel performed by an unknown surgeon. Note full neck, obtuse cervicosubmental contour, and "double-chin" appearance that is exacerbated when the patient looks down in before views. Palpation of the lateral submental triangle revealed a firm mobile mass consistent with an enlarged submandibular salivary gland. Note paucity of subcutaneous neck fat suggesting submental liposuction had been performed at her previous procedure.

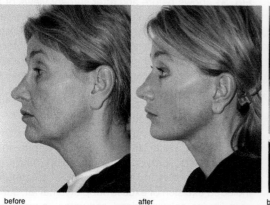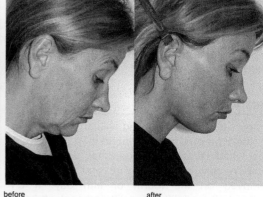

before   after   before   after

Fig. 32. Before and after surgery views of a woman, age 46, who has had no prior surgery. Surgical procedure performed by Timothy J. Marten, MD, FACS. (*Courtesy of* Timothy J. Marten, MD, FACS, Marten Clinic of Plastic Surgery, San Francisco, CA.)

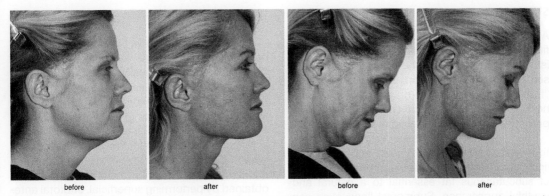

Fig. 33. Before and after surgery views of a woman, age 55, who has had prior eyelifts and a peri-oral chemical peel performed by an unknown surgeon. Surgical procedure performed by Timothy J. Marten, MD, FACS. (*Courtesy of* Timothy J. Marten, MD, FACS, Marten Clinic of Plastic Surgery, San Francisco, CA.)

Fig. 33 also shows the same patient 1 year and 4 months after facelift, neck lift, forehead lift, upper and lower eyelifts, peri-oral dermabrasion, and facial fat injections. The neck lift procedure included excision of a large amount of subplatysmal fat, submandibular salivary gland reduction, superficial digastric myectomy, anterior platysmaplasty, and full-width platysma myotomy. Note well-defined jaw line and attractive, youthful-appearing neckline even when the patient looks down. The double-chin deformity has been corrected by releasing the submental retaining ligaments and blending the fat of the chin and the submental area.

Patient Example 4

Fig. 34 shows before and after surgery views of a man, age 68, who has had no prior plastic

surgery. Note poor cervicosubmental contour and "double-chin" appearance when the patient looks down in before views. An enlarged submandibular salivary gland can be seen beneath the skin in the lateral view and confirmed on palpation. Note paucity of subcutaneous neck fat that is typical for patients in older age groups. Platysma bands are visible in the anterior neck.

Fig. 34 also shows the same patient 1 year and 9 months after facelift, neck lift, forehead lift, upper and lower eye lifts, partial facial fat transfer, and ear lobe reduction. The neck lift procedure included excision of amount of subplatysmal fat, submandibular salivary gland reduction, superficial digastric myectomy, anterior platysmaplasty, and full-width platysma myotomy. Note well-defined jaw line and masculine-appearing neckline even when the patient looks down.

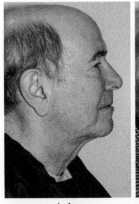
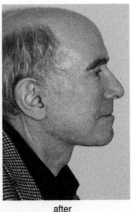
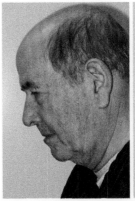
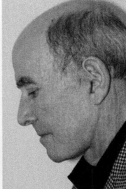

Fig. 34. Before and after surgery views of a man, age 68, who has had no prior plastic surgery. Surgical procedure performed by Timothy J. Marten, MD, FACS. (*Courtesy of* Timothy J. Marten, MD, FACS, Marten Clinic of Plastic Surgery, San Francisco, CA.)

SUMMARY

A well-contoured neckline is essential to a youthful, fit, and attractive appearance. Neck improvement is of high priority to almost every patient who presents for facial rejuvenation, and the results of a "facelift" are often judged on the outcome in the neck. If the neck is not sufficiently improved, our patients will feel we have failed them.

Submental liposuction is an incomplete solution to most patients' neck problems and submental liposuction can result in the inappropriate removal of subcutaneous fat essential to a natural and youthful appearance. Submental liposuction can be particularly problematic when aggressive techniques are used. Overexcision of subcutaneous fat may not be evident at the time of surgery or in the early postoperative period when cervicosubmental tissues are swollen, but can result in problems that appear later that once present, are very difficult to correct. Proper treatment of many necks requires modification of deep layer structures and cannot be limited to submental liposuction and the tightening of skin.

The prominent submandibular gland is large, not ptotic, and aggressive submental liposuction and subplatysmal fat resection can make a large submandibular gland more obvious and objectionable appearing. Experience has shown that submandibular gland reduction is safe and more effective than suture suspension or platysma-tightening techniques.

A subset of patients will be encountered who have objectionably large anterior bellies of their digastric muscles. Typically, large digastric muscles will appear as a linear paramedian fullness lying medial to the rounder and more laterally situated submandibular gland fullness and the difference in appearance of the two problems is a reflection of their differing anatomic origins. When large digastric muscles can be identified, additional improvement in neck contour can be obtained by performing superficial, subtotal anterior digastric myectomy. Failure to identify and treat large digastric muscles will result in objectionable fullness and cervical obliquity in the submental region postoperatively. Digastric muscle reduction is performed *after* subplatysmal fat and protruding portions of the submandibular gland have been removed.

Subplatysmal fat excision, submandibular gland reduction, and superficial digastric myectomy performed in conjunction with each other as indicated provides for the creation of the best neck contour possible, and the skilled neck surgeon must master treatment of all three of these "deep layer" problems and use them in conjunction with each other as indicated, if optimal results are to be obtained.

Reduction Neck Lift
The Importance of the Deep Structures of the Neck to the Successful Neck Lift

Francisco G. Bravo, MD, PhD

KEYWORDS

- Neck lift • Face lift • Facial rejuvenation • Cervicofacial rejuvenation • Jawline definition
- Submental fat • Submandibular gland • Parotid gland

KEY POINTS

- Patients seeking enhancement in jawline definition who present with marked fullness in the submandibular region are best managed through reduction of the deep structures of the neck.
- Facial aging is often associated with perifacial expansion and fullness in the submandibular region.
- Enlarged major salivary glands are common in patients with submandibular fullness and may be responsible for most of the volume laterally and posteriorly.
- The dynamic anatomy of the neck must be considered when planning and evaluating neck lift and facial rejuvenation procedures in order to achieve natural results.
- A thorough analysis of the surface anatomy and features of the young and attractive neck and jawline is essential in order to obtain successful neck lift results.

 Video content accompanies this article at http://www.plasticsurgery.theclinics.com/.

INTRODUCTION

With the growth of nonsurgical or minimally invasive procedures for facial rejuvenation such as neuromodulators, fillers, and skin resurfacing techniques, the neck has gained added attention recently, because an increasing number of patients are seeking solutions in this area that might enhance and complement those obtained in the face.[1]

Despite efforts to achieve adequate results in the neck and jawline nonsurgically,[2] surgery is often the best option in order to obtain long-lasting and both evident and natural outcomes. Physicians looking to modify the anatomy of this region surgically should plan the procedure carefully in order to provide their patients with a technique that meets their expectations, as they will frequently be required to deliver added results to those obtained by other professionals offering nonsurgical options.[3]

The jawline and neck are important features relevant to both perceived age and attractiveness and are also very significant to the perceived body weight of individuals. In a recent study,[4] participants considered subjects with a young perifacial anatomy, despite having a more aged centrofacial appearance, as looking younger than vice versa. Women also consider their jawline as their most disliked feature as they age.[5] Patients have a lower threshold for desire for surgery compared with clinicians with respect to their desired

Disclosure: The author has nothing to disclose.
Clinica Gomez Bravo, Calle Claudio Coello 76, Madrid 28001, Spain
E-mail address: fgbravo@clinicagomezbravo.com

Clin Plastic Surg 45 (2018) 485–506
https://doi.org/10.1016/j.cps.2018.05.002

submental-cervical angle (110° vs 125°, respectively) and consider an attractive submental-cervical angle to be between 90° and 105°,[6] which corroborates the notion that a slim neck without submental fullness is considered a sign not only of youth but also of beauty.

Achieving harmony and balance between the face and the neck is crucial in order to obtain natural-appearing results in cervicofacial rejuvenation procedures. Patients are often undertreated in the neck area.[1] Not providing patients with an adequate solution for their neck deformity while only managing their face may result in an awkward operated look, such as the overdone-face underdone-neck deformity, which is often evident when patients look down in profile view, referred to as the Connell view.[7]

Surgeons committed to providing results in facial rejuvenation must be diligent in the techniques that may best improve the neck and submental region in order to provide their patients with balanced and natural outcomes before undertaking any isolated facial procedures at all.

INDICATIONS FOR MANAGEMENT OF DEEP STRUCTURES

Patients with considerable amounts of submandibular fullness are generally good candidates for management of the deep structures of the neck. Any palpable mass or rapid increase in soft tissue volume around the neck should first be carefully studied in order to discard neoplastic or other pathologic origins. Several other factors, however, may contribute to patients developing fullness in

their cervical region, and surgical intervention may prove valuable in improving this condition.

Weight Gain

Weight gain often results in an increase of volume around the cervical region due to fat accumulation in both the superficial and deep compartments of the neck. Furthermore, fatty deposition in the salivary glands may also contribute to volume increase in the submental area and produce cervical fullness and bulging in the overweight patient.[8] Although there may be differences among men and women in their tendency to accumulate fat around the neck with weight gain, as well as in the location where this cervical fat accumulation is more prevalent, studies have shown that a substantial amount of the fat found in the neck lies in the deep subplatysmal space.[9,10]

It should be noted that patients may present with submandibular and neck fullness and not be overweight. These individuals often have had heavy, thick necks starting at a young age, due to hereditary factors, and complain that their neck conveys them an overweight appearance despite having an adequate body mass index.

Aging

Although many individuals demonstrate a marked cervicofacial thinning and volume loss with aging (type I facial aging) (**Fig. 1**), most persons will experience some degree, if not a profound, volume augmentation around the jawline and neck, with a predominant perifacial expansion (type II

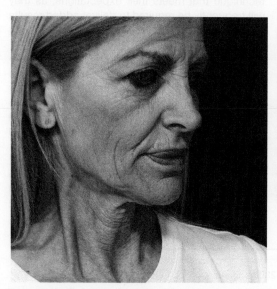
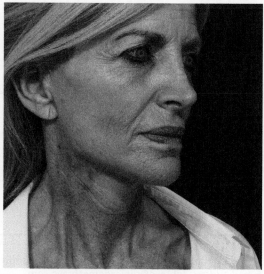

Fig. 1. (*left*) Type I facial aging with predominant facial thinning and volume loss. (*right*) Result after a face and neck lift procedure through a lateral approach only, without opening the neck.

facial aging) (**Fig. 2**), which may account for up to 85% of individuals as they age and may be more prevalent in men.[4]

This perifacial expansion is responsible for the lack of definition of the jawline associated with aging, although it may sometimes be attributed to weight gain alone. Several studies have shown, however, that weight gain may be directly related to aging and often times must be considered an intrinsic part of the aging process itself, defined as age-related weight gain.[11,12]

Although type I facial aging patients with predominant thinning seem to age better and have a simpler surgical solution to their condition, often only requiring mid face volume replacement and tightening of the soft tissue laxity through a lateral approach (see **Fig. 1**), type II facial aging patients with predominant perifacial expansion often show more dramatic signs of aging and require management of the deep structures of the neck through an open neck approach in order to obtain maximal results in their cervicofacial rejuvenation procedure (see **Fig. 2**).

Salivary Gland Hypertrophy

The submandibular and parotid glands may contribute significantly to fullness and bulging in the neck region, with the submandibular glands (SMG) alone accounting for up to 24.5% of the total subcutaneous soft tissue of the neck.[10]

Several conditions may affect the size and position of the salivary glands, and surgeons seeking to enhance the neck should be aware that patients requesting cervicofacial rejuvenation might present with considerably large glands at the time of surgery (**Fig. 3**).

Eating disorders have been associated with enlargement of the major salivary glands.[13] As part of the digestive system, salivary glands may also grow significantly in overweight patients, in the same way other organs of the digestive tract such as the stomach or liver enlarge in individuals with high body mass indexes. Just as it frequently occurs in the liver, fatty deposition of the salivary glands has also been identified histologically in overweight patients.[8] Alcohol consumption has also been related to increase in salivary gland size,[14] and an association between alcohol consumption and aging has also been established.[15]

Finally, the major salivary glands have been shown to increase in size[16,17] and to gradually migrate caudally[18] with aging.

Previous Neck Procedures

Any procedure performed on the neck that may reduce subcutaneous fat, such as radiofrequency,

deoxycholic acid injections, cryotherapy, or liposuction, or surgical tightening procedures of the platysma, may make the deep structures of the neck more evident and visible after treatment, thus requiring surgical management of these structures afterward in order to obtain adequate results (**Fig. 4**).

Furthermore, the decision to undertake the reduction of a deep cervical structure often times requires the surgeon to manage an adjacent subplatysmal structure in order to avoid its visibility postoperatively. Such is the case of the *submandibular triad*,[19] in which the subplatysmal fat, the SMGs, and the anterior belly of the digastric (ABD) muscles are managed sequentially and in that order, to obtain optimal neck contouring.

THE SUCCESSFUL NECK LIFT

Before deciding whether to manage the deep structures of the neck in patients seeking cervical rejuvenation and enhancement, a thorough knowledge of the morphologic characteristics of the young and attractive neck and jawline is essential in order to understand the surgical maneuvers necessary to mimic those features and design a surgical plan accordingly.

Surface Anatomy and Aesthetics of the Neck

Although other anatomic areas subject to modification through aesthetic surgery have seen extensive descriptions of the ideal surface aesthetics and underlying anatomy,[20] the neck and submandibular regions still lack a thorough description of the key surface landmarks that should influence surgical modification.

As with any other anatomic region, differences in the perceived attractiveness of a specific proportion in the neck may vary significantly among different patients and among surgeons themselves. Knowledge of the essential features that constitute a young and attractive neck should be extensively analyzed by specialists performing aesthetic plastic surgery in this region.[21] Furthermore, a thorough discussion should be held with the patient in order to understand their expectations preoperatively.

The submental-cervical angle constitutes the most, if not the only proportion studied in the neck and has been recently defined to be attractive between 90° and 105°, with considerable differences in thresholds for desiring surgery between patients (110°) and clinicians (125°),[6] perhaps manifesting the disparity between what patients desire and what surgeons believe they can provide or achieve through surgery.

A clinically useful surface landmark may be the *submandibular-cervical junction line* (**Fig. 5**), which lies below the border of the jawline and delineates

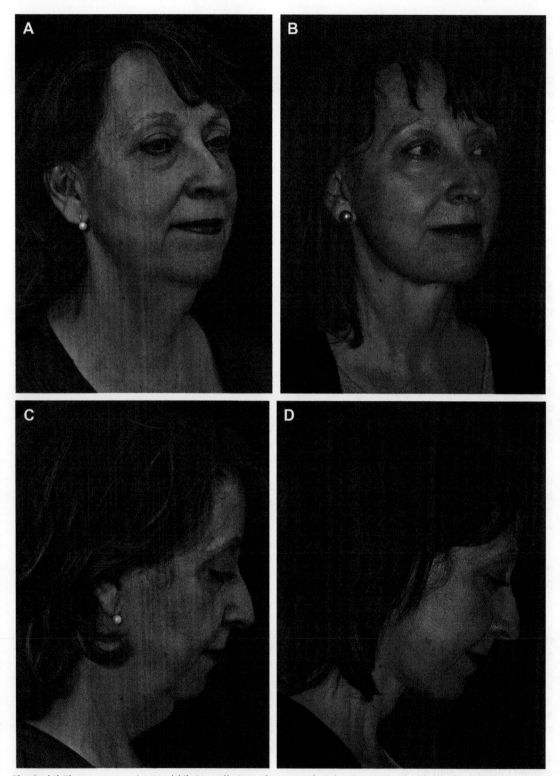

Fig. 2. (*A*) Three-quarter view and (*C*) Connell view of a type II facial aging patient with perifacial expansion and submental fullness. (*B*) and (*D*) Result after reduction neck lift and facelift through a combined lateral and anterior approach, with SMG reduction, subplatysmal fat, and inter-SCMO fat resection. Note the improvement in jawline definition and in the suprasternal notch in the three-quarter view.

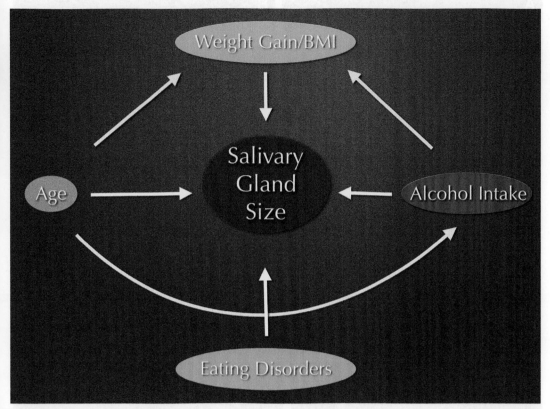

Fig. 3. Conditions that may produce an enlargement of the major salivary glands and their interrelationship. BMI, body mass index.

where the submandibular segment meets the neck. This line serves as the reference point to establish 3 different angles, which have significance in cervical aesthetics: (1) the anterior submandibular-cervical angle (ie, the submental-cervical angle), (2) the lateral submandibular-cervical angle, and (3) the posterior submandibular-cervical angle (see **Fig. 5**). These angles may become progressively and slightly more obtuse from anterior to posterior, but should ideally not surpass 105° anteriorly and 140° posteriorly for optimal jawline definition.

Another useful anatomic landmark of the youthful and attractive neck is a well-defined musculomandibular triangle[22] (**Fig. 6**) demarcated by the anterior edge of sternocleidomastoid (SCM) muscle, the lateral border of the mandible, and the anterior neckline.

In addition, no vertical bands or horizontal skin creases should be present in an ideal neck.

Jawline Definition: Submandibular Shadow

Shadow is the means by which bodies display their form. The forms of bodies could not be understood in detail but for shadow.

— *Leonardo da Vinci*

There is general consensus that achieving a well-defined jawline should be one of the main objectives of a successful surgical cervicofacial rejuvenation procedure. Little has been described, however, on what this actually means visually. Indeed, a well-defined mandible requires that this structure be clearly separated from the underlying neck. This separation or depth beneath the border of the mandible allows a shadow to be cast below the full length of the mandible, which is a key element in the perception of a well-defined jawline (see **Fig. 5**). The way lighting and shadows affect the perceived attractiveness of an anatomic feature was first studied by rhinoplasty surgeons[23,24] and has also been applied to the cleavage area in breast augmentation.[25] Its application to lower face and neck aesthetics is key to understanding jawline definition.

The separation of the mandible from the neck is more evident anteriorly because the chin projects more from the neck than any other area of the mandible. In order to achieve a successful neck lift, however, depth beneath the mandible should be sought along its body and angle as well, by reducing the submandibular structures at these levels, aiming to provide a shadow underneath the entire length of the jawline, which will greatly define it.

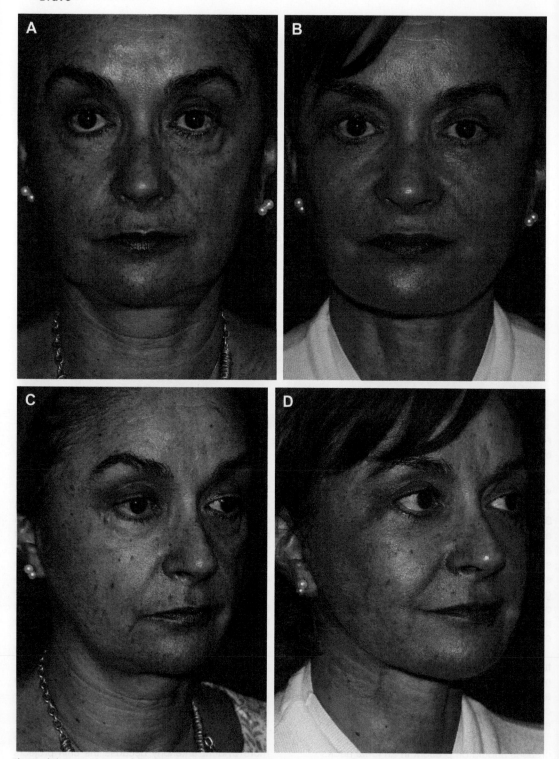

Fig. 4. (A) Front view and (B) three-quarter view of a patient after a previous "minimal" facelift with submental liposuction performed elsewhere. Note the evident SMGs, which the patient mentioned that where made visible after the initial procedure. (B) and (D) Result following SMG reduction, facelift, and facial fat grafting.

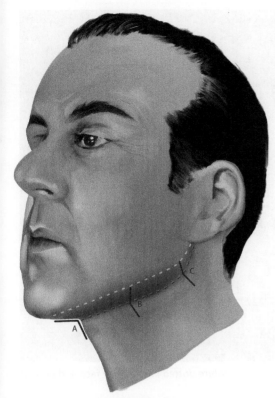

Fig. 5. Surface anatomy of the submandibular region. Notice the shadow under the full extent of the mandible (*white dotted line*), which highlights its definition. The submandibular-cervical junction line (*red dotted line*) delineates the union of the submandibular region with the neck. The anterior (*A*), lateral (*B*), and posterior submandibular-cervical angles (*C*) should be considered when surgically contouring the jawline and neck.

Dynamic Anatomy of the Neck

As stated earlier, a thorough knowledge of the morphologic characteristics of the young and attractive neck is essential in order to achieve successful results in neck lift surgery. This analysis should also be applied to the anatomy of the neck in motion, considering it is one of the most dynamic areas of the human body, and different anatomic configurations of the structures in the submandibular area may be observed when the neck is flexed.

Indeed, considerable differences may be observed between the necks of young and attractive individuals when looking down, as opposed to aged individuals and those with unattractive full necks. The former do not present a double chin when looking down, but maintain a flat straight line beneath the full length of their mandibles, which intersects at a near right angle with their anterior neckline. This downward gaze configuration presents two distinct lines: a first more horizontal line following

the jawline and extending past the neckline and a second more vertical line following the anterior neckline (**Fig. 7**). Defining both succinctly should be one of the goals of a successful neck lift.

Management of the deep structures of the neck is crucial to achieving this type of result in the Connell view after neck lift surgery. This view should be standard in the evaluation and presentation of results after lower facial rejuvenation procedures, because it provides valuable information regarding the effect of the techniques performed in the neck (**Fig. 8**, Video 1).

Failure to acknowledge the importance of this view may contribute to the overdone-face underdone-neck deformity after facial rejuvenation surgery (**Fig. 9**). Natural results are those that are sustained in both static and dynamic positions, and surgeons must realize that their patients will look down eventually at a moment when they will be seen by others (at a restaurant while looking at the menu, in a work meeting while looking at a report, or at any location while using their mobile phones). Achieving well-defined neck contours in this position is crucial to providing patients with a rejuvenated and attractive appearance that will improve their confidence at all times (not only when facing forward or looking up).

Dynamic cadaver dissection studies have shown that the deep structures of the neck play a key role in submental protrusion when looking down in individuals with neck fullness. Analyzing the effect of these structures on neck contour when moving down the mandible and neck of different cadaver specimens (Videos 2 and 3) revealed that there was no place for the submandibular glands to reposition under the mandible, and therefore, were being pushed down and displaced outward when flexing the neck. The ABD muscle also bulged caudally considerably when looking down, pushing the submental superficial soft tissues forward, thus creating a convexity under the chin in this position. These phenomena may also be demonstrated clinically through dynamic MRI studies (**Fig. 10**, Video 4).

MANAGING THE DEEP STRUCTURES OF THE NECK

Individuals with predominant facial thinning (type I facial aging) may achieve excellent results in jawline definition by elevation and traction of the superficial muscular aponeurotic system (SMAS)/platysma muscle and skin through a tightening facelift procedure (see **Fig. 1**). However, in order to achieve jawline definition in patients with any degree of perifacial expansion and submandibular fullness (type II facial aging), a reduction neck lift is better indicated. This procedure has as its main

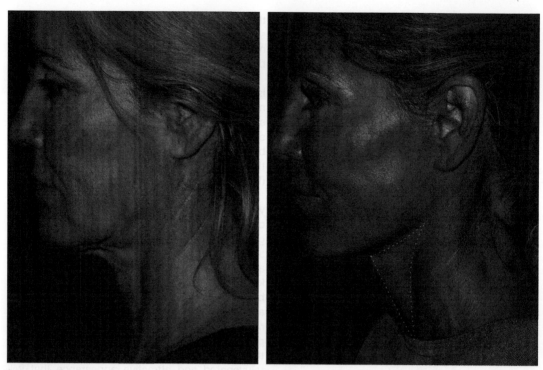

Fig. 6. Achievement of a well-defined musculomandibular triangle (*white dotted line*) after a face and neck lift with SMG reduction.

objective to reduce the volume of the deep structures underneath the mandible in order to achieve a shadow along its full length, which ensures jawline definition (see **Fig. 2**).

It is useful to divide the submandibular region into 3 distinct zones, according to the anatomic structures that need to be addressed in order to approach them systematically (**Fig. 11**).

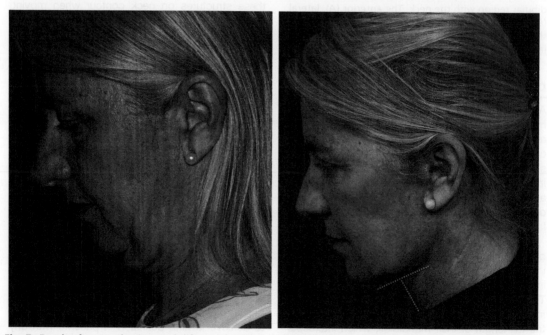

Fig. 7. Result after a reduction neck lift and facelift in the Connell view. Note the more horizontal line in the submental area, which intersects at a near right angle with the more vertical anterior neck line and continues past it following the full extent of the border of the mandible (*dotted lines*). SMG reduction is a key maneuver in order to achieve this outcome.

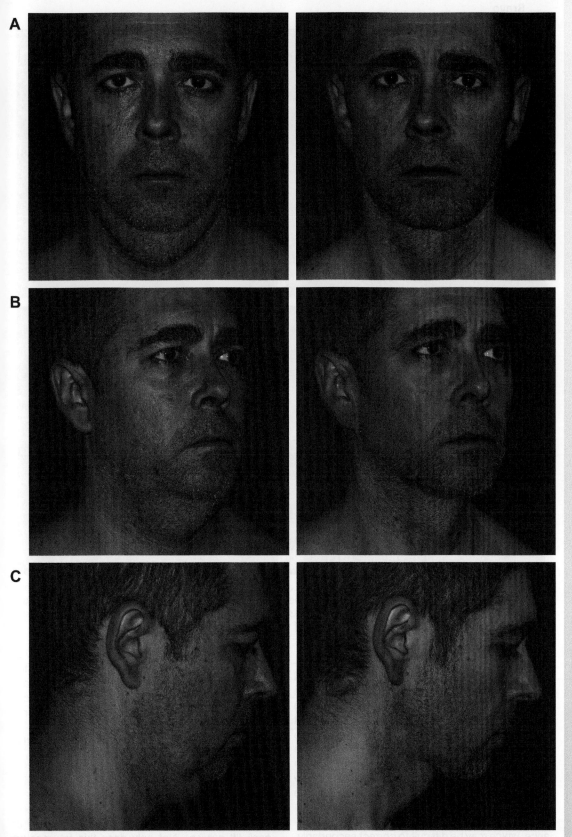

Fig. 8. (*A*) Front view, (*B*) three-quarter view and (*C*) connell view of a reduction neck lift patient before (*left*) and after (*right*) subplatysmal fat excision, ABD muscle reduction, and SMG reduction through an anterior approach and a type I reduction of the TPG through a perilobular lateral short scar approach. Note the maintenance of the clean submental region and definition of the lateral border of the mandible even in the demanding Connell view, due to the management of the deep structures of the neck. see Video 1.

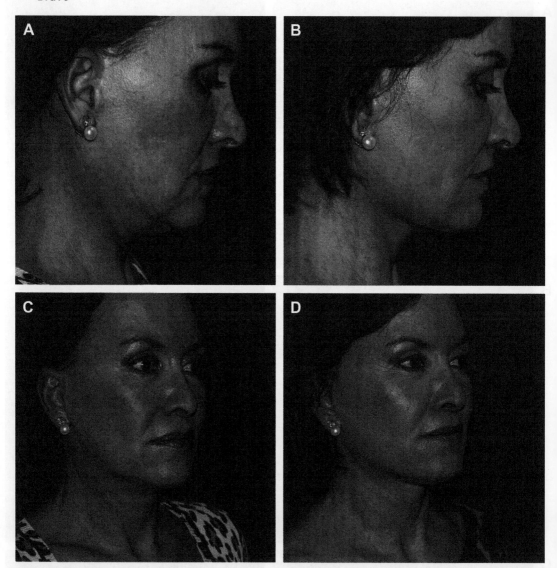

Fig. 9. (*A*) Connell view and (*B*) three-quarter view of a patient with an overdone-face underdone-neck deformity after a previous face and neck lift performed elsewhere. Note the retracted tragus and loss of sideburn in the three-quarter view and the transmandibular crease with submandibular fullness in the Connell view. (*B*) and (*D*) Result after a reduction neck lift procedure with subplatysmal fat excision, ABD muscle reduction, and SMG reduction.

Zone I

Zone I is the zone underneath the parasymphyseal or anterior mental region of the mandible. It is the most frequently treated area in the neck, often times through liposuction, because of the fact that it is where superficial fat accumulation is more prevalent and thus accessible. Aggressive reduction of subcutaneous fat in this area, as in the rest of the neck, should be avoided. It may expose platysma bands, make tissue laxity more evident, and produce irregularities with skin-muscle adherences and a thinned neck appearance, which may be difficult to correct secondarily.

Another superficial structure in this region that may need to be managed is the platysma muscle,

which is quite thick in some patients, especially in men. Resection of excess muscle along the anterior border of the platysma may be necessary before plication in order to avoid adding volume or causing central banding, which could occur if muscle imbrication is performed instead.

Management of several deep structures of the neck in this zone is usually necessary when a reduction neck lift is indicated.

Subplatysmal fat

A substantial reduction of subplatysmal fat is frequently necessary in order to obtain results in neck lift surgery. Not only does this fat account for a large proportion of the overall soft tissue volume of the neck[9,10] but also its management

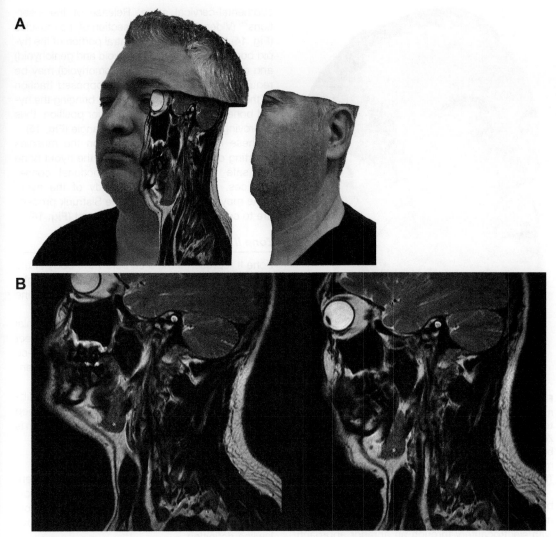

Fig. 10. (*A*) Patient with submandibular fullness in which a parasagittal MRI was performed at the level of Zone II through the submandibular gland. (*B*) MRI of the patient in extended (*left*) and flexed (*right*) position. Note the caudal displacement of the submandibular gland (*marked with a white asterisk*) with neck flexion (Video 4).

through liposuction alone is often not successful, because of its deep location in the neck and due to its much harder and fibrous consistency (**Fig. 12**).

Resection is best carried out through direct excision by means of an anterior open approach using electrocautery. The platysma muscle is identified and its edges elevated to expose the deep cervical fat, which is resected from anterior to posterior, generally up to the level of the hyoid bone (Video 5).

Intersternocleidomastoid origin fat pad
A well-defined and visible origin of the SCM muscles above the sternum is characteristic of young and attractive necks. In many neck lift patients, an added enhancement may be achieved by direct excision through the anterior neck approach of the intersternocleidomastoid origin (SCMO) fat pad

(Video 6), producing a pleasing suprasternal hollow between both origins of the SCM muscles (see **Fig. 2**).

Care should be taken to avoid injury to branches and connections of the anterior jugular veins, which may be large in some patients at this level. Good visualization and use of both long fine-tip scissors and electrocautery are recommended when undertaking this maneuver.

Anterior belly of digastric muscles
Reduction of the ABD muscles may be required in order to achieve a flat surface under the chin in selected patients presenting with submental fullness. Excessive bulkiness of the ABD muscles may be assessed both preoperatively and intraoperatively by tilting the patient's head down or

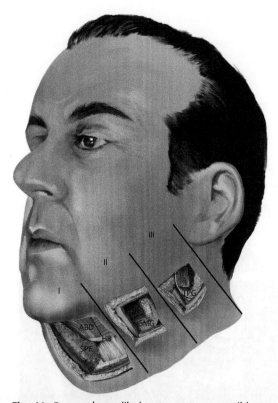

Fig. 11. Deep submandibular structures susceptible to management through a reduction neck lift according to their location underneath and along the mandible. Zone I (parasymphyseal mandible): ABD muscle, hyoid bone (HB), subplatysmal fat (SPF). Zone II (body of the mandible): SMG, and Zone III (angle of the mandible): TPG.

bringing the mandible down toward the neck. If muscular bulging occurs, tangential resection with electrocautery through an anterior approach should be considered (Video 7).

ABD muscle reduction may also be required if both the subplatysmal fat and the SMG have also been reduced. Partial resection of these two latter structures may make more evident the presence of the ABD muscles in the neck postoperatively, therefore making it necessary to reduce these muscles as well.

Usually, only the posterior half of the muscle requires reduction, because this portion protrudes the most, especially when looking down, as demonstrated in dynamic neck anatomy cadaver studies (**Fig. 13**) and in clinical dynamic MRI studies (**Fig. 10**, Video 4). Its management may significantly enhance both the profile and the Connell views in selected patients (see **Fig. 12**).

Hyoid bone

A low-riding hyoid bone in an excessively caudal and anterior position may yield an obtuse

submental-cervical angle. Release of the insertions[26] (Video 8) or partial resection of the muscles (**Fig. 14**) that insert on the central portion of the hyoid bone both cranially (mylohyoid and geniohyoid) and caudally (sternohyoid and omohyoid) may be required in order to allow for unopposed traction of the muscles that insert laterally, bringing the hyoid bone to a higher more posterior position, thus improving the submental-cervical angle (**Fig. 15**).

These maneuvers performed on the muscles inserting on the central portion of the hyoid bone are safe and do not have functional consequences. In fact the whole body of the hyoid bone may be removed as in the Sistrunk procedure to correct a thyroglossal duct cyst (**Fig. 16**).

Zone II

Zone II represents the area below the body of the mandible, between the parasymphysis and angle, and its management is key to improving jawline definition.

The jowl occupies part of this zone at a cranial and superficial level and must be treated by direct excision (jowlectomy), microliposuction (with 1-cc syringes and blunt fine-tip cannulas) or resuspension into the face.

Most of the volume responsible for submandibular fullness at this level is, however, due to a deep subplatysmal cervical structure, the SMG, which is often enlarged[16,17] and caudally displaced.[18]

Submandibular gland

Patients with submental fullness will often present with enlarged SMGs (**Fig. 17**), and partial surgical reduction of the segment of the gland lying below the level of the mandible may significantly improve jawline definition.

Providing depth under the mandible at this level will improve the lateral submandibular-cervical angle, allowing a shadow to appear under the lateral jawline and resulting in a more visible anterior edge of the SCM muscle, which provides a pleasing musculomandibular triangle (**Fig. 18**). This configuration will be maintained when looking down, as it has been shown that untreated protruding submandibular glands are considerably displaced downward and out in this position from cadaver dynamic anatomy studies of the neck (**Fig. 19**) and from clinical dynamic MRI studies (**Fig. 10**, Video 4).

Surgical reduction of the SMGs is better achieved through a short incision posterior to the submental crease (ie open neck or anterior approach),[27–29] although smaller partial reductions may also be performed through a lateral facelift approach only[30,31] (Videos 9–11).

Profuse bleeding may occur during SMG reduction, and several recommendations are warranted

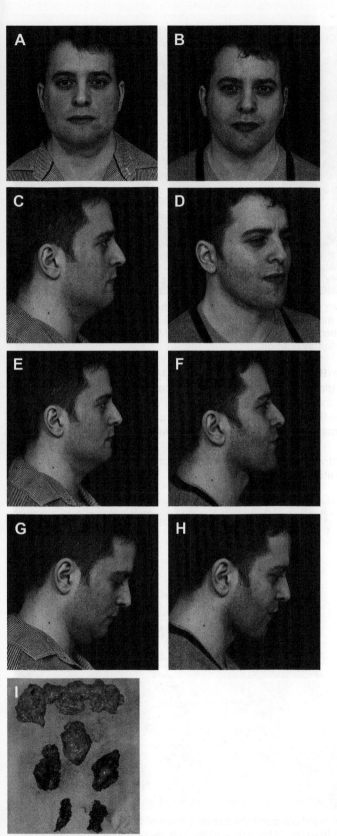

Fig. 12. (*A*) Front view, (*C*) three-quarter view, (*E*) profile view and (*G*) Connell view of a patient unhappy with his jawline definition and submandibular fullness after having undergone a previous submental laser liposuction and placement of silicone implants to the angle of the mandible and chin performed elsewhere. (*B*), (*D*), (*F*) and (*H*) Result after a reduction neck lift through a short scar anterior approach and removal of the angle of the mandible implants through an intraoral approach. (*I*) Specimens removed, from top to bottom: supraplatysmal fat (note its thickness, perhaps due to the thermal effect of the subcutaneous laser liposuction), subplatysmal fat, SMGs, and anterior belly of digastric muscles.

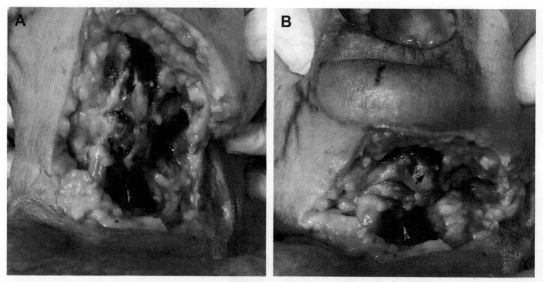

Fig. 13. Dynamic anatomy of the neck cadaver study. The chin is at the top of the image. On the left side of the neck, the skin, supraplatysmal fat, platysma muscle, subplatysmal fat, and SMG have been removed. The arrow points to the ABD muscle. (*A*) Mandible and neck extended, facing forward. (*B*) Mandible and neck flexed, facing down. Note the bulging of the ABD muscle in this position.

in order to safely undertake this procedure (**Box 1**). When a considerable segment of the gland is resected, patients are advised to stay the first night in a hospital setting, to better manage the patient in the rare event of an acute hematoma in the immediate postoperative period.

A sialocele may develop postoperatively,[28] which may require percutaneous aspiration or infiltration of the gland with botulinum toxin to resolve. Several measures, such as the use of drains, tissue sealants, closure of the SMG capsule, intraoperative botulinum toxin gland infiltration, or following a low salivary production diet the first few days after the procedure, may greatly reduce the incidence of this complication.

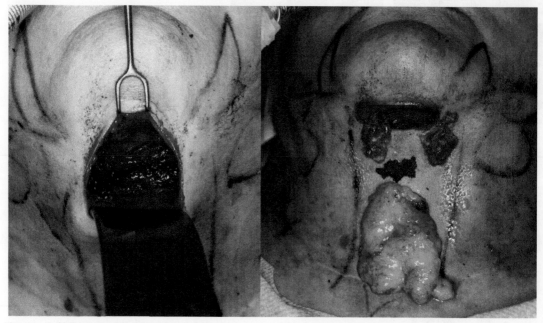

Fig. 14. (*left*) Release of the insertions of the muscles around the central portion of the hyoid bone with partial muscle resection. (*right*) Specimens removed, from top to bottom: ABD muscles, mylohyoid and geniohyoid muscle, and subplatysmal fat.

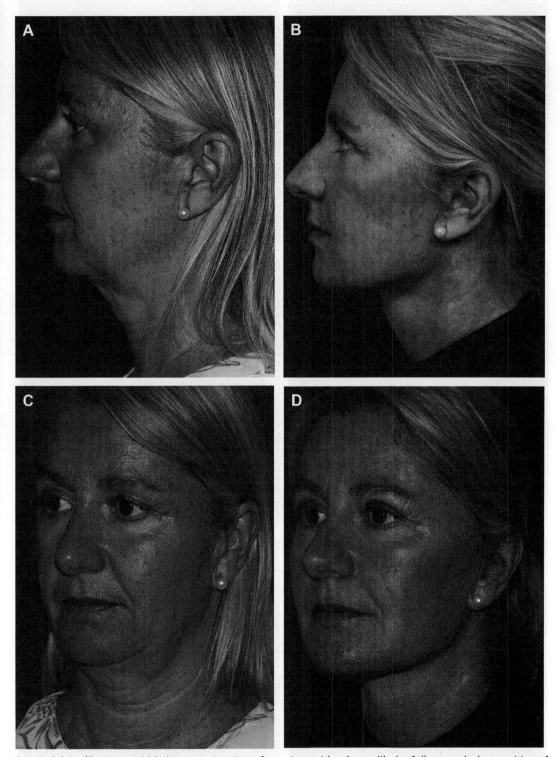

Fig. 15. (*A*) Profile view and (*C*) three quarter view of a patient with submandibular fullness and a low position of the hyoid bone. (*B*) and (*D*) Result after reduction neck lift with hyoid bone release. Note the improvement in the submental-cervical angle and the presence of a shadow underneath the full extent of the mandible, enhancing jawline definition. The patient is also shown in **Fig. 7.**

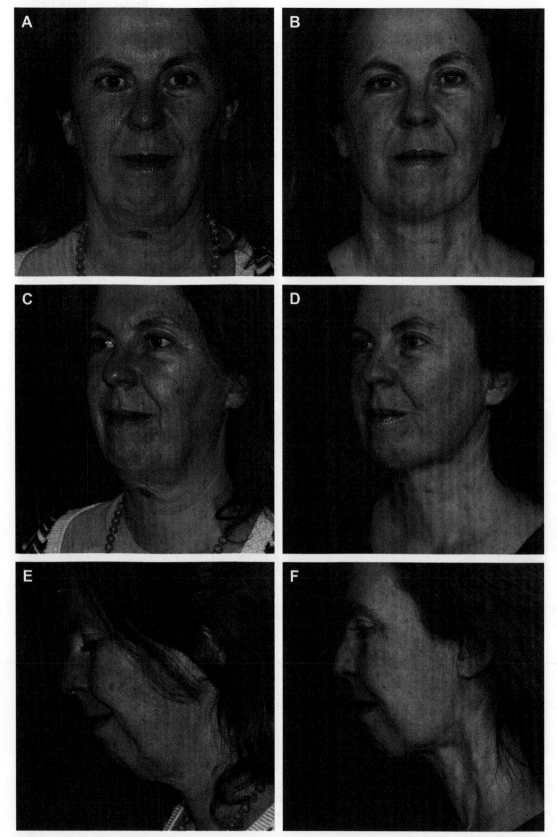

Fig. 16. (*A*) Front view, (*B*) three-quarter view and (*C*) Connell view of a patient with a thyroglossal cyst that was concerned with lack of jawline definition and submental fullness. (*B*), (*D*) and (*F*) Result after a Sistrunk procedure with resection of the central portion of the hyoid bone and SMG reduction. Note the improvement in the submental-cervical angle in the Connell view and the submandibular shadow in the three-quarter view.

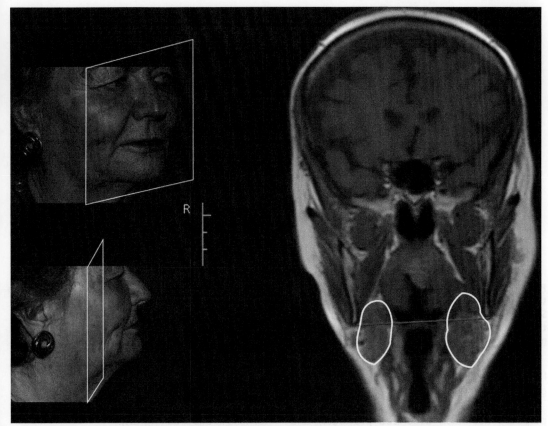

Fig. 17. Patient with submandibular fullness in which most of the volume in the lateral portion of her neck below the mandible is not due to fat, but to large SMGs, outlined in white on the computed tomographic (CT) scan. The red line indicates the inferior border of the mandible.

Zone III

Zone III constitutes the area below and behind the angle of the mandible, and it plays an important role in delineating the posterior edge of the jawline, forming the posterior submandibular-cervical angle (see **Fig. 5**) and creating a retromandibular hollow or groove.

Superficial fat is scarce in this area, and any fullness in this region is most often due to a prominent tail of parotid gland, which is located deep to the SMAS/platysma plane[22] (**Fig. 20**).

Tail of the parotid gland

In order to achieve adequate posterior jawline definition in patients with excessive fullness at this

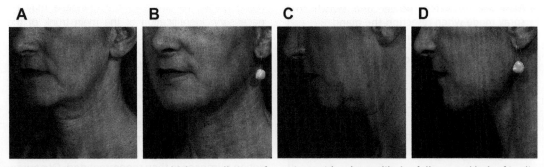

Fig. 18. (*A*) Three-quarter view and (*C*) Connell view of a patient with submandibular fullness and lack of jawline definition. (*B*) and (*D*) Result after SMG reduction. Note the clean and defined musculomandibular triangle in the Connell view and the pronounced shadow in submandibular Zone II in the three-quarter view, increasing jawline definition.

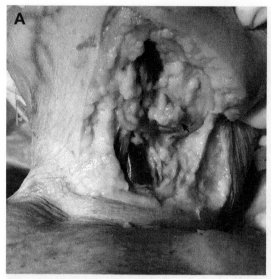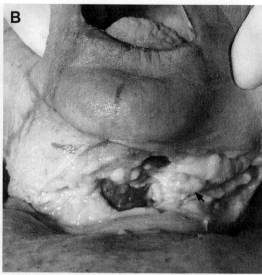

Fig. 19. Dynamic anatomy of the neck cadaver study. The chin is at the top of the image. On the left side of the neck, the skin, supraplatysmal fat, and platysma muscle have been removed. The arrow points to the SMG. (*A*) Mandible and neck extended, facing forward. (*B*) Mandible and neck flexed, facing down. Note the caudal and lateral displacement of the gland in this position after being shifted by the submandibular musculature.

level, partial reduction of the tail of the parotid gland (TPG) may be warranted.

Parotid gland reduction for strictly aesthetic purposes has been described previously and may provide a considerable improvement in select patients.[28,32] Careful SMAS/platysma flap elevation is necessary in order to expose the parotid gland and to adequately cover the resected area to avoid Frey syndrome postoperatively.

Box 1
Recommendations for performing submandibular gland reduction

- Have vascular clips available.
- Use a long paddle-tip electrocautery device.
- Raise electrocautery power and switch to spray mode when resecting the gland.
- Liberate well the gland from its capsule.
- Use DeBakey vascular forceps when handling the gland.
- Use fine-tip suction on nondominant hand when arriving at the central portion of the gland.
- Have 2 assistants scrubbed if possible.
- Use good lighting.
- Use gauze and compression against the mandible for 5 minutes if bleeding is not controlled initially.

The following *clinical classification of parotid reduction in facelift/neck lift patients* may useful in the management of individuals with excessive fullness in this area (**Fig. 21**):

Type I parotid reduction (see **Fig. 8**; Video 12): only the superficial portion of the TPG is removed in order to re-create the desired posterior submandibular-cervical angle. The facial nerve is very deep at this level, making identification and antegrade dissection of the main trunk of the nerve not necessary as long as the reduction is superficial and not extended beyond the anterocaudal border of the gland, where the marginal and mandibular branches of the facial nerve exit it.

Type II parotid reduction (**Fig. 22**, Video 13): in patients with large TPGs, a complete resection of the gland below the angle of the mandible may be necessary. Identification of the main trunk of the facial nerve and antegrade dissection of the inferior division are mandatory to avoid nerve injury.

Type III parotid reduction: patients requiring superficial parotidectomy for tumoral reasons may benefit from an extended SMAS flap dissection through conventional facelift incisions. The SMAS flap may then be split and turned over in order to provide volume (Video 14), and a contralateral-side facelift procedure for symmetrization purposes is then recommended. Of course, identification of the main trunk of the facial nerve and antegrade dissection of all branches of the facial nerve is always necessary in these cases.

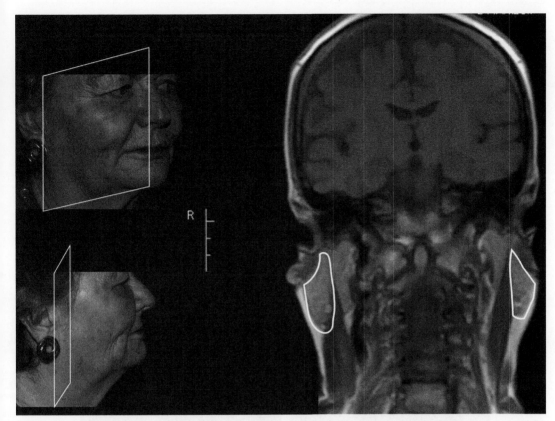

Fig. 20. Patient with fullness in her lateral neck caused by a prominent TPG, outlined in white on the CT scan. Note the near absence of subcutaneous fat in this region.

SUMMARY

A reduction neck lift, in which the main objective is to reduce and contour the deep structures of the neck, should be considered when managing patients with any degree of submandibular fullness in order to achieve long-term results and maximum jawline definition.

Addressing the deep structures of the neck avoids the need to use excessive tightness on the skin and platysma to contour the jawline and neck, because these maneuvers are generally short termed and do not usually provide results in patients with significant submandibular fullness.

Management of the deep structures of the neck provides the added benefit of yielding more

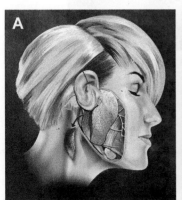
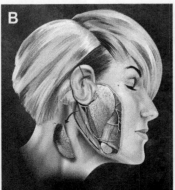
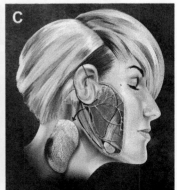

Fig. 21. Clinical classification of parotid reduction in facelift/neck lift patients. (*A*) Type I: superficial resection of the TPG. Facial nerve identification is not necessary. (*B*) Type II: complete resection of the TPG. Facial nerve identification is necessary. (*C*) Type III: superficial parotidectomy. Facial nerve identification is necessary.

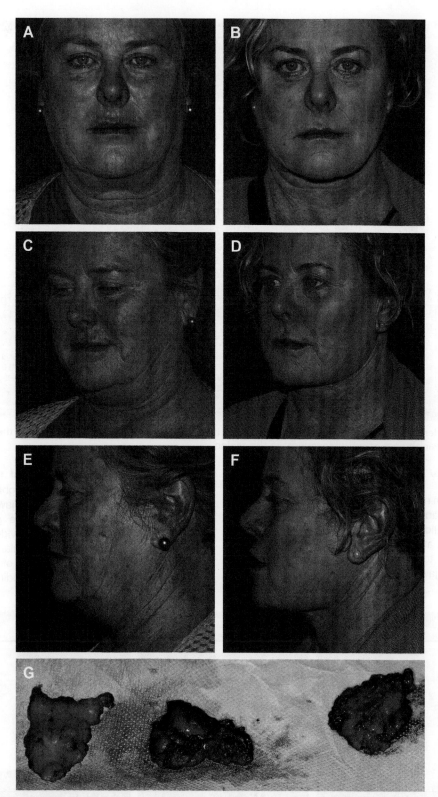

Fig. 22. (*A*) Front view, (*C*) three-quarter view and (*E*) profile view of a patient with submandibular fullness and lack of jawline definition. (*B*), (*D*) and (*F*) Result after a reduction neck lift with type II parotid reduction. Complete excision of the TPG after antegrade dissection of the main trunk and the lower division of the facial nerve (Video 13). Note the improvement in jawline definition in Zone III. (*G*) Specimens removed from the patient's left side, from left to right: subplatysmal fat, SMG, and TPG.

pleasing and natural results when patients move their head forward and look down, as these deep structures are largely responsible for the bulging of the submandibular soft tissues that occurs in this dynamic position.

With the recent increase of nonsurgical and minimally invasive facial procedures, the neck lift has become the cornerstone of facial rejuvenation surgery.[1,33] Specialists offering surgical solutions in this area are expected to deliver results, and these are often best achieved through direct reduction of the deep structures of the neck.

ACKNOWLEDGEMENTS

The author acknowledges radiologist Marina de la Fuente, MD and her staff for valuable contributions in the acquisition of the dynamic MRI presented.

SUPPLEMENTARY DATA

Supplementary data related to this article can be found online at https://doi.org/10.1016/j.cps.2018.05.002.

REFERENCES

1. Stuzin JM. Discussion: a comparison of the full and short-scar face-lift incision techniques in multiple sets of identical twins. Plast Reconstr Surg 2016; 137(6):1715–7.
2. Lawrence WT. Nonsurgical face lift. Plast Reconstr Surg 2006;118(2):541–5.
3. Bravo FG. The aesthetic-health pyramid: a tool for patient education. Plast Reconstr Surg 2010; 126(2):112e–3e.
4. Bravo FG. Perifacial vs. centrofacial morphology on the overall perception of facial aging. ASAPS The Aesthetic Meeting. Montreal, May 2015.
5. Sezgin B, Findikcioglu K, Kaya B, et al. Mirror on the wall: a study of women's perception of facial features as they age. Aesthet Surg J 2012;32(4):421–5.
6. Naini FB, Cobourne MT, McDonald F, et al. Submental-cervical angle: perceived attractiveness and threshold values of desire for surgery. J Maxillofac Oral Surg 2016;15(4):469–77.
7. Connell BF. Contouring the neck in rhytidectomy by lipectomy and a muscle sling. Plast Reconstr Surg 1978;61(3):376–83.
8. Garcia DS, Bussoloti Filho I. Fat deposition of parotid glands. Braz J Otorhinolaryngol 2013;79(2):173–6.
9. Raveendran SS, Anthony DJ, Ion L. An anatomic basis for volumetric evaluation of the neck. Aesthet Surg J 2012;32(6):685–91.
10. Larson JD, Tierney WS, Ozturk CN, et al. Defining the fat compartments in the neck: a cadaver study. Aesthet Surg J 2014;34(4):499–506.
11. Sasaki T. Age-associated weight gain, leptin, and SIRT1: a possible role for hypothalamic sirt1 in the prevention of weight gain and aging through modulation of leptin sensitivity. Front Endocrinol (Lausanne) 2015;6:109.
12. Tian S, Morio B, Denis JB, et al. Age-related changes in segmental body composition by ethnicity and history of weight change across the adult lifespan. Int J Environ Res Public Health 2016;13(8) [pii:E821].
13. Bozzato A, Burger P, Zenk J, et al. Salivary gland biometry in female patients with eating disorders. Eur Arch Otorhinolaryngol 2008;265(9):1095–102.
14. Scott J, Burns J, Flower EA. Histological analysis of parotid and submandibular glands in chronic alcohol abuse: a necropsy study. J Clin Pathol 1988;41(8):837–40.
15. McEvoy LK, Kritz-Silverstein D, Barrett-Connor E, et al. Changes in alcohol intake and their relationship with health status over a 24-year follow-up period in community-dwelling older adults. J Am Geriatr Soc 2013;61(8):1303–8.
16. Mahne A, El-Haddad G, Alavi A, et al. Assessment of age-related morphological and functional changes of selected structures of the head and neck by computed tomography, magnetic resonance imaging, and positron emission tomography. Semin Nucl Med 2007; 37(2):88–102.
17. Saito N, Sakai O, Bauer CM, et al. Age-related relaxo-volumetric quantitative magnetic resonance imaging of the major salivary glands. J Comput Assist Tomogr 2013;37(2):272–8.
18. Lee MK, Sepahdari A, Cohen M. Radiologic measurement of submandibular gland ptosis. Facial Plast Surg 2013;29(4):316–20.
19. Marten T. Neck lift: defining anatomic problems and applying logical solutions. ASAPS Facial and Rhinoplasty Symposium. Las Vegas, February 2018.
20. Çakır B, Öreroğlu AR, Daniel RK. Surface aesthetics and analysis. Clin Plast Surg 2016;43(1):1–15.
21. Ellenbogen R, Karlin JV. Visual criteria for success in restoring the youthful neck. Plast Reconstr Surg 1980;66:826.
22. Feldman J. Neck lift. Stuttgart (Germany): Thieme; 2006.
23. Sheen JH, Sheen AP. Aesthetic rhinoplasty. St Louis (MO): Mosby; 1987.
24. Daniel RK, Hodgson J, Lambros VS. Rhinoplasty: the light reflexes. Plast Reconstr Surg 1990;85(6): 859–66 [discussion: 867–8].
25. Bravo FG. Parasternal infiltration composite breast augmentation. Plast Reconstr Surg 2015;135(4): 1010–8.
26. Guyuron B. Problem neck, hyoid bone, and submental myotomy. Plast Reconstr Surg 1992;90(5): 830–7 [discussion: 838–40].

27. Singer DP, Sullivan PK. Submandibular gland I: an anatomic evaluation and surgical approach to submandibular gland resection for facial rejuvenation. Plast Reconstr Surg 2003;112(4):1150–4 [discussion: 1155–6].

28. Bravo FG. Submandibular and parotid gland reduction in facelift surgery. Plast Reconstr Surg 2013; 132(4S-1):95–6.

29. Mendelson BC, Tutino R. Submandibular gland reduction in aesthetic surgery of the neck: review of 112 consecutive cases. Plast Reconstr Surg 2015;136(3):463–71.

30. Gonzalez R. The LOPP-lateral overlapping plication of the platysma: an effective neck lift without submental incision. Clin Plast Surg 2014;41(1):65–72.

31. Pelle-Ceravolo M, Angelini M, Silvi E. Treatment of anterior neck aging without a submental approach: lateral skin-platysma displacement, a new and proven technique for platysma bands and skin laxity. Plast Reconstr Surg 2017;139(2): 308–21.

32. Thomas DJ, Silfen R, Ritz M, et al. Superficial parotidectomy for rhytidectomy contour refinement. Plast Reconstr Surg 2009;124(5): 255e–6e.

33. Pezeshk RA, Sieber DA, Rohrich RJ. Neck rejuvenation through the lateral platysma window: a key component of face-lift surgery. Plast Reconstr Surg 2017;139(4):865–6.

Management of the Submandibular Gland in Neck Lifts
Indications, Techniques, Pearls, and Pitfalls

André Auersvald, MD, Luiz A. Auersvald, MD*

KEYWORDS

- Submandibular gland • Neck • Neck lift • Face lift • Neck rejuvenation • Subplatysma
- Mandibular nerve • Bleeding

KEY POINTS

- Patients who present for facial rejuvenation often choose to undergo treatment of cervical contour after the initial consultation.
- Physical examination and photographic analysis, including an upward view of the flexed neck, are important surgical planning steps in neck rejuvenation.
- Knowledge of subplatysmal anatomy is crucial for favorable results of neck rejuvenation. The authors introduce novel techniques for management of the submandibular salivary glands.
- The authors describe safety maneuvers to avoid and manage bleeding while treating structures in the subplatysmal region.
- If carefully planned and conducted, partial removal of the submandibular salivary glands is a helpful and safe technique in neck rejuvenation.

 Video content accompanies this article at http://www.plasticsurgery.theclinics.com/.

INTRODUCTION

Deformities of the cervical region can exacerbate the appearance of facial aging.[1] However, patients who seek facial rejuvenation typically do not specify the neck as the primary concern. We have found that a thorough interview and examination of the patient—involving photographic analysis in various views—often has the effect of shifting the patient's chief concern to the neck. Adequate diagnosis and treatment of this area are paramount to achieve patient satisfaction.

The cervical region generally is regarded as a stratified structure comprising layers of skin, subcutaneous tissue, and platysma, much like the middle third of the face. However, findings of anatomic and surgical studies have indicated that subplatysmal structures, such as the digastric muscles, mylohyoid muscle, hyoid, subplatysmal fat, and bilateral submandibular salivary glands (SMSGs), affect the 3-dimensional shape of the neck (**Fig. 1**).[2] These structures may interfere with the criteria for a youthful cervical appearance, as described by Ellenbogen and Karlin[3]: a distinct inferior mandibular border, an identifiable subhyoid depression, a visible thyroid cartilage bulge, a discernible anterior border of the sternocleidomastoid muscle, and a cervicomental angle between 105° and 120° (**Fig. 2**). Furthermore, the neck is an articular region, which distinguishes it

Disclosure Statement: The authors have nothing to disclose.
Clínica Auersvald de Cirurgia Plástica, Alameda Presidente Taunay, 1756, Curitiba, Paraná 80430-000, Brazil
* Corresponding author.
E-mail address: luizauersvald@uol.com.br

Clin Plastic Surg 45 (2018) 507–525
https://doi.org/10.1016/j.cps.2018.06.001
0094-1298/18/© 2018 Elsevier Inc. All rights reserved.

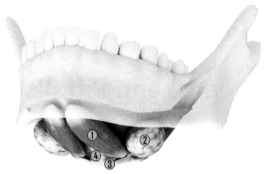

Fig. 1. Subplatysmal structures that affect neck contour. (1) Anterior belly of the digastric muscle, (2) submandibular salivary gland, (3) hyoid, and (4) mylohyoid muscle. Subplatysmal fat (not depicted) is distributed around these structures and also may contribute to contour deformities.

from the front and middle third of the face. Neck flexion may yield increased skin flaccidity and intensify the appearance of aging.

Herein, we describe a safe and effective subplatysmal technique of neck rejuvenation in which

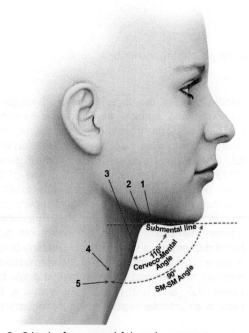

Fig. 2. Criteria for a youthful neck appearance, as described by Ellenbogen and Karlin[3]: (1) a distinct inferior mandibular border, (2) a subhyoid depression, (3) a visible thyroid cartilage bulge, (4) a visible anterior sternocleidomastoid border, and (5) a 90° sternocleidomastoid–submental angle and a cervicomental angle between 105° and 120°.

special attention is given to the SMSGs. We explain how to diagnose hypertrophy and ptosis of the SMSGs and how to determine whether partial resection is indicated.

CONSULTATION

Patients who present for facial rejuvenation often indicate the eyelids and brows as the primary concerns. However, after surgical consultation with photographic analysis, the patient's primary concern frequently becomes the neck (our unpublished findings; **Table 1**).

Before consultation in our practice from April 2016 to September 2016, 98 patients were asked to specify whether the eyelids and brows, cheeks and nasolabial folds, or neck caused them to seek facial rejuvenation. Most (49.0%) chose the eyelids and brows as their chief concern, followed by cheeks and nasolabial folds (36.8%) and neck (14.2%; see **Table 1**). Patients then were photographed in 4 views: front, profile with neck in neutral position, profile with flexed neck, and upward view with flexed neck. When asked again, 53.0% of patients indicated the neck as the chief concern. We have found that a patient usually evaluates his or her face in frontal view, rather than in profile, which may explain these findings. We now routinely include photographic evaluation during the first consultation to ensure that patients' presenting concerns are addressed effectively.

PHYSICAL EXAMINATION

Palpation of subplatysmal structures is valuable for predicting intraoperative findings. Several maneuvers may help with determining the size and position of these structures (**Fig. 3**).

Table 1
Chief concern of patients before and after receiving consultation with photographic analysis

Chief Concern	Before Consultation, n (%)	After Consultation, n (%)
Eyelids and brows	48 (49.0)	28 (28.6)
Cheeks and nasolabial folds	36 (36.8)	18 (18.4)
Neck	14 (14.2)	52 (53.0)

Data represent a series of 98 patients who were evaluated from April 2016 to September 2016.

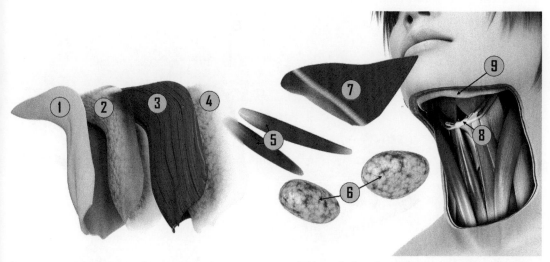

Fig. 3. Structures that contribute to an aging appearance of the neck that should be addressed on physical examination: (1) skin, (2) subcutaneous fat, (3) platysma, (4) subplatysmal fat, (5) digastric muscle, (6) submandibular salivary gland, (7) mylohyoid muscle, and (8) hyoid. The mandible (9) is also shown.

By pinching the submental region, the surgeon may be able to detect subplatysmal structures (**Fig. 4**). The density of interdigastric and subplatysmal fat and the width of the anterior belly of the digastric muscles also can be evaluated with this maneuver. With the patient's neck flexed, palpation of the submental area enables assessment of subplatysmal structures, including the SMSGs, the digastric muscles and the hyoid (**Fig. 5**), because this position relaxes the anterior aspect of the neck. Palpation also allows for evaluation of flaccidity of the platysma and skin and determination of dermal creases that need to be released during surgery (**Fig. 6**).

The SMSG is located in the submandibular triangle, the sides of which comprise the anterior and posterior bellies of the digastric muscle and the lower border of the mandible (**Fig. 7**). The size of the SMSGs varies among healthy individuals; patients who are 50 or more years of age—or sometimes younger—usually present with hypertrophy and ptosis of the SMSGs, which interfere with a pleasing contour of the neck.

Radiologic evaluation of the neck may be indicated based on the patient's medical history and physical examination findings.

PHOTOGRAPHIC ANALYSIS

Easy access to digital cameras has changed the way patients perceive and monitor their physical features. In our experience, patients who undergo

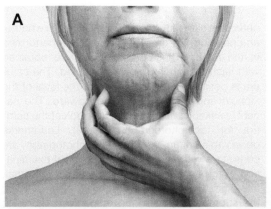
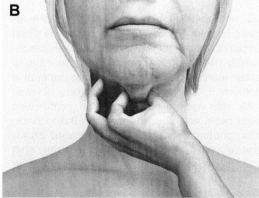

Fig. 4. Palpation of the submental region. (*A*, *B*) The bidigital pinch test allows the surgeon to assess the density of the interdigastric and subplatysmal fat and the width of the anterior bellies of the digastric muscles.

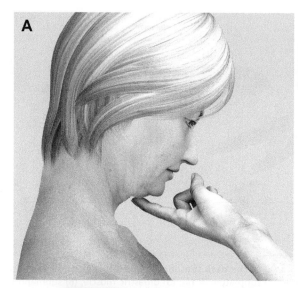

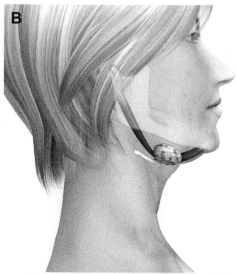

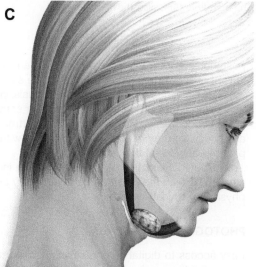

Fig. 5. (*A*) Digital palpation of the submental region with the patient's neck flexed. (*B*) Subplatysmal structures, especially the submandibular salivary gland, the digastric muscle, subplatysmal fat, and the hyoid, are less accessible when the neck is in neutral position. (*C*) Flexing allows for better assessment of neck anatomy by palpation.

facial rejuvenation often monitor postoperative recovery by taking photographs of themselves and comparing these images with those taken preoperatively. The surgeon should exercise care to obtain routine preoperative and postoperative photographs in numerous views: front, oblique, profile with neck in neutral position, profile with flexed neck, and upward view with flexed neck. These photographs should be referenced intraoperatively because anatomic structures may shift when the patient is in the Trendelenburg or supine position.

These authors determined recently that imaging in upward view with the patient's neck flexed helps the surgeon to identify submental structures,

define the skin redundancy, and ascertain whether an open surgical procedure should be performed in the neck.[4] These photographs are obtained with flash and zoom features disabled. The camera is positioned approximately at the level of the xiphoid appendix and oriented upward. The patient is asked to flex the neck and look at the camera for the photograph (**Fig. 8**). Landmarks observable in an upward-view photograph are consistent with findings of the physical examination of the neck (**Fig. 9**) regarding interplatysmal, interdigastric, and subplatysmal fat; the SMSGs; the submental crease; the mandibular ligament; mental fat; and skin redundancy and creases. The submental crease is difficult to evaluate in

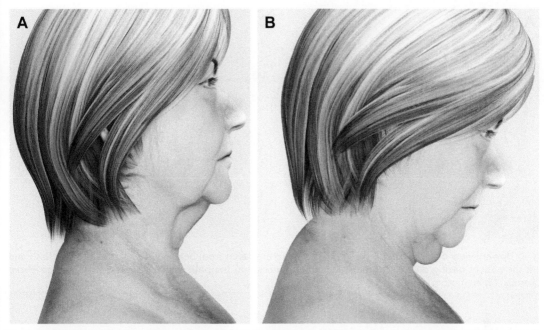

Fig. 6. Evaluation of the skin of the cervical region and platysma. (*A*) The neck in neutral position. (*B*) The neck in flexion allows for improved assessment of skin and platysma redundancies.

other photographic views, but is depicted well in an upward view. Patients who are younger tend to have a minimal crease or no crease; those who are older usually have a noticeable submental crease that extends to the submandibular ligament (**Fig. 10**).

INDICATIONS AND LEARNING CURVE

For neck rejuvenation involving submental access and treatment of subplatysmal structures, the surgeon should consider the patient's degree of

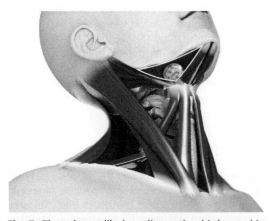

Fig. 7. The submandibular salivary gland is located in the submandibular triangle (depicted in *yellow*), which is defined by the anterior and posterior bellies of the digastric muscle and the lower border of the mandible.

concern with his or her neck as well as physical examination findings. Because the technique involves treatment of disparate structures, open surgical rejuvenation of the neck can be complex and challenging, but also rewarding. Feldman's textbook on neck rejuvenation offers an excellent and detailed description of this subject.[5] We have found that assisting in oncologic neck dissection and examining fresh cadavers are helpful to enhance the plastic surgeon's knowledge of neck anatomy. Surgeons who lack experience in neck procedures should start with patients for whom flaccidity of the platysma is the main indication and subsequently consider cases involving the digastric muscles. Treatment of the SMSGs should be undertaken only after significant experience has been gained.

TREATMENT OF THE SUBMANDIBULAR SALIVARY GLANDS

Treatment of the SMSGs involves resection of the bulging superficial lobe. Alternatively, repositioning may be considered for small ptotic glands. Dissection of the neck to the SMSGs should proceed in a specific sequence. Video 1 depicts an edited process of SMSG treatment. For this operation, general intravenous anesthesia with orotracheal intubation is achieved by means of remifentanil, propofol, and dexmedetomidine.[4,6] To improve pain control and facilitate skin

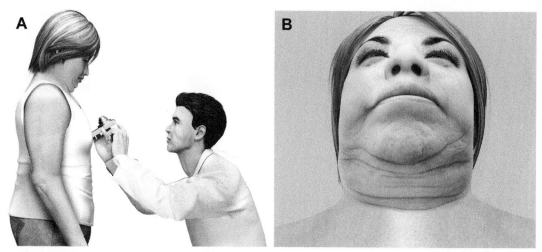

Fig. 8. Upward view of the flexed neck. (*A*) Photographs are taken from below, with no zoom and no flash and with the patient gazing down. The camera should be placed on the patient's chest at the level of the xiphoid appendix. (*B*) A photographic result.

dissection, tumescent local anesthesia is used (1 L of saline, 40 mL of 2% lidocaine, 20 mL of 1% ropivacaine, and epinephrine [1:1,000,000]). The following surgical instruments are necessary for this operation: a lighted retractor, long insulated forceps with delicate teeth, DeBakey forceps, long cautery tips, and a powerful Yankauer suction tip.

With the patient in Trendelenburg position, an incision is made 1.0 to 1.5 cm anterior to the hyoid to facilitate access to the submandibular triangle (**Fig. 11**).[1] The average distance from the midline of the incision to the most lateral part of each SMSG is 5.5 cm, and the average distance to the midline of the submental crease is 7 cm (personal communication, Dr T. Gerald O'Daniel). This incision placement allows for direct access to subplatysmal structures and brings the SMSGs close to the surgical field. In particular, visualization of the posterolateral portion of the gland's superficial lobe, which contains the central perforating artery, is facilitated with this approach.

NECK LAYERS AND THE SUBCUTANEOUS UNDERMINING

The surgeon should be comfortable identifying and dissecting the strata of the neck (**Fig. 12**). Initial subcutaneous undermining should be limited to the area in which the SMSGs are located (**Fig. 13**). This undermining may expose major veins, including the anterior jugular vein and its collaterals. Further dissection should be avoided at this stage because it may encourage bleeding.

In addition, care should be given to prepare a skin flap with adequate thickness to avoid skin slough.

INTERPLATYSMAL AND INTERDIGASTRIC FAT RESECTION

Evaluation and resection of the interplatysmal and interdigastric fat proceed after undermining (**Fig. 14**). Enough fat should be removed to reduce the submental bulge and allow identification of the anterior bellies of the digastric muscles. The authors advise against liposuction in this step because the consistency of this fat typically is fibrous and difficult to suction and because liposuction may traumatize the skin flap. The platysma then is lifted by pulling its medial border and temporarily affixing it to the skin flap with a 5-0 nylon suture (**Fig. 15**). Gentle blunt dissection is performed to further detach the platysma from subjacent structures until the infrahyoid region is reached. At this point, the surgeon should be able to see the anterior belly of the digastric muscle.

CERVICAL TRIAD

The cervical triad comprises the anterior belly of the digastric muscle (and intermediate digastric tendon), the SMSG, and the hyoid (**Fig. 16**) and is an important reference for locating the SMSGs. The digastric muscle is identified and followed to the hyoid. The SMSGs are predictably positioned lateral to this junction.

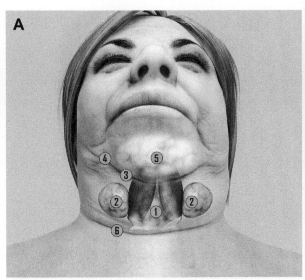

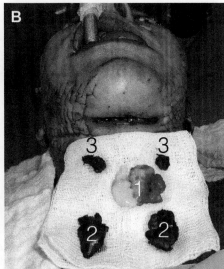

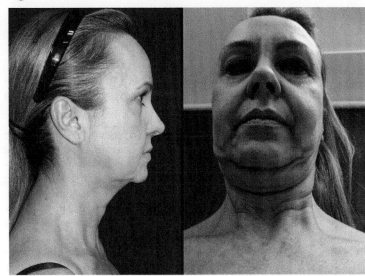

Fig. 9. Upward view of the flexed neck. (*A*) Structures that may be assessed on physical examination and in photographic analysis include (1) the interplatysmal and interdigastric fat and anterior bellies of the digastric muscles, (2) the submandibular salivary glands, (3) the submental crease, (4) the mandibular ligament, (5) the mental fat compartment, and (6) the cervical skin redundancy. (*B*) Intraoperative view with the following structures resected: (1) interplatysmal and interdigastric fat, (2) submandibular salivary glands, and (3) anterior bellies of the digastric muscles. (*C*) Preoperative views of this 53-year-old woman with the neck in neutral position (*left*) and on upward view with the neck flexed (*right*).

HYOID REPOSITIONING

After removal of interplatysmal and interdigastric fat, the surgeon should examine the deep investing cervical fascia and determine whether to reposition the hyoid. The superficial layer of the deep investing fascia is a whitish covering in the midline that envelopes the suprahyoid, perihyoid, and infrahyoid regions. The investing fascia extends posteriorly and attaches to several ligamentous and bony structures, including the cervical spine.[5,7] This fascia can be applied to reposition the hyoid. Specifically, the investing fascia is released and partially removed in the suprahyoid region to facilitate elevation of the hyoid. The anterior bellies of the digastric muscles then are approximated with 1 or 2 stitches in the adjacent area of the intermediate tendon and pulley tissues. In the infrahyoid region, the fascia is preserved. Plication of this fascia at the level of the hyoid and inferiorly repositions it more superiorly and posteriorly, thereby improving the contour of the neck (**Fig. 17**). The strong bony attachments of the fascia help to ensure the durability of the surgical result. Moreover, plication brings the SMSGs closer to the midline, which facilitates visibility and accessibility for resection.

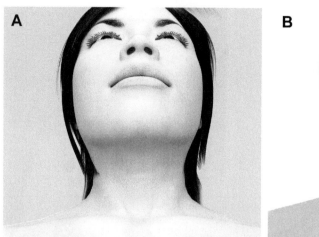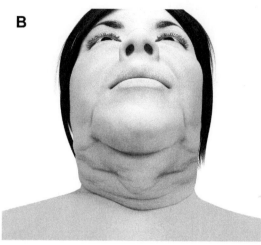

Fig. 10. Upward views of the flexed neck. (*A*) A young woman with a subtle submental crease. (*B*) An older woman with a deep submental crease and skin flaccidity.

PARTIAL RESECTION AND PLICATION OF THE ANTERIOR BELLIES OF THE DIGASTRIC MUSCLES

Hypertrophy of the anterior bellies of the digastric muscles can yield excessive submental volume. With the patient's neck flexed, the surgeon can identify these structures and estimate volume preoperatively by palpation. If hypertrophy is confirmed intraoperatively, wedge resection of 30% to 40% of the anterior bellies can be undertaken with a Mixter forceps and electrocautery. To manage the remaining anterior bellies and reshape the mouth floor, a digastric corset technique can be performed, as described by Labbé and colleagues.[8] We perform this procedure routinely (**Fig. 18**). The attachments of the mylohyoid muscle to the digastric muscle account for the strength and durability of this plication.

SUBMANDIBULAR SALIVARY GLAND CAPSULE AND THE MARGINAL MANDIBULAR NERVE

The SMSG is initially seen as a whitish aponeurotic structure because it is enclosed in a capsule that originates from the splitting of the investing fascia.[5] In neck rejuvenation, the capsule is opened by blunt dissection with Metzenbaum scissors, and the gland is detached; this step is a necessary precursor to partial resection of the superficial lobe. The gland then is released from its medial attachments and mobilized with fine-tip electrocautery (see **Fig. 18**). This region is devoid of crucial nerve structures, so release is relatively easy. Blood vessels encountered during the procedure should be progressively cauterized as the gland is freed. We advise expansion of the inferior capsule, especially if the surgeon determines that there is insufficient space to manipulate the gland (**Fig. 19**).

The marginal mandibular nerve is located superiorly and external to the capsule. Therefore, the nerve is not at risk of direct injury during release of the gland inside the capsule (**Fig. 20**). The authors have found transient weakness of the lower lip depressor muscle in 5.6% of patients who undergo this procedure, a similar rate observed by other surgeons.[4,5] The cause of this temporary weakness has not been ascertained, but may be attributed to the use of monopolar cautery, the narrow space for dissection, and/or direct

Fig. 11. For neck rejuvenation with a subplatysmal approach, incision placement is approximately 1.0 to 1.5 cm anterior to the hyoid; this method enables direct access to the submandibular salivary glands.

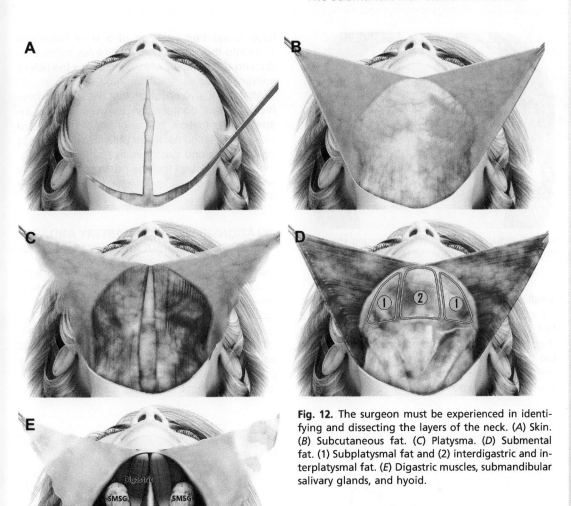

Fig. 12. The surgeon must be experienced in identifying and dissecting the layers of the neck. (*A*) Skin. (*B*) Subcutaneous fat. (*C*) Platysma. (*D*) Submental fat. (1) Subplatysmal fat and (2) interdigastric and interplatysmal fat. (*E*) Digastric muscles, submandibular salivary glands, and hyoid.

trauma by the light retractor. Bilateral injection of botulinum toxin in the lower lip depressor muscle can be offered to alleviate the patient's concerns regarding asymmetric movement of the mouth during the recovery period, which takes up to 90 days (Video 2).

PARTIAL REMOVAL OF THE SUBMANDIBULAR SALIVARY GLAND

With the SMSG freed, the surgeon should analyze whether its volume justifies partial resection. We suggest an anatomic parameter to help determine the resection volume. A line is drawn between the lowest point of the anterior belly of the digastric muscle and the inferior border of the mandible. The portion of each SMSG that bulges below this line is resected (**Fig. 21**).[4]

The most inferior and anterior portion of the superficial lobe of each SMSG is removed with fine-tip electrocautery and forceps (**Fig. 22**). Horizontal and vertical passes of the electrocautery device help to control bleeding. Two assistants should participate in this step. One assistant manages the light retractor and applies a hook to pull the chin upward. The other assistant handles the Yankauer suction tip. The gland should be removed in an oblique or transverse plane in relation to the mouth floor. The result can be refined by removing additional

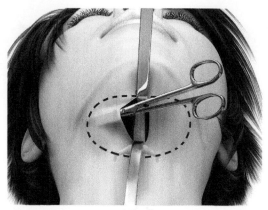

Fig. 13. Initial subcutaneous undermining should be limited to the area within the dashed line.

small portions of the gland. Subsequently, 1.5 mL of 0.75% ropivacaine is injected with a fine needle into the raw surface of the gland (**Fig. 23**) and into the anterior belly of the digastric muscle (Dr Ozan Sozer's personal recommendation). This technique has been found to greatly reduce postoperative pain. We also

have found that injection of 5 U of botulinum toxin into the gland helps to diminish saliva production temporarily, which decreases the risk of salivary fistula.

After partial removal of the SMSG, improvement in neck contour can be confirmed by inspection, palpation, and analysis of the upward view of the flexed neck. For patients who undergo preoperative and postoperative radiologic imaging, we have found that the postresection volume of the gland is decreased postoperatively (**Fig. 24**).

RELATIONSHIP OF FACIAL ARTERY AND VEIN TO THE SUBMANDIBULAR SALIVARY GLAND

Hematoma is the most concerning intraoperative and postoperative complication of SMSG resection.[9] The surgeon should be prepared to manage additional bleeding upon accessing the subplatysmal region. The facial artery and vein enter the SMSG capsule in its posterolateral aspect and small branches of the facial artery penetrate the superficial lobe. The most significant branch is the central perforating artery,

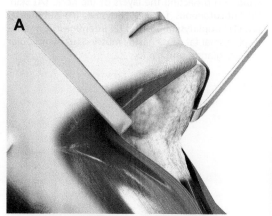

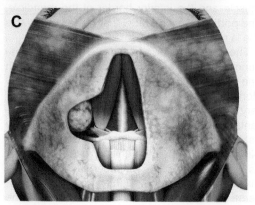

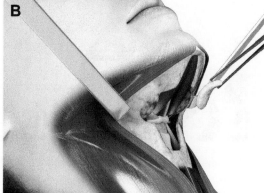

Fig. 14. Removal of interplatysmal and interdigastric fat. (*A*) After subcutaneous undermining, the interplatysmal and interdigastric fat can be examined in the submental area along the midline. (*B, C*) Typically, the surgeon must remove this fat to access the anterior bellies of the digastric muscles.

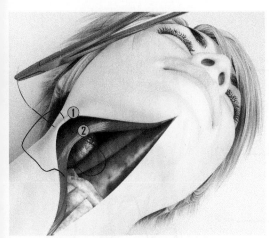

Fig. 15. The platysma (2) is lifted by pulling its medial border and temporarily affixing it to the skin flap (1). This maneuver retracts the platysma from the operating field.

which is located in the most posterior and lateral aspect of this lobe. The facial vein usually is found in the lateral portion of the superficial lobe; however, it is eventually seen in a more medial course over the gland (**Figs. 25–27**).[5,9,10] **Because of the lateral locations of the facial artery and vein, the surgeon should perform blunt dissection when releasing the lateral aspect of the gland.**

Manipulating the SMSG induces pain, which can increase the arterial blood pressure. The anesthesiologist should exercise caution to control blood pressure and pain during this step. In case of intensive arterial bleeding, 2 or 3 gauzes wet with cold saline solution should be applied

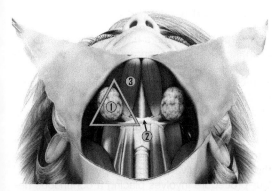

Fig. 16. Subplatysmal structures of the cervical triad. (1) Submandibular salivary gland, (2) hyoid, and (3) anterior belly of the digastric muscle. The submandibular salivary gland is found lateral to the junction of the digastric muscle and the hyoid.

to the SMSG, while the anesthesiologist ensures that arterial blood pressure is controlled. With a long forceps in one hand and the Yankauer suction tip in the other, the surgeon should try to locate and clamp the bleeding vessel so it can be cauterized by the assistant surgeon. Figure-of-8 sutures may be placed to stop arterial bleeding if cauterization alone is not effective.

If the bleeding originates from a vein, the patient should be moved to the reverse Trendelenburg position to lower the venous blood pressure in the head (**Fig. 28**). The vessel then should be located and cauterized (Videos 3 and 4).

Once bleeding is controlled, the surgeon should ensure complete closure of the raw surface of the gland by means of a continuous stitch with a 4-0 absorbable suture. The needle should be placed to encompass approximately 1 cm of the raw edges because the gland is friable. In addition, the thread must be pulled continuously to avoid bleeding owing to needle passage (**Fig. 29**).[4]

INTERMEDIATE DIGASTRIC MUSCLE TENDON AND SUBMANDIBULAR SALIVARY GLAND REPOSITIONING

The intermediate digastric muscle tendon is a stable structure attached to the hyoid. The surgeon can anchor the SMSG to this tendon after partial resection of the gland or as a means to reposition a ptotic, nonhypertrophic gland. The hypoglossal and lingual nerves as well as the lingual artery and Wharton's duct are located posterior to the intermediate digastric muscle tendon (**Figs. 30** and **31**). Dr Fausto Viterbo has taught these authors a straightforward maneuver to locate the tendon. The assistant pulls the patient's chin upward, placing tension on the muscles of the mouth floor. The surgeon then uses an index finger to palpate the tendon (**Fig. 32**), which is rigid and cordlike. A suture is placed that encompasses the gland and the intermediate tendon (**Fig. 33**). Subsequently, the capsule surrounding each SMSG is closed with absorbable sutures. The platysma flap then is sutured over each SMSG with 1 or 2 stiches to further close the area and help to prevent the leakage of saliva.

PLATYSMA CORSET

Once the subplatysmal structures are treated, the surgeon may extend the subcutaneous dissection laterally to allow for plication of the

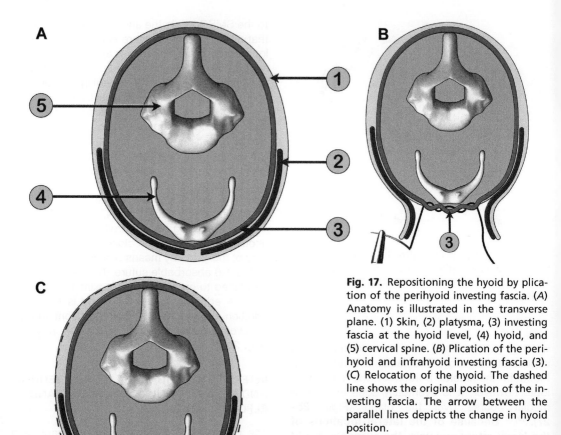

Fig. 17. Repositioning the hyoid by plication of the perihyoid investing fascia. (*A*) Anatomy is illustrated in the transverse plane. (1) Skin, (2) platysma, (3) investing fascia at the hyoid level, (4) hyoid, and (5) cervical spine. (*B*) Plication of the perihyoid and infrahyoid investing fascia (3). (*C*) Relocation of the hyoid. The dashed line shows the original position of the investing fascia. The arrow between the parallel lines depicts the change in hyoid position.

platysma. Plication is carried out by corset suture, preferably in 2 stages. The infrahyoid region is sutured in the first stage. Because the incision is placed close to the hyoid, it is possible to go as low as the sternal notch. In the second stage, the suprahyoid region is closed with a continuous suture that is stopped just before the submental crease. Tumescent infiltration is performed in the chin region to facilitate the release of the submental ligament with Metzenbaum scissors. This procedure enables access to the subcutaneous fat compartment of the chin. By detaching the submental crease, the surgeon also can manage the witch's chin (**Fig. 34**). Chin fat subsequently is trimmed and the platysma corset technique is completed (**Figs. 35** and **36**).

POSTOPERATIVE FINDINGS

Since 2011, the authors have performed subplatysmal neck rejuvenation on 711 patients; 523 of these patients underwent partial resection of the SMSGs. No patient experienced major hematoma from gland resection. Two patients had sialoma, and 1 had a salivary fistula. These complications resolved after treatment with needle aspiration, external compression, and botulinum toxin. We attribute the low incidence of complications to the fact that saliva drains by a pressure gradient. Our procedure involves placing a continuous hemostatic suture over each SMSG and closing each capsule; these steps force the saliva to drain into the mouth. We also apply botulinum toxin, which temporarily decreases saliva production

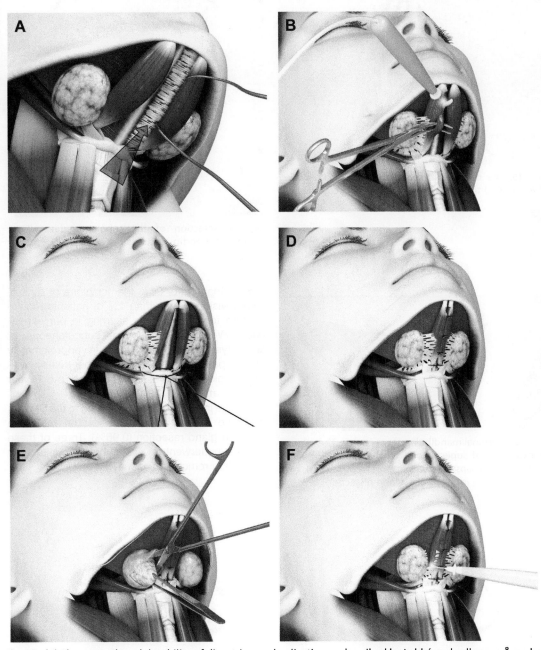

Fig. 18. (*A*) The strength and durability of digastric muscle plication as described by Labbé and colleagues[8] can be attributed to attachments of the mylohyoid muscle to the digastric muscle (*arrow*). (*B*) The anterior bellies of the digastric muscles are resected by 30% to 40% using a Mixter forceps and electrocautery. (*C*) The first stitch in plication of the digastric muscles is placed in the tendinous region of the tissue pulleys. (*D*) Corset plication of the anterior bellies of the digastric muscles. (*E*) Blunt dissection to open the submandibular salivary gland capsule. Freeing the submandibular salivary gland from its capsule is required for resection of the gland. (*F*) Medial gland adhesions are released by fine-tip electrocautery.

from the SMSGs. We do not drain the SMSG space. We have found that partial removal of the SMSGs does not yield dry mouth, as described previously in studies of large series of patients.[4,5]

In our experience, the position and aspect of the submental scar is acceptable to patients. The incision is made in an inconspicuous, shadowed area. In case of hypertrophic scarring, the patient can be treated with serial injections of

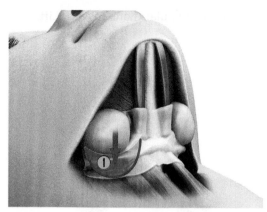

Fig. 19. The capsule is expanded inferiorly (1, *pink shaded area*) to enable manipulation of the gland.

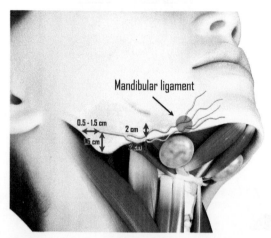

Fig. 20. Marginal mandibular nerve course. The nerve is external and superolateral to the submandibular salivary gland capsule and therefore is at low risk of damage during intracapsular gland dissection.

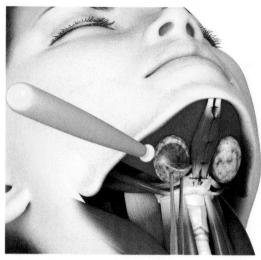

Fig. 22. Resection of the submandibular salivary gland with fine-tip electrocautery.

dexamethasone or 20% triamcinolone or by surgical revision. Fewer than 1% of patients require revision for hypertrophic scarring in our experience. We have found that subcutaneous or subplatysmal fibrosis occurs in approximately 5% of patients. This also may be treated with triamcinolone, but usually resolves by 1 year postoperatively.

A bulge in the neck contour owing to the SMSGs persisted in only 5 patients of the 523 who received gland resection (0.96%). Three of these patients underwent revision subplatysmal surgery to partially remove the gland.

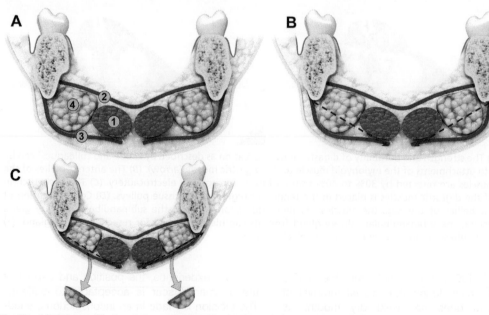

Fig. 21. (*A*) Submandibular anatomy depicted in the frontal plane. (1) Anterior belly of the digastric muscle, (2) mylohyoid muscle, (3) platysma, and (4) submandibular salivary gland. (*B*) The submandibular salivary gland area that bulges below a line drawn between the lowest point of the anterior belly of the digastric muscle and the inferior border of the mandible (*dashed arrow*) is considered for resection. (*C*) The submandibular salivary gland after resection.

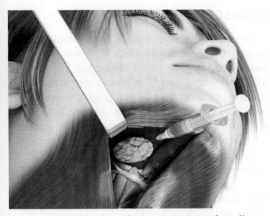

Fig. 23. Injection of a solution containing botulinum toxin and ropivacaine into the raw surface of the submandibular salivary gland. This maneuver reduces the likelihood of salivary fistula and helps to control pain in the early postoperative period.

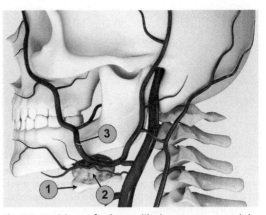

Fig. 25. Positions of submandibular structures and the facial vein and tributaries. (1) Hyoid, (2) submandibular salivary gland, and (3) facial vein.

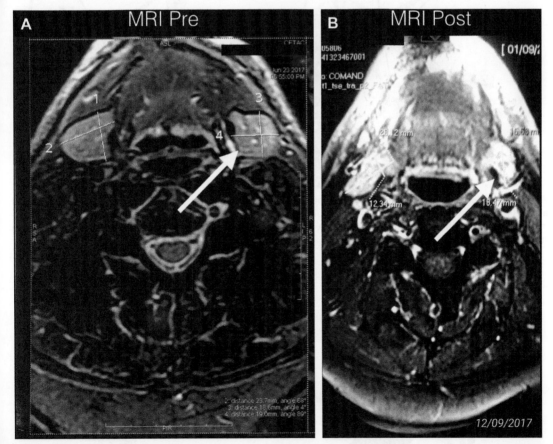

Fig. 24. MRI of the neck of this 48-year-old man who underwent surgical neck rejuvenation. (*A*) Preoperatively. (*B*) Six months postoperatively. Radiologic findings indicated an approximate volume reduction of 2.2 mL in the submandibular salivary gland (from 7.6 to 5.4 mL).

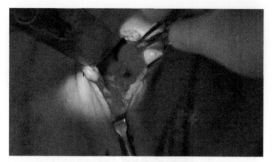

Fig. 26. Collateral vein on the medial aspect of the submandibular salivary gland at the superficial level. In the authors' experience, this occurs in approximately 8% of patients.

HEMOSTATIC NET

In open surgical rejuvenation of the neck, hematoma is a major concern.[11] Previously, we described closure of all dissected areas with the hemostatic net,[12] a series of columns of running sutures that encompass the skin flap and subjacent muscle (**Figs. 37** and **38**). Since its introduction in 2010, nearly 1000 patients have received the hemostatic net and no instance of hematoma has been recorded in the first 48 hours after surgery. The hemostatic net also has usefulness for skin redraping, especially for patients with severe skin redundancy.

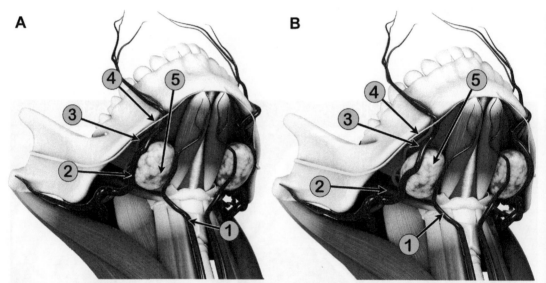

Fig. 27. (*A, B*) Circulatory anatomy in the submandibular area. (1) Anterior jugular vein, (2) facial vein, (3) facial artery, (4) marginal mandibular nerve, and (5) submandibular salivary gland. In most patients, the facial vein occurs lateral to the superficial lobe, as in (*A*). However, the facial vein has a more medial course over the gland in some patients, as in (*B*).

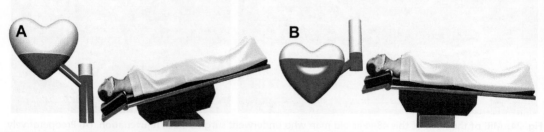

Fig. 28. (*A*) In neck rejuvenation surgery, venous blood pressure usually is high when the patient is in the Trendelenburg position. (*B*) Elevating the head may help to control bleeding.

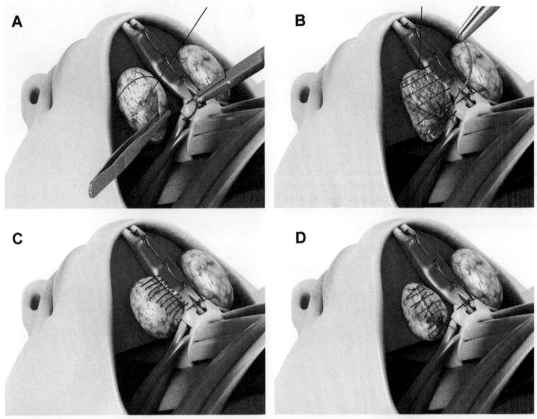

Fig. 29. (*A, B*) For hemostatic control, the raw surface of the submandibular salivary gland is closed. Continuous double-layer absorbable sutures are placed. (*C*) The submandibular salivary gland subsequently is sutured to the lateral portion of the anterior belly of the digastric muscle. (*D*) Affixing the submandibular salivary gland to the intermediate tendon of the digastric muscle helps to prevent ptosis of the gland.

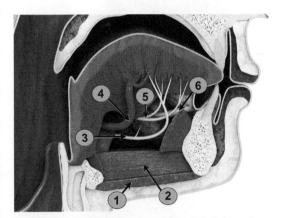

Fig. 30. Schematic anatomy of the subplatysmal region in the sagittal plane. (1) Platysma, (2) digastric muscle, (3) hypoglossal nerve, (4) lingual artery, (5) lingual nerve, and (6) Wharton's duct. When repositioning the submandibular salivary gland by anchoring it to the intermediate tendon of the digastric muscle, caution should be exercised to avoid damaging the hypoglossal nerve.

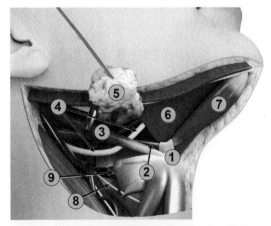

Fig. 31. Schematic anatomy of the subplatysmal region. (1) Hyoid, (2) intermediate tendon of the digastric muscle, (3) stylohyoid muscle, (4) hypoglossal nerve, (5) submandibular salivary gland, (6) mylohyoid muscle, (7) anterior belly of the digastric muscle, (8) superior laryngeal nerve, and (9) superior thyroid vein.

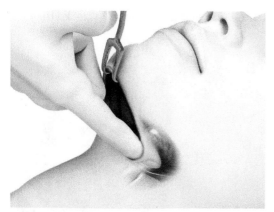

Fig. 32. Maneuver to locate the intermediate tendon of the digastric muscle. The assistant surgeon pulls the chin upward with a hook. The surgeon then locates the tendon either through blind palpation or direct vision. The tendon is rigid and cordlike.

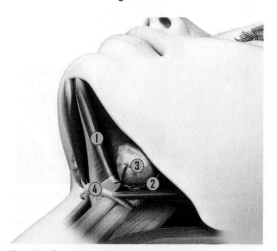

Fig. 33. The submandibular salivary gland may be repositioned by suturing it to the tendon. (1) Anterior belly of the digastric muscle, (2) intermediate tendon of the digastric muscle, (3) submandibular salivary gland, and (4) hyoid.

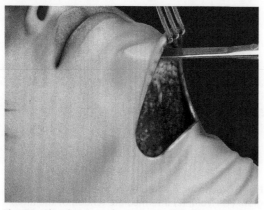

Fig. 34. The skin is undermined in the chin area after plication of the lower part of the neck by the platysma corset technique. This dissection allows for detachment of the submental crease in the treatment of the so-called witch's chin.

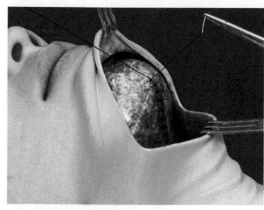

Fig. 35. Completed platysma plication over the chin.

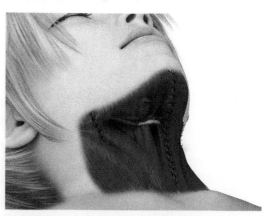

Fig. 36. Suture placement on completion of subplatysmal neck rejuvenation.

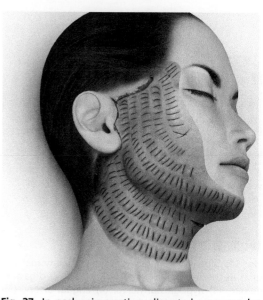

Fig. 37. In neck rejuvenation, dissected areas can be closed with the hemostatic net, a series of columns of running sutures that encompass the skin flap and subjacent muscle. This closure maneuver helps to avoid hematoma.

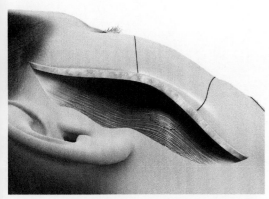

Fig. 38. Detailed depiction of the suture encompassing the skin and subjacent muscle during hemostatic net placement.

SUMMARY

For patients seeking facial rejuvenation, a thorough physical examination and photographic analysis (including of upward view of the flexed neck) allow for a precise determination of structures to be treated. Improving cervical contour frequently becomes the primary aim. Hypertrophy and/or ptosis of the SMSGs is a common cause of contour deformities. With advanced knowledge of neck anatomy and surgical expertise, the SMSGs can be resected safely and reproducibly to yield favorable results of neck rejuvenation.

SUPPLEMENTARY DATA

Supplementary data related to this article can be found online at https://doi.org/10.1016/j.cps.2018.06.001.

REFERENCES

1. Connell BF. Neck contour deformities. The art, engineering, anatomic diagnosis, architectural planning, and aesthetics of surgical correction. Clin Plast Surg 1987;14(4):683–92.

2. Ramirez OM. Multidimensional evaluation and surgical approaches to neck rejuvenation. Clin Plast Surg 2014;41(1):99–107.

3. Ellenbogen R, Karlin JV. Visual criteria for success in restoring the youthful neck. Plast Reconstr Surg 1980;66(6):827–37. Available at: https://journals.lww.com/plasreconsurg/Citation/1980/12000/Visual_Criteria_for_Success_in_Restoring_the.3.aspx.

4. Auersvald A, Auersvald LA, Uebel CO. Subplatysmal necklift: a retrospective analysis of 504 patients. Aesthet Surg J 2017;37(1):1–11. Available at: https://academic.oup.com/asj/article/37/1/1/2623842.

5. Feldman JF, editor. Neck lift. 1st edition. St Louis (MO): Quality Medical Publishing, Inc; 2006.

6. O'Daniel TG, Shanahan PT. Dexmedetomidine: a new alpha-agonist anesthetic agent for facial rejuvenation surgery. Aesthet Surg J 2006;26(1):35–40.

7. Marten TJ, Feldman JJ, Connell BF, et al. Treatment of the full obtuse neck. Aesthet Surg J 2005;25(4):387–97.

8. Labbé D, Giot JP, Kaluzinski E. Submental area rejuvenation by digastric corset: anatomical study and clinical application in 20 cases. Aesthetic Plast Surg 2013;37(2):222–31.

9. Mendelson BC, Tutino R. Submandibular gland reduction in aesthetic surgery of the neck: review of 112 consecutive cases. Plast Reconstr Surg 2015;136(3):463–71. Available at: https://journals.lww.com/plasreconsurg/fulltext/2015/09000/Submandibular_Gland_Reduction_in_Aesthetic_Surgery.4.aspx.

10. Singer DP, Sullivan PK. Submandibular gland I: an anatomic evaluation and surgical approach to submandibular gland resection for facial rejuvenation. Plast Reconstr Surg 2003;112(4):1150–4 [discussion: 1155–6]. Available at: https://journals.lww.com/plasreconsurg/Abstract/2003/09150/Submandibular_Gland_I__An_Anatomic_Evaluation_and.32.aspx.

11. Grover R, Jones BM, Waterhouse N. The prevention of haematoma following rhytidectomy: a review of 1078 consecutive facelifts. Br J Plast Surg 2001;54(6):481–6.

12. Auersvald A, Auersvald LA. Hemostatic net in rhytidoplasty: an efficient and safe method for preventing hematoma in 405 consecutive patients. Aesthetic Plast Surg 2014;38(1):1–9.

Extended Deep Plane Facelift

Incorporating Facial Retaining Ligament Release and Composite Flap Shifts to Maximize Midface, Jawline and Neck Rejuvenation

Andrew Jacono, MD[a,b,]*, Lucas M. Bryant, MD[a]

KEYWORDS

- Rhytidectomy • Face lift • Deep plane facelift • Facial retaining ligaments • SMAS • Platysma
- Neck lift

KEY POINTS

- Deep plane facelifting targets the mobile medial superficial muscular aponeurotic system, bypassing the lateral fixed superficial muscular aponeurotic system dissected in these techniques.
- Releasing facial and cervical retaining ligaments allows greater redraping of the superficial muscular aponeurotic system and platysma during rhytidectomy.
- Extending the deep plane flap inferiorly into the neck and incorporating a platysmal myotomy creates a platysma hammock to define the inferior mandibular contour and support the submandibular gland.
- Deep plane composite flaps of skin, the superficial muscular aponeurotic system, and malar fat can be repositioned to volumize the midface and gonial angle.

INTRODUCTION

To better understand the rationale behind deep plane facelifting and how it differs from lateral superficial muscular aponeurotic system (SMAS) facelifting (high or low), an understanding of the complex anatomy of the SMAS and soft tissues of the face is necessary. The SMAS layer was first described by Mitz and Peyronie in 1976.[1] The SMAS layer is continuous with the platysma muscle inferiorly and the temporoparietal fascia and galea aponeurotica superiorly. In the face, the SMAS lies between the subcutaneous adipose tissue, which compromises the superficial fat compartments of the face, and the underlying parotidomasseteric fascia, within which lies the facial nerves. The thickest SMAS is found in the lateral face overlying the parotid gland. The SMAS attenuates as it travels from lateral to medial in the midface, terminating at the lateral border of the zygomaticus major muscle[2] (**Fig. 1**).

Sub-SMAS dissection techniques, first introduced by Skoog in 1974,[3] tend to allow for both improvement of aesthetic change as well as increased longevity. The variance of SMAS mobility in different facial regions is important

Disclosure: The authors have nothing to disclose.
[a] New York Center for Facial Plastic and Laser Surgery, 630 Park Avenue, New York, NY 10065, USA; [b] Department of Otolaryngology/Head and Neck Surgery, Albert Einstein College of Medicine, 1300 Morris Park Avenue, Bronx, NY 10461, USA
* Corresponding author. New York Center for Facial Plastic and Laser Surgery, 630 Park Avenue, New York, NY 10065.
E-mail address: drjacono@gmail.com

Clin Plastic Surg 45 (2018) 527–554
https://doi.org/10.1016/j.cps.2018.06.007
0094-1298/18/© 2018 Elsevier Inc. All rights reserved.

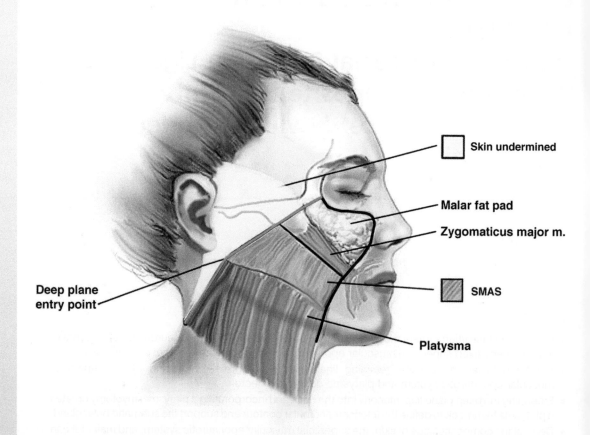

Skin undermined

Malar fat pad

Zygomaticus major m.

SMAS

Platysma

Deep plane
entry point

Fig. 1. The superficial muscular aponeurotic system (SMAS) is found in the lateral face overlying the parotid gland, is contiguous with the platysma inferiorly, and terminates at the lateral border of the zygomaticus major muscle. Medial to this point the malar fat pad overlies the zygomaticus musculature.

when considering the optimal areas for surgical manipulation during facial rejuvenation. The lateral SMAS overlying the parotid gland is generally fixed by the parotid cutaneous fascial attachments connecting it to the underlying parotid gland. We refer to this area as the "lateral fixed SMAS." Release of these attachments is required for successful mobilization and redraping of the SMAS. SMAS plication or imbrication techniques do not release these tissue attachments, so that redraping the jawline and medial facial tissues is more difficult. In contrast, surgical procedures that release the lateral SMAS from its deep attachments allow for more effective redraping of ptotic facial tissues.

As the SMAS extends medial to the parotid gland, it is not firmly adherent. A transition zone can be seen topographically in the aging face where the medial mobile SMAS descends and the lateral fixed SMAS does not (**Fig. 2**). The area of the lateral fixed SMAS involutes, creating a scalloping or concavity over the gonial angle, and the neck and jawline lie in the same plane with no

distinct mandibular border. As we will discuss elsewhere in this article, deep plane facelifting adds volume and contour to the gonial angle through composite flap shifts, improving the definition of the jawline.

The deep plane facelift enters the sub-SMAS plane at a line that traverses from the angle of the mandible to the lateral canthus. This approximates the transition zone between the fixed and the mobile SMAS. Traditional low SMAS and high lateral SMAS techniques elevate the fixed SMAS that has not descended with age to access the mobile SMAS that has. The deep plane facelift bypasses lifting the lateral fixed SMAS and targets the descended mobile SMAS and medial soft tissues (**Fig. 3**). The fixed lateral SMAS is fibrous, adherent, and difficult to dissect. The mobile SMAS is areolar in nature and easier to dissect. We believe this variation in SMAS mobility makes facelifting procedures that place traction on the medial mobile SMAS instead of the fixed lateral SMAS more

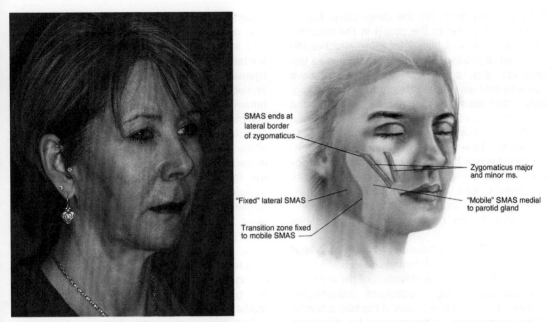

Fig. 2. Preoperative view of a 51-year-old woman demonstrating the "fixed" superficial muscular aponeurotic system (SMAS) overlying the lateral face and parotid with a transition zone to the "mobile" SMAS medial to the parotid where the jowl and lower face descends more readily.

effective in restoring a youthful appearance. This is true for both sub-SMAS and superficial SMAS plication, imbrication, and SMAS-ectomy techniques.

The deep plane facelift also has biomechanical advantages when lifting the medial soft tissue ptosis of aging compared with lateral SMAS procedures. The sub-SMAS entry point and thus the

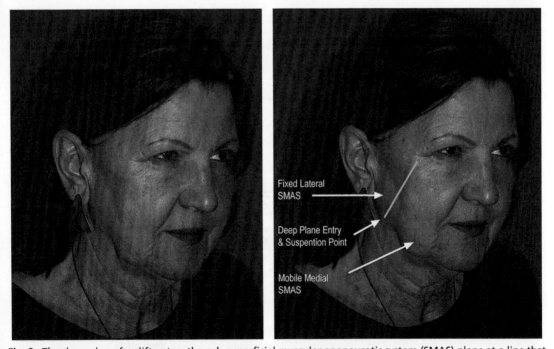

Fig. 3. The deep plane facelift enters the sub-superficial muscular aponeurotic system (SMAS) plane at a line that traverses from the angle of the mandible to the lateral canthus, which exists approximately at transition zone between the fixed and mobile SMAS. Traditional low SMAS and high lateral SMAS techniques elevate the fixed SMAS that has not descended to access the medial mobile SMAS that has.

point of suspension for the deep plane flap is anterior and closer to the ptosis in the midface, jowl, and neck so it allows for more effective lifting of facial ptosis. Hooke's law helps us to understand this concept. Facial tissues have elasticity and are put on stretch during facelifting, thus acting like a spring. Hooke's law states that the force, or in this case lift, on the spring (the elastic facial tissues) is inversely proportional to the length of the spring. The deep plane suspension point is one-half the distance from the drooping midface and jowl when compared with the suspension point of lateral SMAS approaches. This means that anteriorly based suspension exerts twice the lift on the medial facial tissues (**Fig. 4**).

Another difference between lateral SMAS and deep plane techniques is that the deep plane facelift allows for soft tissue elevation of the midface, whereas SMAS flap procedures anatomically cannot. The SMAS terminates at the lateral border of the zygomaticus in the midface (as described elsewhere in this article); therefore, elevation and traction on this tissue layer cannot effectively exert force medial to this point (see **Fig. 1**). The upper and medial midface where the SMAS is absent is occupied by the cheek fat. Rohrich and Pessa[4] divided the cheek fat into the malar and nasolabial

superficial facial fat compartments. The malar fat pad was further subdivided into medial, middle, and lateral anatomic divisions. These fat pads are tethered by the zygomatic cutaneous retaining ligaments.[5] The nasolabial fat compartment lies immediately lateral to the nasolabial fold and is tethered by fascial attachments to the zygomaticus major muscle. As aging progresses, the prominence over the malar region flattens with descent of the cheek fat. Volume loss becomes noticeable in the upper and lateral midface, and hollowing of the lower lid–cheek junction is evident. This descended cheek fat creates a synchronous increase and relative widening of the midfacial tissues just lateral to the nasolabial folds (see **Fig. 7**). The advance of these aging changes converts the heart-shaped face of youth into an inverted triangle shape. These heterogenous changes of the different facial fat compartments has been confirmed in cadaveric and imaging studies.[6–8]

The deep plane rhytidectomy creates a composite flap of skin, subcutaneous fat, and malar fat medial to the zygomaticus major muscle after releasing the zygomatic cutaneous ligaments. When this composite flap is repositioned vertically, it can be used to volumize the upper midface (**Fig. 5**). The senior author performed volumetric

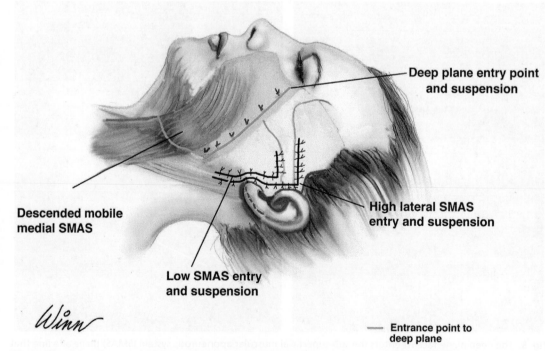

Fig. 4. The deep plane suspension point is one-half the distance from the drooping midface and jowl when compared with the suspension point of lateral superficial muscular aponeurotic system approaches. This anteriorly based suspension can exert more lift on the medial facial tissues. SMAS, superficial muscular aponeurotic system.

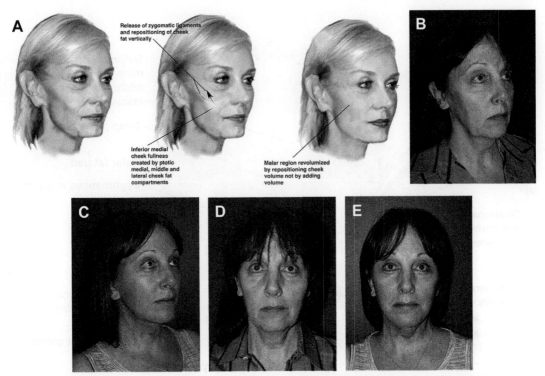

Fig. 5. (A) Midface volume augmentation can be achieved by elevating the descended malar fat pads without addition of facial volume. This requires release of the zygomatic cutaneous ligament and vertical vector lifting. (B, D) Preoperative and (C, E) 9-month postoperative views of a 59-year-old woman who underwent an extended deep plane facelift. Notice the volumizing of the midface with repositioning of the cheek fat compartments.

analysis after vertical vector deep plane rhytidectomy with a 23-month follow-up and demonstrated that patients gain an average of 3.2 mL of midface volume per side. This is the consequence of full composite flap release, allowing tension-free redraping of cheek fat compartments.[9] There is no statistical difference between the cheek volume gain from vertical vector deep plane rhytidectomy, and that achieved 16 months after 10 mL of autologous fat transfer per cheek for midfacial rejuvenation[10] (see **Fig. 7**). When patients have insufficient volume reservoir to reposition, volume supplementation with fat grafting, injectable fillers, or implant placement may be used as an adjunctive procedure.

Since the original description of deep plane rhytidectomy in 1990 by Sam Hamra,[11] the senior author has developed modifications to further improve rejuvenation of the midface, jawline, and neck. This article describes our volumizing extended deep plane facelift (**Fig. 6**). In brief, skin flap elevation is performed anteriorly up to a preoperatively marked line traveling obliquely from the angle of the mandible to the lateral canthus. The zygomatic–cutaneous ligaments are lysed similar to Hamra's technique, but a more extensive release of other facial retaining ligaments is performed as well. Additional ligamentous release includes the medial aspects of the zygomaticus major, the anterior extensions of the masseteric cutaneous ligaments, and the mandibular cutaneous ligaments. We have also extended the deep plane dissection below the angle of the mandible inferiorly. In the neck, the platysma is elevated from its posterior fascial attachments to the sternocleidomastoid muscle to approximately 5 cm below the inferior body of the mandible and anteriorly to the fascia overlying the submandibular gland. This maneuver releases the cervical retaining ligaments that would otherwise limit platysmal redraping. Incorporating a platysmal myotomy inferior to the mandibular border extending medially to the fascia overlying the submandibular gland creates a platysmal sling or hammock that supports ptosis of the gland and defines the submandibular contour. This extended sub-SMAS and subplatysmal approach can also mitigate the need to open the central neck in patients with mild to moderate neck laxity. Last, we have modified the redraping and suspension of the composite deep plane flap to volumize the midface and gonial angle, which

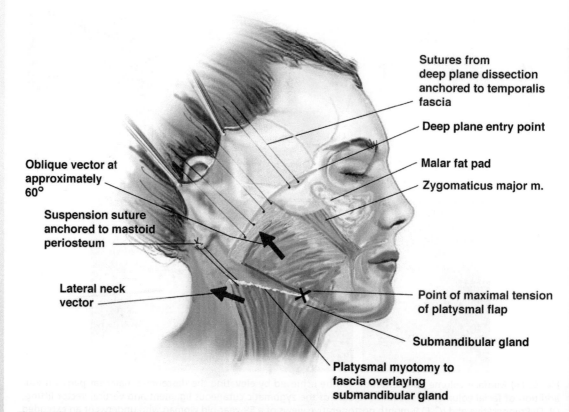

Sutures from
deep plane dissection
anchored to temporalis
fascia

Deep plane entry point

Oblique vector at
approximately
60°

Malar fat pad

Zygomaticus major m.

Suspension suture
anchored to mastoid
periosteum

Lateral neck
vector

Point of maximal tension
of platysmal flap

Submandibular gland

Platysmal myotomy to
fascia overlaying
submandibular gland

Fig. 6. Planes of dissection of the deep plane facelift, with a deep plane entry point from the angle of the mandible to the lateral canthus, and our modification extending the deep plane for 5 cm below the angle of the mandible with a platysma myotomy to the submandibular gland.

atrophy with age, thus improving cheek and jawline contour.

RELEVANT ANATOMY
Retaining Ligaments

Fully understanding the function and anatomy of the facial retaining ligaments is paramount to successful rejuvenation of the aging face. If not released, the mobility of facial tissues will be greatly inhibited. With ligamentous release, any applied traction to the lateral rhytidectomy flap can be fully transmitted to the medial facial soft tissues, allowing a natural and complete redraping. These concepts can be viewed as a natural extension to the same reconstructive principles used when soft tissues surrounding cutaneous defects are widely undermined and mobilized during local flap closure. In such cases, it is well-known that wide release allows for successful tissue redraping and a durable, tension-free closure.

Retaining ligaments are strong, fibrous attachments that secure defined dermal regions to deeper structures. They are present both within

the face and cervical regions (**Fig. 7**). Two types of ligaments have been described. Osseocutaneous ligaments run from the periosteum to the dermis. These include the zygomatic and mandibular ligaments. The second type of ligament is formed from a coalescence of superficial and deep facial fascia. Examples of this type of ligament are the parotid cutaneous and masseteric cutaneous ligaments.[12]

The zygomatic retaining ligaments originate from the periosteum of the zygoma body and extend through the malar fat pad and insert into the overlying dermis. The zygomatic retaining ligaments fix the aging midface and cheek fat. Biomechanical studies have shown that the zygomaticocutaneous ligament is the strongest of all of the facial retaining ligaments, elongating by a mere 9 mm.[13] Additional tendinous attachments run from the zygomaticus major and minor through the malar fat to the skin, reaching the nasolabial fold overlying the maxilla medially. This is called the premaxillary space.[14]

The mandibular cutaneous ligaments originate from the periosteum of the parasymphyseal

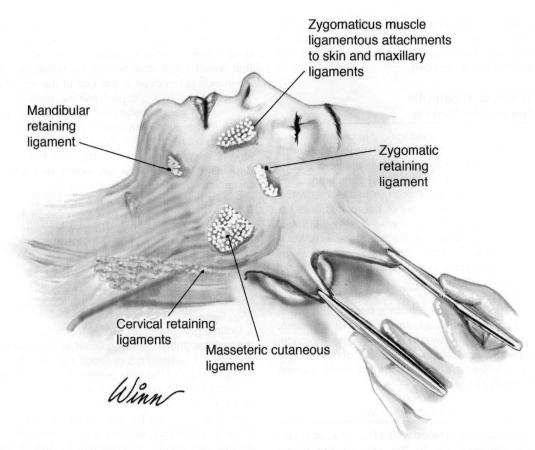

Zygomaticus muscle ligamentous attachments to skin and maxillary ligaments

Mandibular retaining ligament

Zygomatic retaining ligament

Cervical retaining ligaments

Masseteric cutaneous ligament

Fig. 7. Ligamentous attachments released in the extended deep plane face lift include the zygomatic cutaneous ligaments, the maxillary ligaments, the anterior extensions of the masseteric cutaneous ligaments, the mandibular cutaneous ligaments, and the cervical retaining ligaments.

region of the mandible. They similarly traverse superficially and insert into the overlying dermis. The mandibular retaining ligaments limit the mobility of the skin and soft tissue around the prejowl sulcus. By tethering the skin at the mandibular border, it prevents anterior submental neck skin redraping during rhytidectomy. The further posterior the ligament is displaced from the symphysis the greater tethering effect it has in the neck. In our study of 108 patients, we found the average tethering point to be 5 cm lateral to the symphysis. This means the surgeon would note a restriction of anterior cervical skin redraping starting approximately 5 cm posterior to the pogonion (Jacono AA: Limitation of neck redraping due to mandibular ligament tethering, personal communication, 2013).

Masseteric cutaneous ligaments lie along the anterior border of the masseter muscle. This ligamentous confluence acts to tether the jowl posteriorly. Complete ligamentous release requires

elevation of the SMAS to the anterior border of the masseter.[12] The parotidocutaneous ligament lies along the parotid gland, and are bypassed as the sub-SMAS dissection in deep plane surgery begins anterior to their point of termination.[15]

The cervical retaining ligaments of the neck are reproducibly found along the posterior border of the platysma at its junction with the sternocleidomastoid muscle, along the anterior inferior portion of the parotid gland, and along the posterior body of the mandible.[16,17] They tether the platysma to the deeper cervical fascia along the angle of the mandible and along the anterior border of the SCM. Just like facial ligaments, the cervical retaining ligaments restrict the surgeon's ability to mobilize and redrape the platysma if not released. Extending the deep plane subplatysmal dissection inferiorly into the neck requires a lateral platysmal dissection to release the cervical retaining ligaments.[18,19] We have performed anatomic studies that demonstrated that the cervical retaining ligaments extend for 1.5 cm medial to the anterior border of the SCM.[20] Complete redraping of the platysma thus requires extended platysma flap elevation past this point.

SURGICAL TECHNIQUE
Preoperative Marking

The patient is positioned upright to be marked pre-operatively (**Fig. 8**). The rhytidectomy incision is marked as well as the path of the temporal branch of the facial nerve, and the deep plane entry point. The deep plane entry point is marked as a line extending from the angle of the mandible to the lateral canthus. This places the area of SMAS manipulation anterior to the fixed lateral SMAS. A horizontal line is drawn across the neck at the level of the cricoid to mark the minimal inferior extent of neck skin elevation. We council male patients about the potential for transposition of bearded skin into the ear canal with a retrotragal incision and discuss a preauricular incision as an option. The patient is allowed to decide on the approach. In our practice, approximately 75% of men choose the retrotragal approach for improved incision camouflage.

Incision and Skin Flap Elevation

Skin incision is initiated with a No. 10 scalpel cutting perpendicular to the skin at the dense

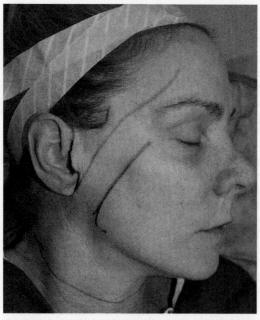

Fig. 8. Important landmarks drawn preoperatively include the trajectory of the temporal branch of the facial nerve, the deep plane entry point, incision lines, and inferior extent of neck skin elevation.

hairline of the temporal hair tuft. We use a temporal hair tuft–sparing incision because the deep plane technique causes large flap shifts that would result in removing the temporal hair when skin is removed at the end of the surgery. The temporal and occipital hairline portions of the incision can be extended during the operation if further skin redraping is needed. When a beveled trichophytic incision was used, the long-term outcome commonly resulted in a depressed incision in a significant percentage of cases. We believe this occurs because the skin of the anterior temporal region is thin and the skived edge of the beveled incision tends to become devitalized and heal in a contracted fashion. This is different from the thicker anterior forehead/scalp skin in the area of the frontal hairline, where trichophytic incisions were first described. We have noted temporal scars that are barely perceptible with this modification (**Fig. 9**).

Coursing inferiorly from the temporal region, the incision should not be placed at the anterior edge of the helical crus cartilage because it can make the root of the helix seem to be unnaturally wide. It should be placed at the natural highlight, which reflects the apparent width of the helical crus. It should then traverse along the posterior edge of the tragus, but not on its inner surface as this can create an unnatural folding of the cheek skin that blunts the tragus and can be a tell-tale sign of a facelift incision. A small step in the incision is placed at the inferior tragus to preserve the natural depression at the intertragic incisure. Around the earlobe, the incision should continue 2 mm inferior to the lobule cheek junction to preserve the natural sulcus between the lobe and the cheek. Posteriorly, the incision should continue a few millimeters onto the posterior conchal cartilage rather than directly in the postauricular crease. This step helps to minimize later inferior descent of the posterior auricular scar into a more visible location with age. In patients with less neck laxity, the incision ends here. If the surgeon is uncertain of the amount of neck skin that will need excision, the incision can always be extended to remove redundancy. In cases of more significant neck skin excess, the incision is transitioned at the level of the triangular fossa down the anterior aspect of the occipital hairline posteroinferiorly. In the past, we used a high transverse incision that was hidden in the occipital hair. This incision requires that the neck skin flap be shifted anteriorly and vertically to prevent hairline margin step offs, which limits the amount of redundant neck skin that can be removed.

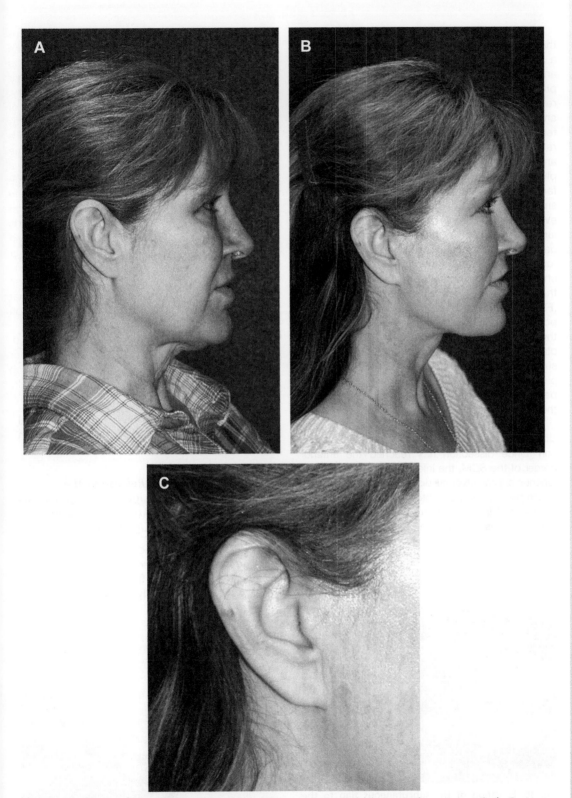

Fig. 9. Postoperative preauricular facelift incision. (*A*) Preoperative and (*B*) 12 months postoperatively. Postoperative views of a 53-year-old woman who underwent an extended deep plane facelift. (C) Notice well-healed temporal scar and well-camouflaged retrotragal incision with preservation of infratragal hollow.

After the initial rhytidectomy incision is made, the facial subcutaneous flap is elevated with a No. 10 scalpel. The skin flap is elevated anteriorly approximately 2 cm to allow for placement of an Anderson multiple prong retractor. The retractor is used to place superior and lateral tension on the flap. Direct counter-tension is placed by an assistant manually retracting the skin in the opposite direction and the flap is backlit to visualize the subdermal plexus (**Fig. 10**). Flap elevation continues with facelift scissors, tips pointed upward, making small, forward-snipping motions to create an even-thickness flap. The intensity of the transilluminated light gives the surgeon the ability to gauge the thickness of the flap and create a uniform depth. Subcutaneous elevation in the cheek ends approximately 2 to 4 mm beyond the marked line of the deep plane entry point (**Fig. 11**). The deep plane facelift approach poses no risk to the frontal branch because the dissection is superficial in the subcutaneous plane where the frontal branch exists, and the sub-SMAS dissection is begun at the deep plane entry point, which is 2 cm anterior and parallel to the course of the frontal branch of the facial nerve.

The postauricular skin is then dissected in a similar fashion and connected to the facial dissection. Once dissection has reached the anterior border of the SCM, the inferior and medial subcutaneous/supraplatysmal dissection in the neck is accomplished with a lighted retractor to provide tension and facelift scissors using a vertical blunt spreading. Dissecting on top of the supraplatysmal fascia during the medial neck skin elevation preserves a blanket of fat on the skin flap that prevents irregularities and adhesions between the deep dermis of the skin and the platysma postoperatively.

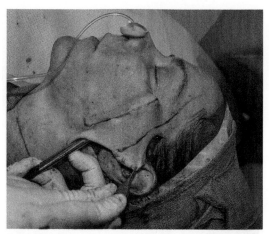

Fig. 11. The preauricular subcutaneous flap ends at the marked line of the deep plane entry point.

This dissection is continued to the midline and inferiorly to just below the level of the cricoid (**Fig. 12**).

Attention is directed to the mandibular cutaneous ligaments. The mandibular cutaneous ligaments are released using the same backlit skin-under tension method as the rest of the skin flap, releasing the ligaments in a subcutaneous plane. In cases with more fibrous and dense ligaments, dissection can be aided through the submental incision and a sharp curved iris sharp scissor can be used instead of facelifting scissors (**Fig. 13**).

Deep Plane Dissection: Release of the Zygomatic–Cutaneous Ligament, Zygomaticus Major Muscle Fibrous Attachments, and Masseteric Cutaneous Ligaments

An Anderson 5-prong retractor is placed at the anterior extent of the skin dissection parallel to the deep plane entry point line. The flap is held under vertical tension away from the body and a No. 10 scalpel is

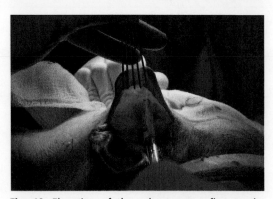

Fig. 10. Elevation of the subcutaneous flap to the deep plane entry point is performed with a facelift scissor with the flap back lit with an operating room light to visualize the subdermal plexus and maintain uniform flap thickness.

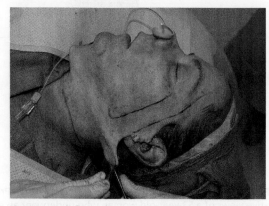

Fig. 12. Neck flap subcutaneous dissection is continued to the midline using a longer lighted retractor and long facelift scissors.

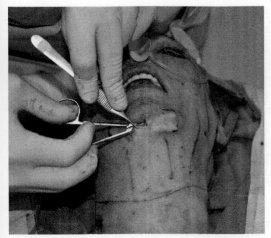

Fig. 13. Release of the mandibular ligaments requires dissection to the posterior edge of the tethering point and inferiorly to the lower edge of the mandible as it transitions to neck.

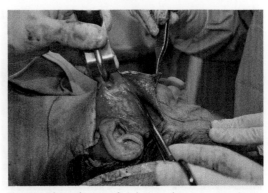

Fig. 15. The sub-superficial muscular aponeurotic system dissection continues anteriorly with vertical spreading motion with a facelift scissor until the masseteric cutaneous ligaments are released to the anterior border of the masseter.

used to incise the SMAS layer and expose the deep plane (**Fig. 14**). The incision extends from the mandible to the to the orbital rim near the lateral canthus. A lighted retractor is again used to create vertical tension away from the body and vertical blunt dissection with facelift scissors is performed to elevate the composite flap of skin and SMAS off the parotid–masseteric fascia. The masseteric cutaneous ligaments are released, allowing for more complete repositioning of the jowl (**Fig. 15**). Complete ligamentous release requires elevation of the composite flap to the anterior border of the masseter.[12] Another dissection endpoint is the facial artery, which can be palpated and visualized in the sub-SMAS plane. Elevation of this flap continues superiorly until resistance is reached at the zygomatic osteocutaneous ligament. Blunt

dissection through the inferior part of the deep plane flap is continued under the platysma below the mandibular border and onto the neck to facilitate later release of the platysma from the sternocleidomastoid muscle.

The zygomatic ligaments are isolated by blunt dissection of the superior extent of the deep plane entry point in the prezygomatic space.[14] Here, the dissection plane lies superficial to the orbicularis oculi muscle. Once the lateral border of the orbicularis is identified, the prezygomatic space can be easily dissected with blunt finger dissection. This dissection is carried medially into the premaxillary space, ending at the nasal facial crease. This technique was originally described as the FAME or finger-assisted malar elevation by Aston[21–24] (**Fig. 16**). Because SMAS is not present medial to the zygomaticus major, the composite flap in this area is composed of skin and the malar fat pad.

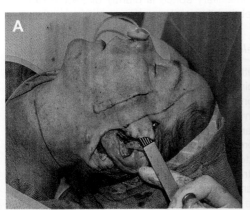
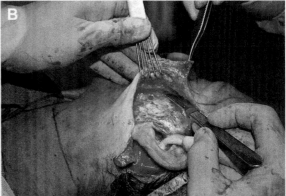

Fig. 14. (*A*) An Anderson 5-prong retractor is placed at the anterior extent of the skin dissection parallel to the deep plane entry point line. (*B*) With vertical tension on the retractor, a No. 10 scalpel is used to make the incision into the deep plane.

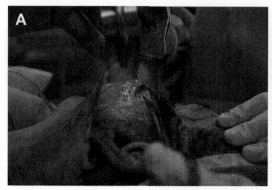
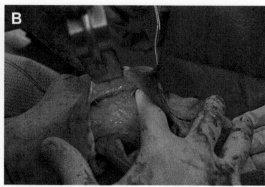
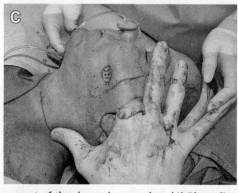

Fig. 16. Elevation of the superior aspect of the deep plane pocket. (*A*) Blunt dissection at the superior extent of the deep plane entry point, creating a plane superficial to the orbicularis oculi muscle (*B*). (*C*) Blunt finger dissection medially to free it to the deep plane to the nasal facial crease. Note the circular hashed marking that identifies the location of the zygomatic ligaments.

At this point, the zygomatic osteocutaneous ligaments have been isolated between the upper and lower composite deep plane flaps. These ligaments tether the SMAS/platysma complex to the malar bone and must be released to accomplish vertical elevation of the composite flap. Sharp dissection of the ligaments is initiated with a No. 10 scalpel staying superficial to the zygomaticus musculature (**Fig. 17**). Staying

superficial to the zygomaticus protects the facial nerve branches, which innervate the zygomaticus muscle from its deep surface. After sharp release of the dense ligaments, blunt dissection continues along the plane of the zygomaticus major and minor until the premaxillary space and nasolabial fold is reached (**Fig. 18**). A dense maxillary ligament at the inferior border of the premaxillary space is bluntly dissected to complete midface release.[14]

Release of the Cervical Retaining Ligaments

With the deep plane now free, the only remaining point that tethers the SMAS–platysma complex from moving vertically is the cervical retaining ligaments. The deep plane flap in the neck is marked from the gonial angle to the anterior border of the sternocleidomastoid muscle extending 5 cm inferiorly into the neck. A lighted retractor provides countertraction and the platysma muscle is partially incised. After incision, the remaining fibrous and ligamentous attachments at the anterior border of the sternocleidomastoid muscle are released with gentle, blunt scissor dissection. This dissection continues

Fig. 17. Release of the deep plane flap with sharp dissection of the zygomatic ligaments using a No. 10 scalpel cutting from superior to inferior and staying superficial to the zygomaticus musculature.

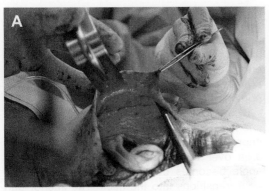
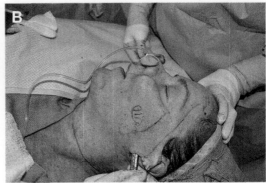

Fig. 18. (*A*) Deep plane flap is released through the zygomatic ligaments and (*B*) elevated to the nasolabial fold.

anteriorly and connects with the subplatysmal dissection plane that was previously created during the facial dissection. The anterior limit of the platysma flap is the anterior border of the submandibular gland so that the platysma flap can suspend gland ptosis (**Fig. 19**).

The dissection plane immediately below the platysma ensures that the marginal mandibular and cervical branches of the facial nerve down remain deep, on the superficial cervical fascia.

Dissection immediately under the platysma in the neck below the gonial angle is a safe plane protecting the marginal branch of the facial nerve, analogous to dissection just underneath the SMAS in the cheek is a safe plane protecting the facial nerves. The nerves above the gonial angle are in the parotidomasseteric fascia and below it in the superficial cervical fascia. These layers are contiguous. The marginal branch would be at risk if dissection under the SMAS

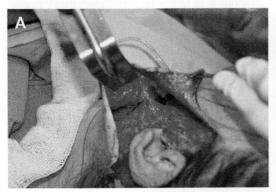
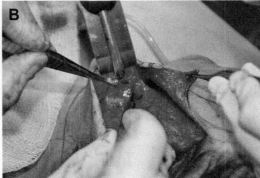
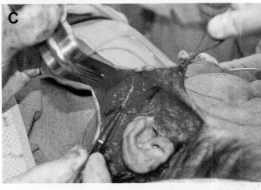

Fig. 19. Release of the cervical retaining ligaments. (*A*) Surgical marking of the lateral platysmal border at its connection to the sternocleidomastoid muscle extending 5 cm below the angle of the mandible. (*B*) A No. 15 scalpel is used to make a broad and gentle incision until a lip of tissue is obtained, the edge grasped and sharp dissection within the sternocleidomastoid muscle fascia is continued for approximately 1 cm, (*C*) Subplatysmal flap freed after bluntly dissect through the ligaments 3 cm anterior to the sharply elevated flap.

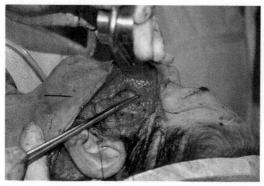

Fig. 20. The deep plane flap is typically sutured at 5 to 7 nearly equidistant points along the cuff formed at the deep plane entry point to the preauricular and deep temporal fascia.

and platysma is continued medial to the facial artery where the nerves become more superficial. Therefore, dissection in this region should be avoided.

Deep Plane Flap Suspension

Because the skin flap was raised slightly beyond the deep plane entry point in the face, this cuff of SMAS tissue is used for suture suspension. Five to 7 suspension sutures are placed (the author's preference is 4-0 nylon with PS-2 needle in most cases). The angle of flap suspension transitions from vertically dominant at the mandibular angle to horizontally dominant near the orbit (**Fig. 20**). This maximizes elevation of the cheek fat pads while preventing distortion of tissues in the temple region and lateral to the eye. The vector of lift for the composite flap in deep plane rhytidectomy is vertical oblique. The individual's anatomy dictates the exact angle. In a study of more than 300

patients, the average vector approached 60° relative to the Frankfort horizontal plane[25] (**Fig. 21**). Suture suspension begins with a half-mattress suture connecting the SMAS cuff at the deep plane entry point to the parotid masseteric fascia in the preauricular region for suspension of the inferior portion of the flap.

It is important to note that redraping of the inferior deep plane composite flap create improved mandibular contour. With age, the area over the lateral fixed SMAS and gonial angle becomes concave, blunting the jawline as it transitions into the neck. The inferior part of the composite skin and SMAS deep plane flap is fixated at the level of the gonial angle. This volumizes the gonial angle and creates a more distinct mandibular/jawline contour (**Fig. 22**).

The superior portions of the flap in the upper cheek are suspended to the deep temporal fascia. Importantly, the point of flap suspension for the upper flap is to the deep temporal fascia 2 cm above the zygomatic arch, similar to the high and lateral SMAS facelift. Repositioning the ptotic midface revolumizes the upper cheek over the zygoma. Volumetric analysis with 23 months of follow-up has shown that this suspension technique give patients an average gain of 3.2 mL of volume in each hemi midface[9] (**Figs. 23 and 24**).

Lateral Platymsa Suspension in the Neck and Skin Closure

After resuspension of the composite flap in the face is finished, attention is directed to redraping of the cervical platysma. A horizontal myotomy of the platysma is performed parallel to the inferior margin of the mandible for approximately 4 cm,

A

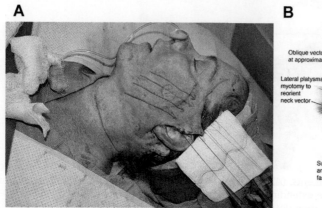

B

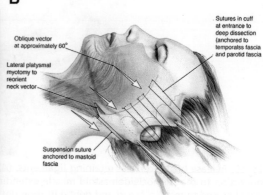

Fig. 21. (*A*) The flap is suspended vertically at an angle that maximizes elevation of the cheek fat pads and revolumizes the midface. (*B*) Suture suspension along vertically oblique vector of 60°.

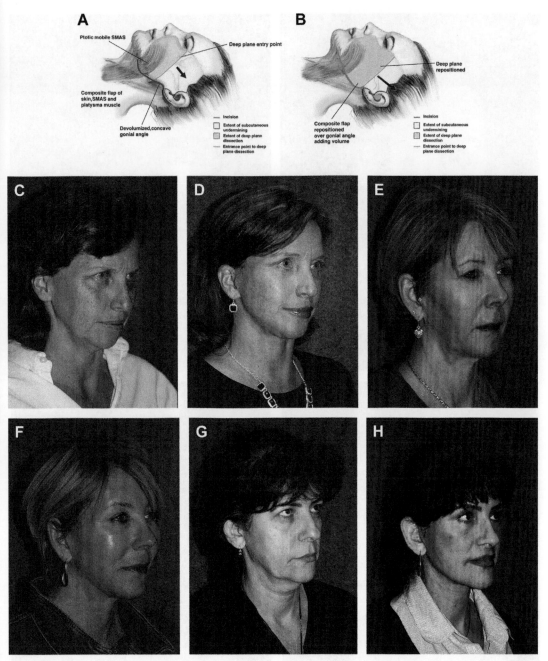

Fig. 22. (*A, B*) The inferior part of the composite skin and superficial muscular aponeurotic system (SMAS) deep plane flap is fixated at the level of the gonial angle. This volumizes the gonial angle and creates a more distinct mandibular/jawline contour. Preoperative view of (*C*) a 56-year-old woman, (*E*) a 57-year-old woman, and (*G*) a 58-year-old woman. (*D, F, H*) The same patients at 12 months postoperative after volumizing extended deep plane rhytidectomy with composite flap repositioning to augment the gonial angle.

ending at the area over the submandibular gland. The inferior platysmal tab is anchored to the mastoid fascia with a 3-0 nylon suture and positioned just below the margin of the mandible (**Fig. 25**). The vector of pull runs along the submandibular region and away from the cervicomental angle. This platysmal flap places its maximal tension at the most anterior extent of the myotomy, allowing for support of the submandibular region, elevating any ptotic

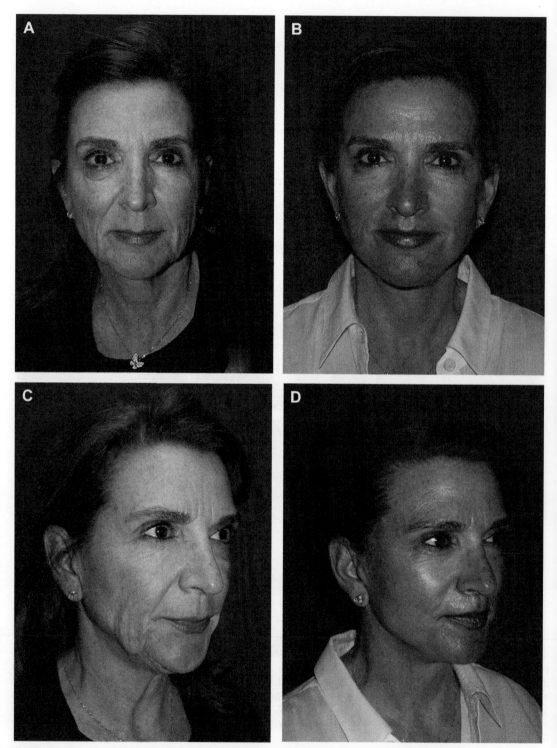

Fig. 23. (*A, C*) Preoperative and (*B, D*) 9 months postoperative views of a 57-year-old woman who underwent an extended deep plane facelift with zygomatic ligament. Notice the volumizing of the midface with repositioning of the cheek fat compartments.

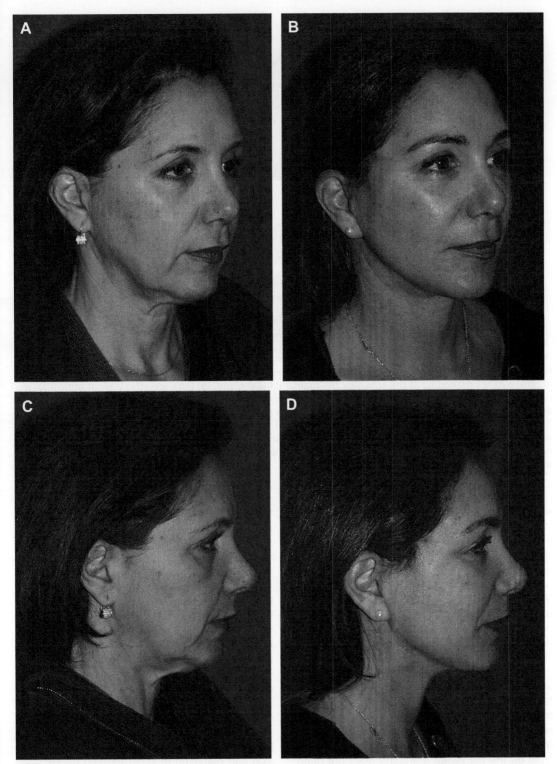

Fig. 24. (*A, C*) Preoperative and (*B, D*) 15 months postoperative views of a 62-year-old woman who underwent an extended deep plane facelift with zygomatic ligament. Notice the volumizing of the midface with repositioning of the cheek fat compartments.

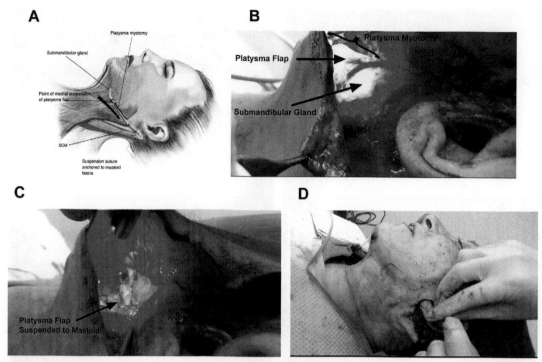

Fig. 25. (A) Horizontal myotomy of the platysma performed parallel to the inferior margin of the mandible for approximately 4 cm ending at the area over the submandibular gland. (B) Intraoperative view of horizontal myotomy of the platysma performed parallel to the inferior margin of the mandible for approximately 4 cm ending at the area over the submandibular gland. (C) The inferior platysmal tab is anchored to the mastoid fascia with a 3-0 nylon suture and positioned just below the margin of the mandible creating a platysma hammock that elevates the ptotic submandibular gland. Mandibular contour. (D) Note contour improvement of jawline and upper neck with tension placed on platysmal hammock. The circle marked on the skin is the location of the submandibular gland.

submandibular tissues, while concomitantly increasing a hollow below the angle of the mandible that exists in youth. Interestingly, this also places more traction on the platysma anteriorly and can help to smooth out platysmal bands, avoiding the need to open the neck (**Figs. 26–28**). Additional sutures are used to redrape the incised platysmal edge over the sternocleidomastoid muscle. A Jackson-Pratt drain is placed in the hairline, and positioned in the lower neck until the next morning.

After resuspension of the face and neck, attention is turned to redraping of the skin. The facial skin is suspended in the same plane as the composite flap. The majority of the skin is removed vertically in the temporal region (**Fig. 29**). Because the cervical skin has been lifted off the platysma, redraping does not need to equate the platysmal lift vector. Adequate elevation of the temporal skin in the subcutaneous plane avoids bunching. In patients with more significant laxity, the temporal incision must be carried along the hairline superior to

the lateral brow to avoid a dog ear deformity. Deep, everting 4-0 Vicryl sutures are placed along the temporal incision prevent depression and spreading of the scar over time. Skin closure is completed with everting 5-0 nylon vertical mattress sutures. The remainder of the incision is closed with 5-0 nylon sutures anteriorly, 5-0 nylon sutures behind the ear, and 4-0 nylon sutures in the occipital hairline (**Fig. 30**). The majority of anterior sutures are removed after 4 to 5 days.

We perform subcutaneous liposuction in the neck in less than 10% of our patients, and only when they have significant supraplatysmal fat excess, which can be grasped and clearly identified before injection. In general, we prefer to leave the natural blanket of fat between the skin and platysma to avoid forming depressions from adhesions and retraction. When performing submental liposuction we use modern techniques that mitigate the chance of commonly noted irregularities.[26–35] In general, we have found that elevating the neck skin flap before

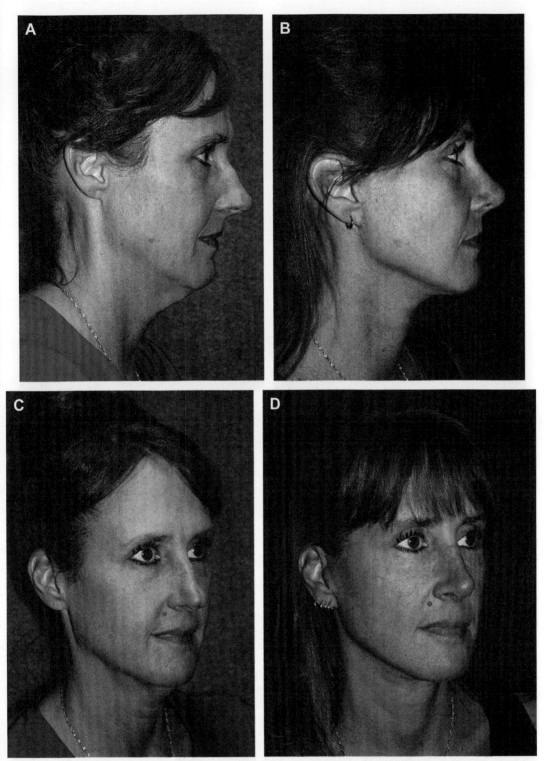

Fig. 26. (*A*, *C*) Preoperative and (*B*, *D*) 12 months postoperative views of a 51-year-old woman who underwent an extended deep plane facelift. Note improvement in anterior neck cording without opening the neck.

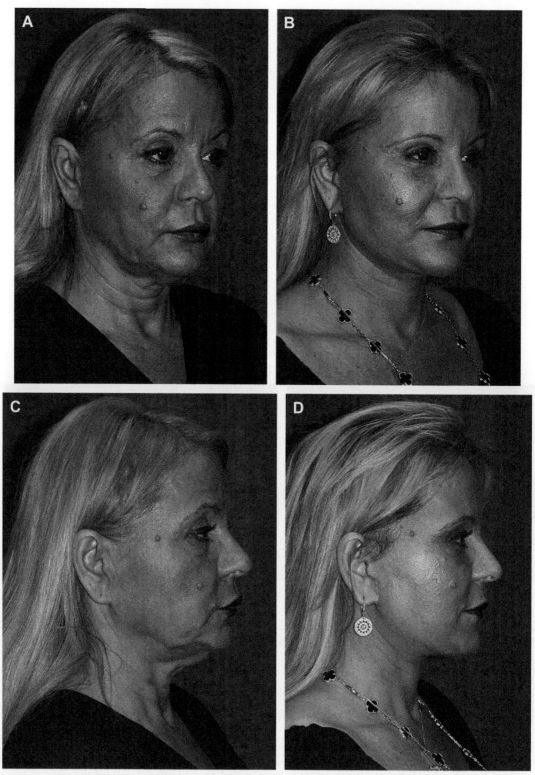

Fig. 27. (*A, C*) Preoperative and (*B, D*) 12 months postoperative views of a 61-year-old woman who underwent an extended deep plane facelift with platysma hammock suspension of the submandibular gland and improvement in anterior neck cording without opening the neck.

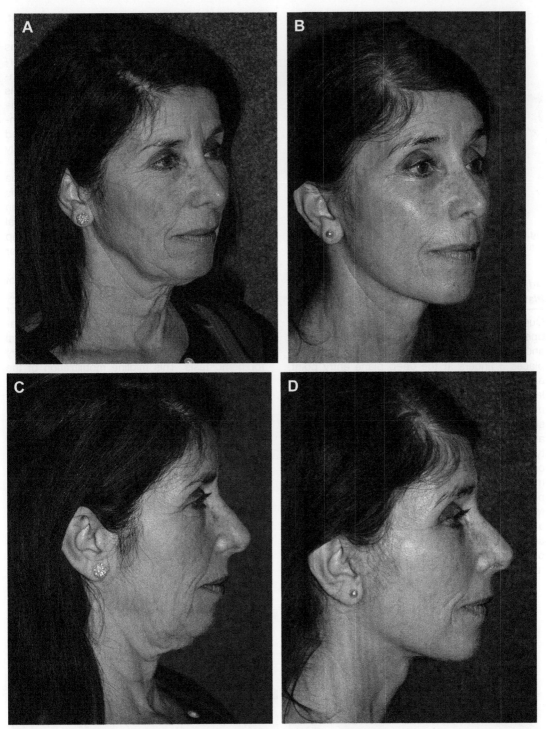

Fig. 28. (*A, C*) Preoperative and (*B, D*) 12 months postoperative views of a 58-year-old woman who underwent an extended deep plane facelift with platysma hammock suspension of the submandibular gland and improvement in anterior neck cording without opening the neck.

liposuction controls the amount of fat on the neck skin and decreases the risk of postoperative topographic irregularities. After flap elevation we use a 3-mm flat-tipped liposuction cannula to then remove supraplatysmal fat and sculpt the neck (**Fig. 31**).

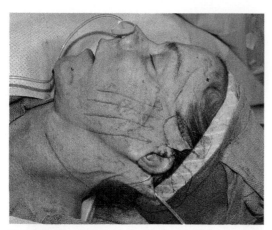

Fig. 29. The majority of the skin redundancy is removed vertically in the temporal region.

Adjunctive Submental Procedures and Platysmaplasty

Our main indications for rhytidectomy without opening the neck is if the submental platysmal and skin laxity is corrected when the surgeon places 3 fingers at the deep plane entry point, a line from the angle of the mandible to the lateral canthus, on both sides of the face and moves the skin vertically. If the patient still has significant neck redundancy with this maneuver and platysmal cording exists, then a midline platysmaplasty is indicated in addition to the vertical neck lift. We use 3 other indications for a midline approach. If widely separated midline platysma bands exist, midline plication is used to bridge their dehiscence. This is described as a DeCastro type III decussation pattern.[36] Additionally, a midline approach is used when subplatysmal surgery, such as subplatysmal fat removal, is performed to prevent cobra neck

deformity occurring postoperatively. Last, midline plication is indicated when intraoperatively the midline platysmal redundancy remains after the lateral platysmal lift is performed bilaterally. If it is determined preoperatively that the patient will require anterior platysmaplasty, this is performed before rhytidectomy. Increasing the number of procedures performed in the submentum increases the chances of irregularities, and each maneuver must be performed precisely and in a metered fashion.

A small submental incision is made and the submental skin is dissection with a curved iris scissor. Once an entry skin flap has been made, a skin hook is used to place the cervical skin under traction, while subcutaneous flap elevation continues using a blunt curved scissor (Metzenbaum).

At this point, the medial edges of each side of the platysma muscle are identified. The subplatysmal plane is extended laterally to the anterior border of the submandibular gland. The intraplatysmal fat is dissected away from the platysmal borders using blunt dissection and bipolar cautery for hemostasis. This midline mobilization of the platysma is extended approximately to the inferior border of the cricoid. The interplatysmal and subplatysmal fat is then removed from the submental area using suction monopolar cautery. Once the fat is removed, the subplatysmal flap is extended laterally.

The anterior belly of the digastric muscle is identified, and is sculpted with monopolar suction cautery if it contributes to submental fullness as identified on preoperative photographs. The neck is irrigated, and the midline platysmaplasty is closed using interrupted, buried 4-0 Vicryl sutures. There are key sutures used when closing the midline platysma. The first

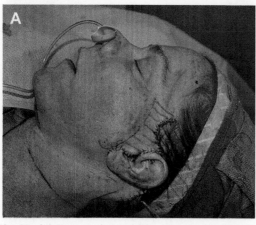

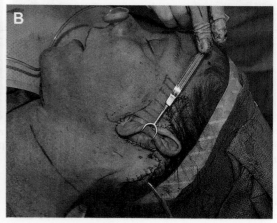

Fig. 30. (*A*) Preauricular and (*B*) postauricular skin closure.

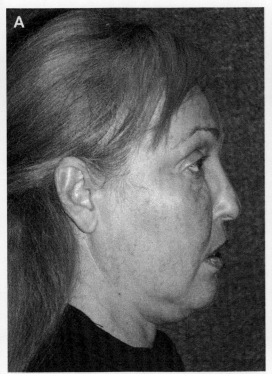 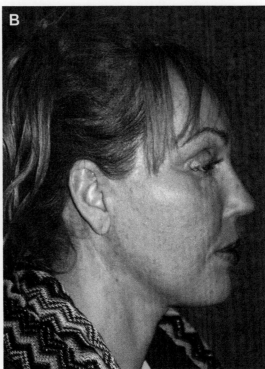

Fig. 31. (*A*) Preoperative and (*B*) 12 months postoperative views of a 59-year-old woman who underwent a modified, extended deep plane facelift without midline platysmaplasty but requiring supraplatysmal liposuction after skin flap elevation.

suture is placed at the cervicomental region. Here, the platysmal edges are sutured to the midline hyoid fascia to prevent separation and a midline banding after healing.[37] Additional interrupted 3-0 Vicryl sutures similarly adhere the platysmal edges to the deep submental tissues along the length from the chin to the hyoid to aid in cervical definition. The platysmal corset continues inferiorly to the level of the cricoid (**Figs. 32–34**).

Special Considerations in Deep Plane Rhytidectomy

Efficacy

There is a paucity of data comparing efficacy of rhytidectomy by technique. Short-term follow-up has shown higher efficacy in techniques using more aggressive SMAS manipulation, boasting fewer secondary procedures and happier patients.[38] The need for tuck up varies widely among rhytidectomy techniques and surgeons. SMAS plication and imbrication techniques have been shown to carry the highest tuck up rates of up to 21%[39] and up to 50% at 2 years.[40] More extensive skin flaps with extended SMAS dissections have a lower tuck up rate of 11%.[41] The deep plane

rhytidectomy reproducibly carries substantially lowered tuck up rates of 3% to 4%, which is statistically significant.[18,41]

Studies on medium-term efficacy show that less invasive SMAS approaches have a greater recurrence of neck laxity than jowl reformation.[38] There are few long-term follow-up data available for review. Patients presented for secondary facelifts after primary SMAS plication rhytidectomy on average 9 years later.[42] Secondary facelifts were sought after primary SMAS flap rhytidectomy on average 11.9 years later, suggesting this is a slightly more durable procedure; however, the data remain too limited to draw conclusions and the significance of this information is unclear.[43]

Complications

It is important to clarify that more aggressive dissection with deep plane techniques does not portend an increased risk to the patient. The rates of facial nerve damage and hematoma in deep plane rhytidectomy has been shown to be equal to those of less invasive techniques.[18,41] Our incidence of temporary facial nerve injury with an extended deep plane approach is 1.2% in a prior study reviewing

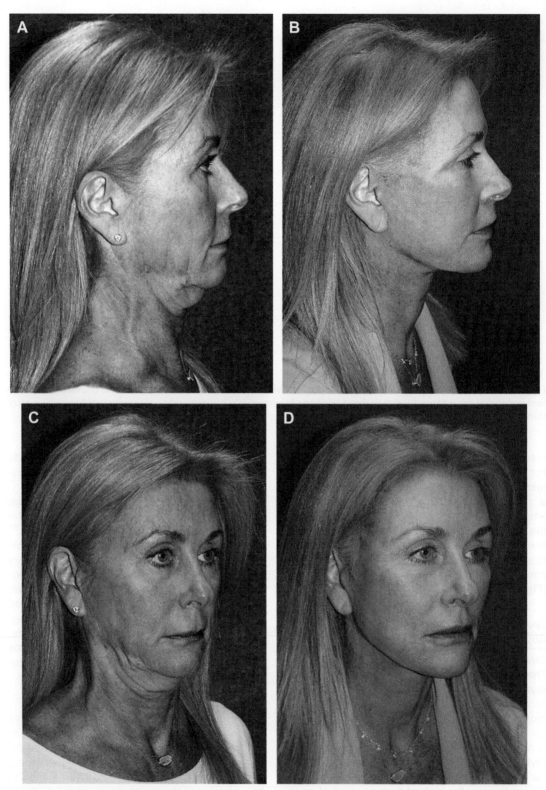

Fig. 32. (*A*, *C*) Preoperative and (*B*, *D*) postoperative views of a 62-year-old woman with excessive platysmal redundancy. She required a concomitant midline corset platysmaplasty suspended to the hyoid fascia with an extended deep plane facelift.

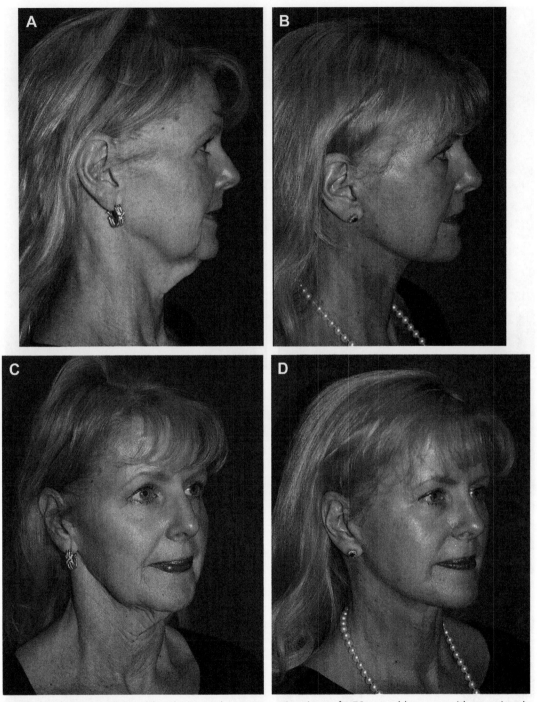

Fig. 33. (*A, C*) Preoperative and (*B, D*) 12 months postoperative views of a 56-year-old woman with excessive platysmal redundancy. She required a concomitant midline corset platysmaplasty suspended to the hyoid fascia with an extended deep plane facelift.

323 patients who underwent this technique with the primary author,[44] and has remained stable on follow-up review of more than 800 cases. This temporary facial nerve injury rate is the same as less invasive SMAS plicating and suturing techniques that can cause temporary traction injury.[45]

Deep plane surgery bears an improved risk profile in some aspects when compared with the traditional less extensive surgeries. It is associated

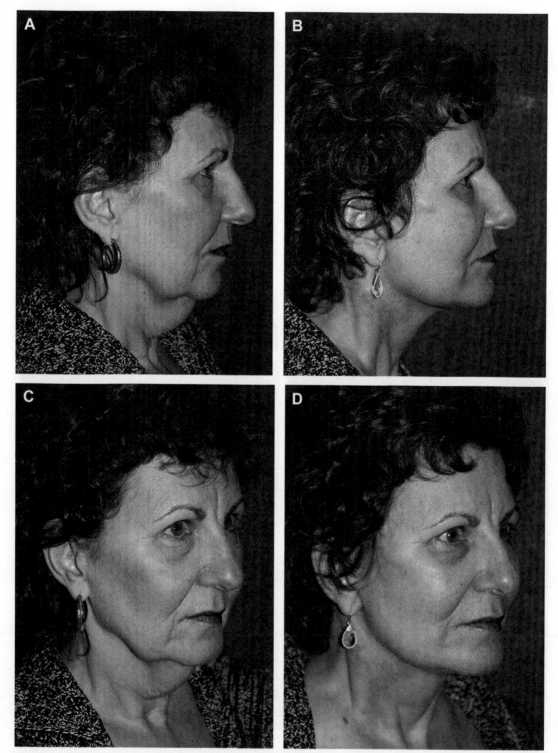

Fig. 34. (A, C) Preoperative and (B, D) 12 months postoperative views of a 70-year-old woman with poor submental contour requiring concomitant subplatysmal lipectomy, digastric reduction and midline corset platysmaplasty suspended to the hyoid fascia with an extended deep plane facelift.

with lower rates of skin flap sloughing and need for tuck up procedures.[18,41]

SUMMARY

The volumizing extended deep plane rhytidectomy is a safe procedure with superior outcomes in facial rejuvenation. A comprehensive understanding of the facial anatomy and pathophysiology of aging is imperative to incorporate this procedure successfully. The extended deep plane facelift incorporates additional ligamentous release of the face and neck to create durable redraping of face and neck ptosis redraping. This includes the zygomatic cutaneous, masseteric cutaneous, mandibular cutaneous, and cervical retaining ligaments. Deep plane dissection creates composite flaps that can be redraped to volumize the midface and gonial angle along the jawline, thus improving cheek and jawline contour.

REFERENCES

1. Mitz V, Peyronie M. The superficial musculo-aponeurotic system (SMAS) in the parotid and cheek area. Plast Reconstr Surg 1976;58(1):80.
2. Gassner HG, Rafii A, Young A, et al. Surgical anatomy of the face: implications for modern face-lift techniques. Arch Facial Plast Surg 2008; 10(1):9–19.
3. SKoog T. Plastic surgery: new methods and refinements. Philadelphia: Saunders; 1974.
4. Rohrich RJ, Pessa JE. The fat compartments of the face: anatomy and clinical implications for cosmetic surgery. Plast Reconstr Surg 2007;119(7):2219–27 [discussion: 2228–31].
5. Alghoul M, Codner MA. Retaining ligaments of the face: review of anatomy and clinical applications. Aesthet Surg J 2013;33(6):769–82.
6. Rohrich RJ, Pessa JE. The retaining system of the face: histologic evaluation of the septal boundaries of the subcutaneous fat compartments. Plast Reconstr Surg 2008;121(5):1804–9.
7. Gosain AK, Amarante MT, Hyde JS, et al. A dynamic analysis of changes in the nasolabial fold using magnetic resonance imaging: implications for facial rejuvenation and facial animation surgery. Plast Reconstr Surg 1996;98(4):622–36.
8. Gosain AK, Klein MH, Sudhakar PV, et al. A volumetric analysis of soft-tissue changes in the aging midface using high-resolution MRI: implications for facial rejuvenation. Plast Reconstr Surg 2005;115(4):1143–52 [discussion: 1153–5].
9. Jacono AA, Malone MH, Talei B. Three-dimensional analysis of long-term midface volume change after vertical vector deep-plane rhytidectomy. Aesthet Surg J 2015;35(5):491–503.
10. Gerth DJ, King B, Rabach L, et al. Long-term volumetric retention of autologous fat grafting processed with closed-membrane filtration. Aesthet Surg J 2014;34(7):985–94.
11. Hamra ST. The deep-plane rhytidectomy. Plast Reconstr Surg 1990;86(1):53–61 [discussion: 62–3].
12. Stuzin JM, Baker TJ, Gordon HL. The relationship of the superficial and deep facial fascias: relevance to rhytidectomy and aging. Plast Reconstr Surg 1992; 89(3):441–9 [discussion: 450–1].
13. Brandt MG, Hassa A, Roth K, et al. Biomechanical properties of the facial retaining ligaments. Arch Facial Plast Surg 2012;14(4):289–94.
14. Wong CH, Mendelson B. Facial soft-tissue spaces and retaining ligaments of the midcheek: defining the premaxillary space. Plast Reconstr Surg 2013; 132(1):49–56.
15. Furnas DW. The retaining ligaments of the cheek. Plast Reconstr Surg 1989;83(1):11–6.
16. Feldman JJ. Neck lift my way: an update. Plast Reconstr Surg 2014;134(6):1173–83.
17. Connell BF. Contouring the neck in rhytidectomy by lipectomy and a muscle sling. Plast Reconstr Surg 1978;61(3):376–83.
18. Jacono AA, Parikh SS. The minimal access deep plane extended vertical facelift. Aesthet Surg J 2011;31(8):874–90.
19. Jacono AA, Parikh SS, Kennedy WA. Anatomical comparison of platysmal tightening using superficial musculoaponeurotic system plication vs deep-plane rhytidectomy techniques. Arch Facial Plast Surg 2011;13(6):395–7.
20. Jacono AA, Malone MH. Characterization of the cervical retaining ligaments during subplatysmal facelift dissection and its implications. Aesthet Surg J 2017; 37(5):495–501.
21. Aston SJ. The FAME facelift: finger assisted malar elevation. In The Cutting Edge: Aesthetic Surgery Symposium. New York, December 5, 1998.
22. Graf R, Groth AK, Pace D, et al. Facial rejuvenation with SMASectomy and FAME using vertical vectors. Aesthetic Plast Surg 2008;32(4):585–92.
23. Ferreira LM, Horibe EK. Understanding the finger-assisted malar elevation technique in face lift. Plast Reconstr Surg 2006;118(3):731–40.
24. Aston SJ, Walden JL. Facelift with SMAS techniques and FAME. In: Aston SJ, Walden JL, editors. Aesthetic plastic surgery. London: Saunders Elsevier; 2009. p. 73–86.
25. Jacono AA, Ransom ER. Patient-specific rhytidectomy: finding the angle of maximal rejuvenation. Aesthet Surg J 2012;32(7):804–13.
26. Adamson PA, Cormier R, Tropper GJ, et al. Cervicofacial liposuction: results and controversies. J Otolaryngol 1990;19(4):267–73.
27. Bank DE, Perez MI. Skin retraction after liposuction in patients over the age of 40. Dermatol Surg 1999;25(9):673–6.

28. Chrisman BB. Liposuction with facelift surgery. Dermatol Clin 1990;8(3):501–22.

29. Daher JC, Cosac OM, Domingues S. Face-lift: the importance of redefining facial contours through facial liposuction. Ann Plast Surg 1988;21(1):1–10.

30. Dedo DD. Liposuction of the head and neck. Otolaryngol Head Neck Surg 1987;97(6):591–2.

31. Goodstein WA. Superficial liposculpture of the face and neck. Plast Reconstr Surg 1996;98(6):988–96 [discussion: 997–8].

32. Grotting JC, Beckenstein MS. Cervicofacial rejuvenation using ultrasound-assisted lipectomy. Plast Reconstr Surg 2001;107(3):847–55.

33. Jacob CI, Berkes BJ, Kaminer MS. Liposuction and surgical recontouring of the neck: a retrospective analysis. Dermatol Surg 2000;26(7):625–32.

34. Koehler J. Complications of neck liposuction and submentoplasty. Oral Maxillofac Surg Clin North Am 2009;21(1):43–52, vi.

35. O'Ryan F, Schendel S, Poor D. Submental-submandibular suction lipectomy: indications and surgical technique. Oral Surg Oral Med Oral Pathol 1989;67(2):117–25.

36. De Castro CC. Anatomy of the neck and procedure selection. Clin Plast Surg 2008;35(4):625–42, vii.

37. Yousif NJ, Matloub HS, Sanger JR. Sanger, hyoid suspension neck lift. Plast Reconstr Surg 2016;138(6):1181–90.

38. Jones BM, Lo SJ. How long does a face lift last? Objective and subjective measurements over a 5-year period. Plast Reconstr Surg 2012;130(6):1317–27.

39. Kamer FM, Parkes ML. The two-stage concept of rhytidectomy. Trans Sect Otolaryngol Am Acad Ophthalmol Otolaryngol 1975;80(6):546–50.

40. Prado A, Andrades P, Danilla S, et al. A clinical retrospective study comparing two short-scar face lifts: minimal access cranial suspension versus lateral SMASectomy. Plast Reconstr Surg 2006;117(5):1413–25 [discussion: 1426–7].

41. Kamer FM, Frankel AS. SMAS rhytidectomy versus deep plane rhytidectomy: an objective comparison. Plast Reconstr Surg 1998;102(3):878–81.

42. Beale EW, Rasko Y, Rohrich RJ. A 20-year experience with secondary rhytidectomy: a review of technique, longevity, and outcomes. Plast Reconstr Surg 2013;131(3):625–34.

43. Sundine MJ, Kretsis V, Connell BF. Longevity of SMAS facial rejuvenation and support. Plast Reconstr Surg 2010;126(1):229–37.

44. Jacono AA, Rousso JJ. The modern minimally invasive face lift: has it replaced the traditional access approach? Facial Plast Surg Clin North Am 2013;21(2):171–89.

45. Barton FE Jr. Aesthetic surgery of the face and neck. Aesthet Surg J 2009;29(6):449–63 [quiz: 464–6].

Management of the Platysma in Neck Lift

Timothy Marten, MD*, Dino Elyassnia, MD

KEYWORDS

- Neck lift • Platysmaplasty • Platysmamyotomy • Platysmapexy • Platysma bands
- Platysma hyperfunction • Full-width platysma transection • Postauricular transposition flap

KEY POINTS

- Traditional treatment of platysma bands has consisted of corset tightening of the anterior platysma muscle borders or suspension of the lateral platysma borders to sternocleidomastoid or periauricular fascia. Despite numerous variations and modifications of these maneuvers they have largely failed, and treating platysma bands remains a frustrating and perplexing problem for many surgeons.
- Experience has confirmed that platysma tighening will not universally correct "platysma bands", and that our traditional view that all platysma bands were a homogenous problem and simply a product of horizontal platysmal laxity was conceptually flawed and the underlying cause of many decades of failed treatment.
- "Platysma bands" comprise a heterogeneous group of distinct problems and can be seen to be the product of not only horizontal laxity but longitudinal platysmal hyperfunction. As such, are often refractory to horizontal pulling. Proper treatment in such situations requires horizontal platysma transection to disrupt longitudinal muscle hyperfunction.
- Examination of the neck with and without platysmal activation allows one to distinguish between "hard" dynamic and "soft" adynamic platysma bands and their differing origins.
- Soft, adynamic bands change little during platysma activation and are predominantly a problem of loose skin or horizontal platysmal laxity. Hard dynamic bands become tight or exaggerated upon platysmal activation and indicate a problem of platysmal hyperfunction. These problems represent two disticnt enities, and as such will require different and specific treatment.

FUNDAMENTAL CONCEPTS IN THE TREATMENT OF PLATYSMA IRREGULARITIES

As surgeons have pursued improved outcomes in treating the neck and platysma, our understanding of the origin of platysma muscle irregularities has improved and platysma muscle treatment techniques have evolved. Experience has since shown that the traditional notion that platysma tightening will correct deep layer neck problems, including accumulations of subplatysmal fat, large submandibular glands, and protruding digastric muscles, was misguided, and that proper treatment of these problems requires deep layer procedures that address the actual anatomic problems present.

Over time, surgeons have come to understand and accept that improved neck contour is not created by platysma tightening, but by deep layer maneuvers (subplatysmal fat excision, submandibular gland reduction, and partial digastric myectomy) that specifically target these problems, and these issues are discussed (see Timothy Marten and Dino Elyassnia's, "Neck Lift: Defining Anatomic Problems and Choosing Appropriate Treatment Strategies," and Timothy Marten and Dino Elyassnia's, "Short Scar Neck Lift: Neck Lift Using a Submental Incision Only," in this issue).

Experience has also confirmed that platysma tightening will not universally correct platysma bands, and that our traditional view that all

Disclosure: The authors have nothing to disclose.
Marten Clinic of Plastic Surgery, 450 Sutter Street, Suite 2222, San Francisco, CA 94108, USA
* Corresponding author.
E-mail address: tmarten@martenclinic.com

platysma bands were a homogenous problem and simply a product of age associated horizontal platysmal laxity was conceptually flawed and the underlying cause of many decades of failed treatments. In reality platysma bands comprise a heterogeneous group of distinct problems, and for many patients they can be seen to be the product of not only horizontal laxity but longitudinal platysmal hyperfunction and, as such, are refractory to horizontal pulling. Proper treatment of these problems requires horizontal platysma transection to disrupt longitudinal hyperfunction or treatment by other like means.

The fundamental flaw in the platysma tightening approach is that it fails to recognize or address the underlying differences and differing functional origins of platysma bands. Examination of the cervicosubmental region with and without platysmal activation allows one to distinguish between hard dynamic and soft adynamic cervical bands and their differing physiologic origins (**Fig. 1**). Soft, adynamic bands change little during platysma activation and are predominantly a problem of loose skin or horizontal platysmal laxity. Hard dynamic bands become tight or exaggerated upon platysmal activation and indicate a problem of longitudinal platysmal hyperfunction. These problems represent two distinct entities, and as such require different and specific treatments.

Planning Treatment of the Platysma

Assessing platysma deformity

The cervicosubmental region of each patient must be carefully examined both at rest and during platysma activation if complete assessment of platysma condition is to be made. This examination is best accomplished by asking the patient to push the jaw forward and tighten the neck. It is often helpful if the surgeon demonstrates this maneuver first for the patient to be sure it is correctly performed. Frequently, an insignificant appearing irregularity at rest will be obvious upon muscle activation (see **Fig. 1**). Failure to recognize and appropriately correct these dynamic irregularities is the reason too many facelift patients seem to be improved in repose, but unnatural or bizarre in conversation, animation, and during other activities that result in platysma muscle activation.

Examination of the cervicosubmental region with and without platysma activation as outlined allows one to distinguish between hard dynamic and soft adynamic cervical bands. Soft, adynamic bands change little during platysma activation and are predominantly a problem of loose skin or horizontal platysmal laxity (**Fig. 2**A). Hard dynamic bands become tight or exaggerated upon platysma activation and indicate a problem of longitudinal platysma hyperfunction (**Fig. 2**B).

Treatment of horizontal platysma laxity and soft bands

If submental support is poor owing to horizontal platysma laxity or platysma diastasis and optimal improvement in the anterior neck is desired, an anterior platysmaplasty is planned (**Fig. 3**). Anterior platysmaplasty is the procedure in which the medial borders of the platysma muscle are sutured together to help consolidate the neck, reduce

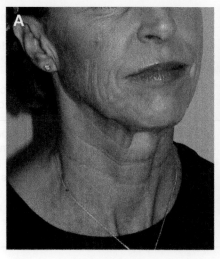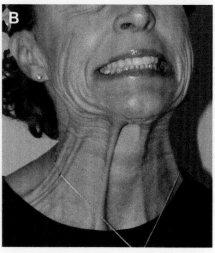

repose   platysma contraction

Fig. 1. Dynamic assessment of the cervicosubmental region. The neck is examined in repose (*A*) and as the platysma is contracted (*B*). Dynamic platysma muscle irregularities as seen in (*B*) are often referred to as hard platysma bands.

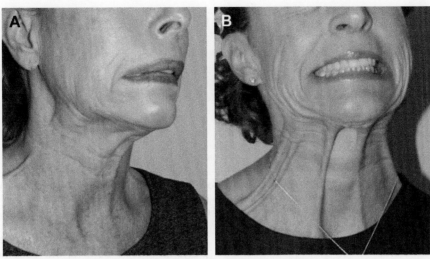

Fig. 2. Soft and hard platysma bands. Examination of the cervicosubmental region during platysma activation allows one to distinguish between hard dynamic and soft adynamic cervical bands. (*A*) A patient's neck seen during platysma activation. Soft, adynamic bands change little during platysma activation and are predominantly a problem of loose skin or horizontal platysmal laxity. (*B*) A different patient's neck seen during platysma activation. Hard dynamic bands become tight or exaggerated upon platysma activation and indicate a problem of longitudinal platysma hyperfunction.

horizontal platysma laxity, and improve neck appearance when patients flex their neck and look down (**Fig. 4**). It is not, however, adequate or effective treatment of excess subplatysmal fat, prominent submandibular glands, protruding anterior bellies of the digastric muscles, or for the treatment of hard dynamic platysma bands. Not

recognizing and acknowledging this fact, and well-intended but misguided attempts to treat these problems by medial or lateral platysmal tightening, have led to frustration for many surgeons treating the aging neck. Treatment of these problems require that other maneuvers be performed.

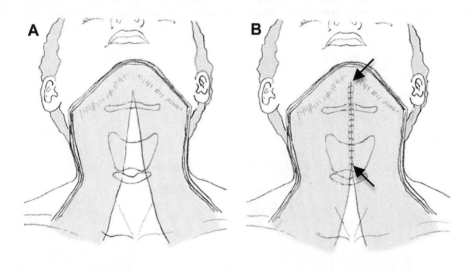

before   after

Fig. 3. (*A*, *B*) Anterior platysmaplasty reduces horizontal platysma laxity, improves submental support, consolidates the neck, and is the primary treatment for soft platysma bands. It is not an adequate or effective treatment of dynamic hard platysma bands or excess subplatysmal fat, prominent submandibular glands, and protrusion of the anterior bellies of the digastric muscles, however. Suturing is made in an interrupted fashion with absorbable suture from menton to thyroid cartilage as shown (*arrows*).

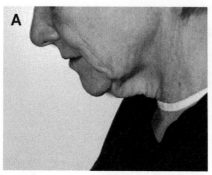
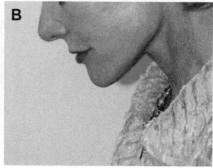

Fig. 4. (*A, B*) Anterior platysmaplasty. Platysmaplasty improves submental support and enhances neck appearance when the patient looks down. Procedures performed by Timothy J. Marten, MD, FACS. (*Courtesy of* Timothy J. Marten, MD, FACS, Marten Clinic of Plastic Surgery, San Francisco, CA.)

Treatment of platysma hyperfunction and dynamic hard bands

It is important to distinguish between soft adynamic playsma bands and hard dynamic bands because the treatment varies depending on the type present. Patients with soft bands are usually adequately treated with skin excision or skin excision and platysmaplasty alone as outlined elsewhere in this article. Patients with hard bands, however, require transverse platysma myotomy or some other procedure that disrupts longitudinal platysma muscle hyperfunction. The result of platysma myotomy is typically long-lasting and superior to any suture, suture suspension, lateral suspension of the platysmal border, or corset platysma tightening technique (**Fig. 5**). The length of transection required can be varied depending on the location and configuration of bands present and may, thus, differ from patient to patient.

Platysma bands are generally seen to lie in medial and lateral locations and are often referred to as anterior and lateral platysma bands (**Fig. 6**).

Each band is situated near the medial and lateral platysma muscle borders, but does not usually correlate precisely with them. Patients with anterior platysma bands only can be treated with partial transverse platysma myotomy by dividing the muscle medially and subtotally through and beyond the section of it in which the band is present low in the neck at the level of the cricoid cartilage (**Fig. 7**A, B). The platysma muscles need not arbitrarily be completely transected when an anterior band only is present, just the region where the platysma band is located.

If lateral, as well as anterior bands are present, the myotomy is carried more laterally to include them as well (**Fig. 8**). If poor definition is present over the lateral mandibular border, in addition to anterior and lateral neck bands, or if comprehensive improvement is desired, the platysma myotomy is planned to continue full-width superolaterally up to the anterior border of the sternocleidomastoid muscle (**Fig. 9**). A similar full-width myotomy of this type may also indicated in a firm

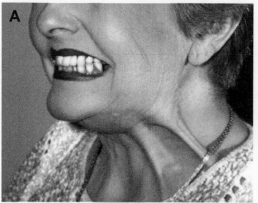
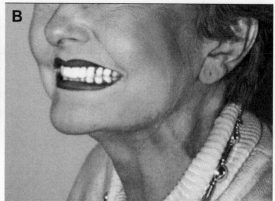

Fig. 5. (*A, B*) Platysma myotomy. (*A*) Patient seen preoperatively with objectionable appearing hard dynamic platysma bands before platysma myotomy. (*B*) The same patient after platysma myotomy. The result of platysma myotomy is typically dramatic, long-lasting, and superior to any suture, suture suspension, lateral suspension of the lateral platysmal border, or corset platysma tightening technique.

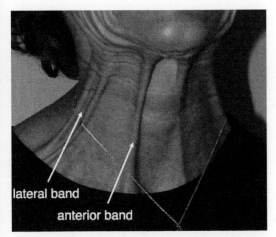

Fig. 6. Anterior and lateral platysmal bands. Platysma bands are generally seen to lie in medial and lateral locations and are often referred to as anterior and lateral platysma bands. Each band is situated near the medial and lateral platysma muscle borders but does not usually correlate precisely with them.

obtuse neck with a short platysma and poor definition over the mandibular angle, but no bands.

In theory and principle, in many necks a subtotal myotomy only is indicated and need be performed. As a practical matter, however, complete transection of the platysma is often performed when any form of myotomy is indicated to limit the possibility of band reoccurrence or that residual platysma bands will be present. Despite assertions to the contrary, full-width platysma myotomy will not result in an overly thin-appearing neck

(lollipop neck), or reduced support of the submandibular glands.

Medial wedge resections of platysma at the hyoid and vertical excisions of platysma bands, although shown in many textbooks, are not effective in that a large segment of adjacent and more laterally situated muscle remains untreated. Vertical excision of platysma bands, although still advocated by some investigators, has proven to be an ineffective treatment that has largely been abandoned by experienced surgeons. Trying to isolate and specifically excise the responsible muscle segment is difficult at best, and typically incites a new band to form in an adjacent untreated area.

Medial wedge resections of platysma at the hyoid can result in unaesthetic exposure of underlying cervical anatomy and a harsh transition from the submental region to the neck, as well as lower lip dysfunction and asymmetric smile. These procedures are not recommended in the routine treatment of platysma bands, although they may be useful in certain secondary cases and in situations where there has been fibrosis and scarring of the platysma in that area. These problems can result from noninvasive treatment of the neck with radiofrequency, ultrasound therapy, internal tissue heating, cryolipolysis, chemolipolysis, laser liposuction, and the use of inflammatory fillers in the neck area. Similarly, attempts to place rigid support across the cervicomental angle in the form of a mastoid-to-mastoid noose of suture or commercially available straps to lift platysma bands is

A

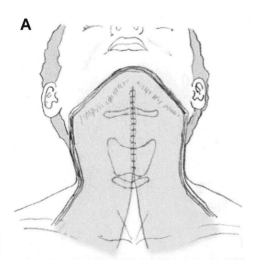

B

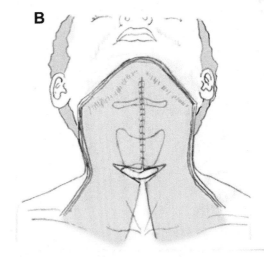

Fig. 7. (*A*, *B*) Plan for treatment of anterior dynamic hard platysmal bands. Transverse platysma myotomy is performed in the region of the platysma muscle where the platysmal band is present. (*A*) Anterior neck after platysmaplasty but before anterior platysma myotomy. (*B*) After anterior platysma myotomy. (Note: Myotomy is most easily and effectively performed after platysmaplasty has been completed; note also that, because uninterrupted muscle is present laterally, the potential for new band formation in that area is possible).

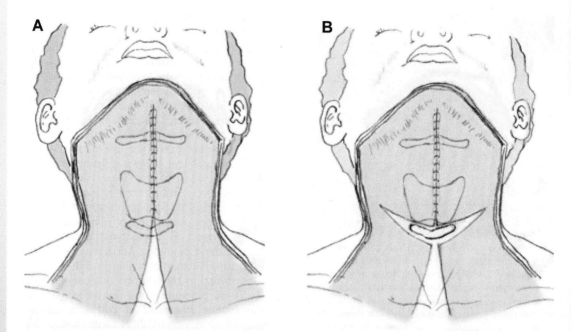

Fig. 8. (*A, B*) Plan for the treatment of anterior and lateral platysmal bands. If lateral bands are present, the myotomy is carried more laterally to include them as well. (*A*) Anterior neck after platysmaplasty but before anterolateral platysmal myotomy. (*B*) After anterolateral myotomy. (Note: Myotomy is most easily and effectively performed after platysmaplasty has been completed; note that, because uninterrupted muscle is present laterally, the potential for new band formation in that area is possible).

conceptually flawed and practically problematic. Experience has shown that these maneuvers do not work and are the source of many patient problems.

Recognizing the origin of neck problems in the submental region

Traditional neck lift techniques do not adequately address many aspects of aging in the submental

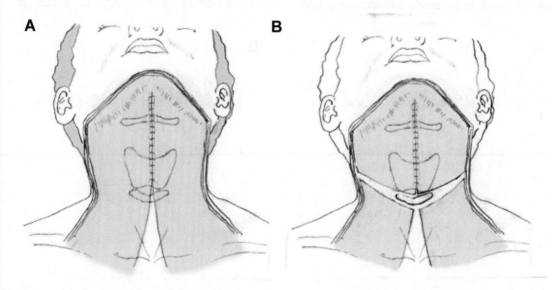

Fig. 9. (*A, B*) Plan for full-width platysmal transection. Full-width myotomy corrects not only anterior and lateral bands, but also provides improved definition over the lateral mandibular border. Note that muscle transection is performed at the level of the cricoid cartilage extending slightly superiorly to the midlateral muscle border as it extends laterally. (*A*) Anterior neck after platysmaplasty but before full-width platysmal myotomy. (*B*) After full-width platysmal myotomy (note: myotomy is most easily and effectively performed after platysmaplasty has been completed).

region and it is not enough in most situations to limit treatment of the neck to preplatysmal lipectomy and platysmaplasty alone. For many patients, subplatysmal fat accumulation, submandibular salivary gland "ptosis" (enlargement), and digastric muscle hypertrophy contribute significantly to the neck deformity present and necessitate specific additional treatments (**Fig. 10** and see Timothy Marten and Dino Elyassnia's, "Neck Lift: Defining Anatomic Problems and Choosing Appropriate Treatment Strategies," in this issue). It must be acknowledged and accepted that simply tightening the platysma and creating a tight platysma corset over these problems will not correct them and will not produce a sustained improvement in neck contour if underlying deep layer problems are not addressed.

Recognizing the presence of subplatysmal fat
In all but the unusual or young patient, the majority of cervical fat accumulation in the full obtuse neck will be present in a subplatysmal location and little if any will need to be removed from the preplatysmal layer. Indeed, as patients age, fat stores generally shift from a preplatysmal location to a subplatysmal one, and the small amount of subcutaneous fat present in the typical patient presenting for a neck lift is necessary and must be preserved if a soft, youthful, and attractive appearance is to be obtained.

Once one recognizes this fact, the futility and undesirability of corset tightening of the platysma as a means of treating excess subplatysmal fat becomes evident. Attempts at tightening the platysma when

subplatysmal fat is present usually results in modest improvement that is short lived. The same is true with the various suture suspension methods that have been proposed and now largely abandoned. If excess subplatysmal fat is present it must be excised if optimal improvement is to be obtained (see Timothy Marten and Dino Elyassnia's, "Neck Lift: Defining Anatomic Problems and Choosing Appropriate Treatment Strategies," in this issue).

Recognizing the presence of the prominent submandibular gland
A preoperative assessment must be made of the submandibular glands in neck lift patients because they often contribute to the appearance of a full, obtuse, lumpy, unattractive neck (**Fig. 11**). Large glands are frequently hidden by submental fat or a lax platysma muscle in the patient with a full neck presenting for a primary procedure, however, and a plan that does not recognize this fact will lead to disappointing and unexpected bulges in the lateral submental regions postoperatively.

Despite claims to the contrary, experience has shown that prominent submandibular glands are actually large, not ptotic, and that the platysma contributes little to their position or support. Attempts at tightening the platysma when a prominent gland is present usually results in modest improvement that is short lived. The same is true with the various suture suspension methods that have been proposed and now largely abandoned. Large, prominent glands will require that the protruding portion be resected if optimal improvement is to be obtained (see Timothy Marten and

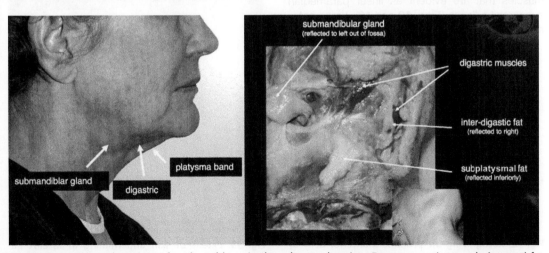

Fig. 10. Recognizing the origin of neck problems in the submental region. For many patients, subplatysmal fat accumulation, submandibular salivary gland ptosis (enlargement), and digastric muscle hypertrophy will contribute significantly to the neck deformity present and necessitate specific treatment. Simply tightening the platysma over these problems will not correct them. Specific additional treatment is necessary if these problems are to be improved. (Note that the presence of submandibular gland and digastric muscle problems can be diagnosed simply by looking at this patient).

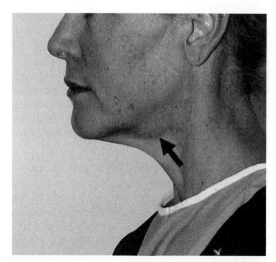

Fig. 11. Recognizing the prominent submandibular gland. For many patients, submandibular salivary gland ptosis (enlargement; *arrow*) contributes significantly to the neck deformity present and necessitates specific treatment. Simply tightening the platysma over this problem will not correct it. Specific additional treatment (resection of the protruding portion) is necessary if this problem is to be improved.

Dino Elyassnia's, "Neck Lift: Defining Anatomic Problems and Choosing Appropriate Treatment Strategies," in this issue).

RECOGNIZING THE PRESENCE OF PROMINENT ANTERIOR BELLY OF THE DIGASTRIC MUSCLE

A significant subgroup of patients will present with large, bulky anterior bellies of their digastric muscles that are evident as linear paramedian submental fullness (**Figs. 10** and **12**). Large anterior bellies of the digastric muscles are most easily

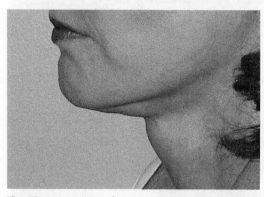

Fig. 12. Recognizing the prominent anterior belly of the digastric muscle. For many patients, a prominent digastric muscle contributes significantly to the neck deformity present and necessitates specific treatment. Simply tightening the platysma over this problem will not correct it. Specific additional treatment is necessary if this problem is to be improved.

seen in the secondary facelift patient who has undergone prior aggressive cervicosubmental lipectomy. Large muscles are frequently hidden by excess submental fat or lax platysma muscle in the patient presenting for primary procedures, however, and failure to identify them may lead to unexpected and objectionable submental bulges postoperatively. When large, prominent digastric muscles are identified subtotal superficial digastric myectomy is indicated (excising the protruding part of the muscle).

Experience has shown and common sense dictates that platysmaplasty is ineffective in treating prominent digastric muscles. Attempts at tightening the platysma when a prominent digastric muscle is present usually results in modest improvement that is short lived. Prominent digastric muscles will require that the protruding portion be resected if optimal improvement is to be obtained (see Timothy Marten and Dino Elyassnia's, "Neck Lift: Defining Anatomic Problems and Choosing Appropriate Treatment Strategies," in this issue).

Surgical Technique

Skin flap elevation

Proper treatment of the platysma by the means discussed here will typically require a complete undermining of the neck skin from mentum to cricoid (**Fig. 13**).

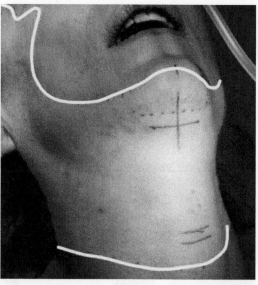

Fig. 13. Extent of skin undermining in facelift patients. Proper treatment of the platysma will typically require a complete undermining of the neck skin from mentum to cricoid. The *dotted line* marks submental crease. Th *solid single line* marks site for submental skin incision. The *double solid line* marks location of cricoid cartilage.

Anterior platysmaplasty

Anterior platysmaplasty (see **Fig. 4**) is performed in the majority of patients and provides an improved result in most necks. The purpose of platysmaplasty is to consolidate the neck, reduce irregularities owing to horizontal platysmal laxity, and enhance neck appearance when it is flexed and the patient is looking down. Contrary to prevailing opinion, it cannot create a sustained improvement in neck contour in and of itself if deep layer problems (subplatysmal fat excess, or submandibular gland and digastric muscle hypertrophy) are present and not appropriately treated, and it is not adequate treatment for longitudinal platysmal hyperfunction and dynamic platysma bands in most patients.

Platysmaplasty is performed by suturing the medial muscle borders of the platysma muscles together from the mentum to the thyroid cartilage (**Fig. 14**). If redundant muscle is present medially, it is gauged and excised before suturing is performed so that a smooth, edge-to-edge approximation of the medial muscle borders can be made without inversion, invagination, or imbrication (**Fig. 15**). Experience has shown that this produces a better and more consistent outcome and decreases the likelihood that objectionable midline fullness or bands will result after healing and relaxation of tissues has occurred than when excess muscle is invaginated and a multilayer plication or corset is performed.

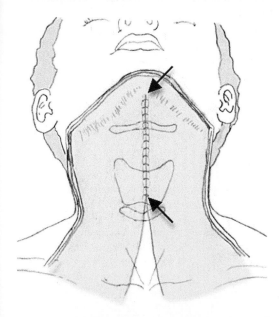

Fig. 14. Anterior platysmaplasty. Repair of platysmal diastasis from mentum to thyroid cartilage (*arrows*) improves submental support and helps consolidate the neck. It is not an adequate or effective treatment of platysmal bands, however.

Typically, platysmaplasty is performed by suturing the medial muscle borders together with interrupted sutures beginning at the mentum and proceeding inferiorly to the hyoid and then down to the level of the midthyroid cartilage. Alternatively, approximation can be started at the hyoid and then extended superiorly to the mentum and then from hyoid to midthyroid level. The approach is not as important as is creating a smooth, well-tailored approximation and reconstitution of the platysmal layer.

When performing a face and neck lift together platysmaplasty should be performed after cheek superficial musculoaponeurotic system (SMAS) flap dissection and suspension to prevent an accentuation of the effects of aging and gravity and compromised improvement on the face (**Fig. 16**). Although raising and suspending cheek SMAS flaps first makes working through the submental incision and platysmaplasty suture placement more difficult, it allows optimal repositioning of the cheek and jowl, and provides for the best overall improvement. If platysmaplasty is performed first, the cheeks and jowls will be pulled inferiorly toward and into the neck and the effectiveness of the SMAS flap will be significantly diminished (**Fig. 17**).

Platysmaplasty is usually performed using multiple simple interrupted sutures of 3-0 polyglycolic acid suture (Vicryl, or suture of choice) on a medium to large tapered needle. Long instruments are needed and patience is required. The platysmaplasty repair should be snug but should not tight. A tight corset and permanent sutures are not necessary and a tight corset will not result in a sustained improvement in cervical contour if deep layer problems are not addressed.

Optimal improvement generally cannot be obtained if repair is performed using a running suture because some gathering and a purse string effect can occur. This maneuver will result in shortening along the line of repair and can cause bowstringing and postoperative midline band formation. If the approximation is made using interrupted sutures, this problem is averted and the platysma is distributed over and into the concave surface created by deep layer neck maneuvers (removal of subplatysmal fat, submandibular gland reduction, and partial digastric myectomy). If partial suturing to the hyoid only is performed in the submental area irregularities may result at the cervicomental angle.

Once the initial approximation has been made with interrupted sutures, the line of repair can be oversewn and reinforced if desired with a simple running or running inverting suture without a purse string and shortening effect. The repair need only be snug and should not be tight. If a permanent suture is used, care should be taken to saturate each

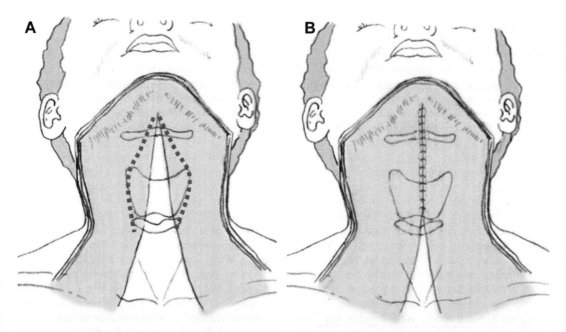

Fig. 15. Anterior platysmaplasty. If redundant muscle is present medially (*A, dashed red line*), it is gauged and excised before suturing is performed so that a smooth, edge-to-edge approximation of the medial muscle borders can be made (*B*). This process produces a better outcome and reduces the likelihood that objectionable midline fullness or bands will result after healing has occurred than when excess muscle is invaginated and a multilayer plication or corset is performed.

suture with antibiotic solution before placement and to bury all knots.

Platysmaplasty should be performed with the neck in a neutral position. If the closure is made with the neck extended, excessive tightness may

result when the patient looks down after surgery. This is particularly the case if platysmaplasty is performed in conjunction with a postauricular transposition flap of the cheek SMAS (see description that follows).

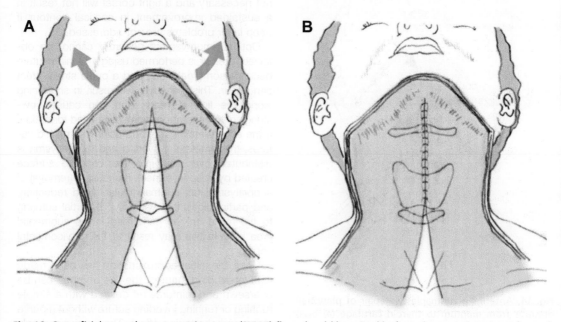

Fig. 16. Superficial musculoaponeurotic system (SMAS) flaps should be raised before platysmaplasty is performed (*green arrows in A*). If the neck lift is done with a facelift the cheek SMAS should be suspended before platysmaplasty is performed.

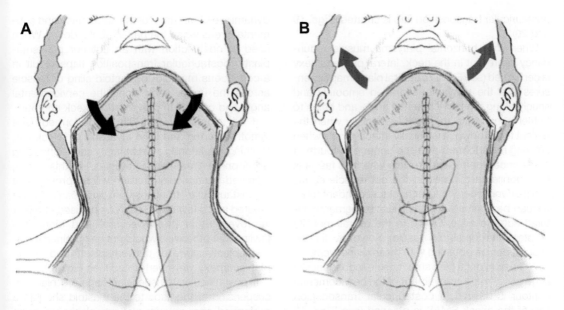

Fig. 17. Superficial musculoaponeurotic system (SMAS) flaps should be raised before platysmaplasty is performed. If platysmaplasty is performed before cheek SMAS suspension (*A, black arrows*), elevation of the cheek SMAS flaps, and improvement in the face will be compromised (*B, red arrows*).

Management of the lateral platysmal border

If a short scar neck lift is performed (submental incision only; see the Timothy Marten and Dino Elyassnia article "Short Scar Neck Lift: Neck Lift Using a Submental Incision Only", in this issue) there is no access to, or option for, lateral platysma suspension. If a neck lift is performed in conjunction with a facelift or if an extended neck lift is being performed (see Timothy Marten and Dino Elyassnia's, "Neck Lift: Defining Anatomic Problems and Choosing Appropriate Treatment Strategies," in this issue), lateral platysmapexy (**Fig. 18**) can be performed or, more typically, a

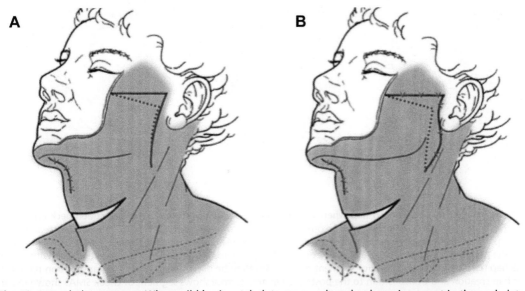

Fig. 18. Lateral platysmapexy. When mild horizontal platysma muscle redundancy is present in the neck, lateral platysmapexy may suffice. (*A*) Before lateral platysmapexy. (*B*) After lateral platysmapexy. The inferior border of the posterior margin of the superficial musculoaponeurotic system flap is advanced laterally and posteriorly and sutured to the upper sternocleidomastoid fascia in a manner that tightens the platysma under the mandibular border and along the cervicomental angle. A lateral platysmapexy should be performed after an anterior platysmaplasty (see **Fig. 14**).

postauricular transposition flap is created (**Figs. 19** and **20**).

When mild horizontal platysma muscle redundancy is present in the neck, lateral platysmapexy is performed (see **Fig. 17**). Lateral platysmapexy ensures that the platysma is draped smoothly and snugly along the cervicomental angle and helps to further consolidate the neck, especially when the patient looks down. It is usually effective only when suturing is performed over the upper one-fourth of the sternocleidomastoid muscle where its fascia is less mobile. In thin necks, the cut muscle edges can be overlapped. In fuller necks, redundant muscle can be trimmed and the muscle segments sutured edge to edge. Owing to the overall mobility of sternocleidomastoid fascia, however, limited support can be obtained with these maneuvers.

When horizontal platysma muscle redundancy is large or optimal improvement of the cervicomental contour is desired, a postauricular transposition flap of the cheek SMAS is planned (see **Figs. 18** and **19**; **Fig. 20**). The postauricular transposition flap is created by splitting off redundant tissue from the posterior margin of the cheek SMAS flap, but leaving it attached inferiorly to the cervicosubmental platysma. If properly constructed and secured, this flap will provide for optimal reduction in horizontal platysma laxity and

dynamic reinforcement of the upper neck and submental areas when the patient looks down. When used in conjunction with an anterior platysmaplasty, postauricular transposition flaps result in a continuous mastoid-to-mastoid sling of muscle across the upper neck along the cervicomental angle and optimal improvement in neck contour.

If an extended neck lift is performed (see Timothy Marten and Dino Elyassnia's, "Neck Lift: Defining Anatomic Problems and Choosing Appropriate Treatment Strategies," in this issue), a limited periauricular incision will be present but a postauricular transposition flap can still be created and a low SMAS flap can be used to effect improvement in the lower face and along the jawline that otherwise would not be obtained if platysmaplasty alone or platysmaplasty and lateral platysmapexy were performed (see **Fig. 18**).

If postauricular transposition flaps are planned, suspension of the flaps to the mastoid should be performed after anterior platysmaplasty has been performed. If the transposition flaps are suspended first, the platysma muscles can be shifted laterally and it may be difficult to join them in the midline (**Fig. 21**). Suspension to the mastoid is performed with interrupted sutures of 4-0 polyglactin (Vicryl, or other suture of choice). The more proximal portions of the flap are secured to the underlying

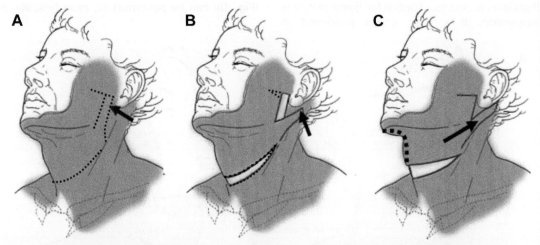

Fig. 19. Postauricular transposition flap when an extended neck lift is performed. If an extended neck lift is performed a limited periauricular incision will be present but a postauricular transposition flap can still be created and a low superficial musculoaponeurotic system (SMAS) flap can be used to effect improvement in the lower face and along the jawline that otherwise would not be obtained. (*A*) Plan for a postauricular transposition flap with a low SMAS flap (*arrow* designates posterior segment of facial SMAS to be used as post-auricular transposition flap). (*B*) After flap creation and transposition to the postauricular area (*arrow* shows segment of cheek SMAS shown in (*A*) after transposition behind the ear to mastoid area). (*C*) After elevation and suturing of low SMAS flap and suturing of postauricular transposition flap to the mastoid fascia. In combination with anterior platysmaplasty (*dashed line*), a mastoid-to-mastoid sling of autologous tissue that defines the cervicomental angle is created (*arrow* shows how traction on the post-auricular transposition flap and suturing to the mastiod fascia deepens the cervicomental angle). The low SMAS flap provides improvement in the lower face and along the jawline that would not be otherwise obtained if platysmaplasty alone, or platysmaplasty and lateral platysmapexy were performed.

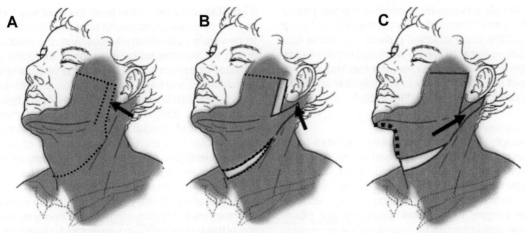

Fig. 20. Postauricular transposition flap when a facelift lift is performed. If a facelift is performed, a postauricular transposition flap can be created from the posterior margin of a high superficial musculoaponeurotic system (SMAS) flap and the high SMAS flap can be used to effect improvement in the cheek and midface region. (*A*) Plan for postauricular transposition flap with high SMAS flap (superior margin of SMAS flap planed at level of zygomatic arch) (*arrow* designates posterior segment of facial SMAS to be used as post-auricular transposition flap). (*B*) After flap creation and transposition to the postauricular area (*arrow* shows segment of cheek SMAS shown in (*A*) after transposition behind the ear to mastiod area). (*C*) After elevation and suturing of a high SMAS flap and suturing of a postauricular transposition flap to the mastoid fascia (typically some shortening of the flap is performed). In combination with anterior platysmaplasty (*dashed line*) a mastoid-to-mastoid sling of autologous tissue that defines the cervicomental angle is created (*arrow* shows how traction on the post-auricular transposition flap and suturing to the mastiod fascia deepens the cervicomental angle). The high SMAS flap provides improvement in the upper face and midface that would not be otherwise obtained if platysmaplasty alone, or platysmaplasty and lateral platysmapexy, or platysmaplasty and low SMAS lift was performed.

fascia with a simple running suture of the same material. This technique consolidates the deep layer repair in the perilobular area and prevents the flap from bunching up or rolling up on itself.

For the postauricular transposition flap to be effective, it must be properly designed and constructed and its intended purpose kept in mind. A common error is for the surgeon to construct it

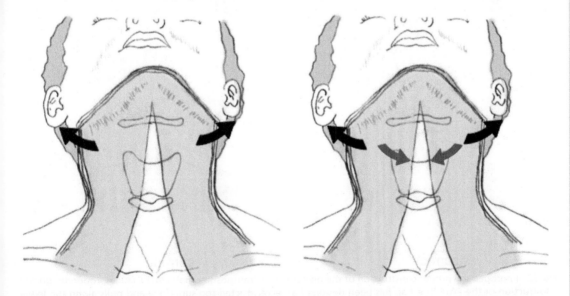

Fig. 21. Anterior platysmaplasty should be performed before lateral platysma suspension. If suspension of the lateral platysmal borders (lateral platysmapexy or postauricular transposition flap) is performed before anterior platysmaplasty (*black arrows*), the platysma muscles may be displaced laterally and approximation of the medial platysma borders (platysmaplasty) may not be possible (*red arrows*).

too timidly and superiorly and in a manner that its pull is placed over and along the mandibular border (**Fig. 22**A). Such a design pulls on the lateral face and does not improve the neck and cervicomental angle. Properly constructed, the flap should exert its pull below and inferior to the mandible and along the cervicomental angle (**Fig. 22**B).

Transverse platysma myotomy

Although anterior platysmaplasty will often result in an attractive neck at rest and on the operating table, objectionable-appearing, hard, dynamic platysma bands and muscle striations are often still evident in conversation and during animation after surgery if additional steps are not taken. These problems can be minimized by performing a transverse platysma myotomy (see **Figs. 7–9**). The extent of platysma transection depends on the type and extend of bands present and thus varies from patient to patient.

Platysma myotomy should be performed after anterior platysmaplasty and lateral platysmal suspension (lateral platysmapexy or postauricular transposition flap) has been completed, because the platysma muscle will be uniformly distributed over the anterior neck and under slight tension. Myotomy should be performed low in the neck at the level of the cricoid cartilage and extended slightly superiorly as it is extended laterally

(**Figs. 23**A and **24**A). At this level, the muscle is thin and will bleed less, and the cut edges are less likely to be visible postoperatively; however, the muscle action will nonetheless be interrupted. In addition, a smooth transition across the cervicomental angle is maintained and lower lip dysfunction is avoided. If the transection is too high, these benefits are typically lost (**Fig. 23**B). This is particularly true when myotomy is performed at the level of the hyoid along the cervicomental angle or when wedges of platysma muscle are removed at that location, as is shown in many plastic surgery textbooks. The platysma muscle is much thicker at that level and the cut edges are more likely to bleed and/or be visible after surgery. In addition, a high transection or resection of this sort can result in a severe and unaesthetic transition from the submental region to the neck, and adversely affect platysma action and result in asymmetrical movement of the lower lip during speaking and expression. Transecting the platysma high along the cervicomental angle laterally also puts both the cervical and marginal mandibular branches of the facial nerve at risk.

Anterior platysma myotomy is best begun working through the submental incision just inferior to the inferior most suture placed when platysmaplasty was performed (see **Fig. 24**A). The medial platysma border is identified over the cricothyroid area and grasped and lifted away from the deep

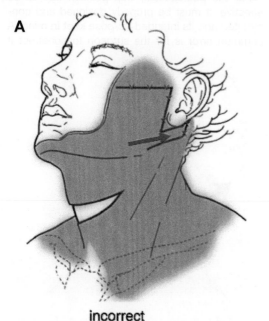

A

incorrect

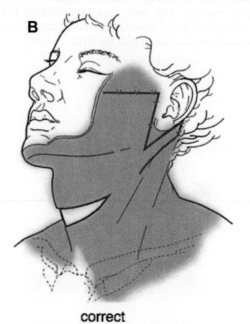

B

correct

Fig. 22. Improper and proper construction of the postauricular transposition flap (PATF). (*A*) Improper design and construction of the PATF. The flap has been designed and constructed too superiorly and pulls along the lower face and lateral mandibular border (*red arrow*). Such a construction does little to improve the neck. (*B*) Correct design and construction of the PATF. The flap has been designed and constructed more inferiorly so that its resultant pull is below the mandible and along the cervicomental angle (*green arrow*). Such a design optimizes the cervicosubmental contour.

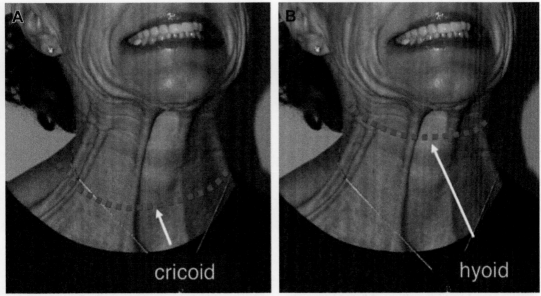

Fig. 23. Correct and incorrect level for platysma myotomy. (*A*) Correct level (level of cricoid cartilage) for platysma myotomy. Myotomy should be performed low in the neck at the level of the cricoid cartilage and extended slightly superiorly as it is extended laterally. At this level, the muscle is thin and will bleed less, and the cut edges are less likely to be visible postoperatively. In addition, a smooth transition across the cervicomental angle is maintained and lower lip dysfunction is avoided. (*B*) Incorrect level (level of hyoid cartilage) for platysma myotomy. The platysma muscle is much thicker and the cut edges are more likely to bleed and be visible after surgery. In addition, a high transection or resection can result in an unaesthetic transition from the submental region to the neck, and result in asymmetrical movement of the lower lip.

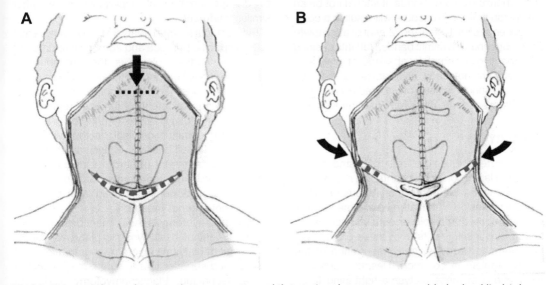

Fig. 24. Sequence for performing platysma myotomy. (*A*) Anterior platysma myotomy (*dashed red line*) is begun working through the submental incision (*black arrow*) just inferior to the inferior most suture placed when platysmaplasty was performed. The medial platysma border is identified over the cricothyroid area and grasped and lifted away from the deep cervical fascia. Myotomy is then made by nibbling through the muscle in small increments with a Metzenbaum scissors or using electrocautery. (*B*) If a full-width division of the platysma is planned, the lateral most portion of the transection is completed through the postauricular incisions (*black arrows*) by identifying the midlateral muscle border, incising it, and incrementally extending the incision until it is brought into continuity with the incision made in the muscle anteriorly through the submental incision (*red dashed lines*).

cervical fascia with a long DeBakey type forceps. Myotomy is then made by nibbling through the muscle in small increments with a Metzenbaum scissors (or alternatively using electrocautery). As the muscle is divided it usually separates a centimeter or more, exposing the fascia beneath it.

Serrated and super-sharp scissors should not be used because they tend to pick up and cut adjacent tissue and this can result in injury to the anterior jugular vein. Unintended injury to the anterior jugular vein results in annoying bleeding that can be difficult to control. Gentle spreading with scissors tips before each cut is made helps to separate the platysma from underlying cervical fascia and facilitates dissection.

Myotomy is continued laterally and slightly superiorly according to the preoperative plan. If a full-width division of the platysma is planned, the lateral most portion of the transection (lateral one-half of the muscle) is completed through the postauricular incisions by identifying the midlateral muscle border, incising it, and incrementally extending the incision until it is brought into continuity with the incision made in the muscle anteriorly through the submental incision using the method previously described (**Fig. 24**B).

Patients should be counseled that the goal of platysma myotomy is a decrease in platysma hyperfunction and a decrease in the prominence of hard, dynamic platysma bands. It should not be an expectation that the procedure will result in a complete absence of platysmal movement or a complete elimination of hard dynamic bands. Patients desiring and expecting a complete absence of platysmal movement are not good candidates for the procedure and should instead be steered toward neuromodulators or some other form of treatment.

SUMMARY

Traditional techniques to treat platysma bands have relied largely on corset tightening of the anterior platysma muscle borders or various methods of rigid suspension of the lateral platysma borders to the sternocleidomastoid or periauricular fascia. Although the initial results from these procedures often seem to be good, early recurrence of the original problem is common. Despite numerous modifications of these platysma-tightening techniques they have largely failed, and for many surgeons treating platysma bands remains one of the most frustrating and perplexing problems in neck surgery.

As surgeons have pursued improved outcomes in treating the neck and platysma, our understanding of the origin of platysma muscle irregularities has improved and platysma muscle treatment techniques have evolved. Experience has shown that the traditional notion that platysma tightening will correct deep layer neck problems, including accumulations of subplatysmal fat, large submandibular glands, and protruding digastric muscles was misguided, and that proper treatment of these problems will require specific, targeted procedures. Gradually, surgeons have come to understand and accept that improved neck contour is not created by platysma tightening, but by deep layer maneuvers (subplatysmal fat excision, submandibular gland reduction, and partial digastric myectomy) that target these problems specifically.

Experience has also confirmed that platysma tightening will not universally correct platysma bands and that our traditional view that all platysma bands were a homogenous problem and simply a product of age associated horizontal platysmal laxity was conceptually flawed and the underlying cause of decades of failed treatment. In reality, platysma bands comprise a heterogeneous group of distinct problems and for many patients they can be seen to be the product of not only horizontal laxity, but also longitudinal platysmal hyperfunction and, as such, refractory to horizontal tightening. Proper treatment of these problems requires horizontal platysma transection to disrupt longitudinal hyperfunction or other similar treatment.

Platysmaplasty and platysma myotomy each have a specific purpose and address two different problems. Platysmaplasty is the procedure in which the medial borders of the platysma muscles are sutured together. The purpose of platysmaplasty is to consolidate the submental region, correct horizontal platysma laxity and soft platysma bands, and enhance cervical contour when the neck is in a flexed position. Platysmaplasty is not an effective treatment of hard dynamic platysma bands and will not produce a sustained improvement in the neck contour if deep layer problems are present and not treated.

Platysma myotomy is the primary procedure for the treatment of hard dynamic platysma bands. The result of platysma myotomy is dramatic, long-lasting, and superior to any suture suspension or corset technique. Platysmamyotomy also optimizes the overall neck contour and accentuation of the cervicomental line. Many patients benefit from both platysmaplasty and platysma myotomy; the key to successful treatment rests in understanding the origins of platysma problems, identifying the type of problem present in a given patient, and using logical solutions to address those problems.

Noninvasive Methods for Lower Facial Rejuvenation

David A. Sieber, MD[a],[*], Jeffrey M. Kenkel, MD[b]

KEYWORDS

- Noninvasive • Nonsurgical • Face • Neck • Rejuvenation • Skin tightening

KEY POINTS

- Proper patient selection and realistic expectations are key for optimal nonsurgical results.
- Thermal energy is responsible for skin tightening.
- Patients should be treated at the lowest energy able to produce a response.
- All nonsurgical devices carry risk for significant complications.

INTRODUCTION

Nonsurgical aesthetic medicine continues to be a growing field, with an increase of 22% in the number of nonsurgical procedures performed in 2015.[1] Demand for noninvasive options is increasing because of the popularity of nonsurgical procedures and industry's focus on direct to consumer marketing. The nature of these types of procedures allows for patients to continue to cycle through a practice and may ultimately lead to surgical conversion for some in the future. Such techniques as nonablative and ablative lasers, intense pulsed light (IPL), radiofrequency (RF), high-intensity focused ultrasound (US), and skin care with peeling agents may also be used in conjunction with surgery to optimize the patient's overall aesthetic results.

Each of these technologies relies on a similar principle of thermal disruption of collagen fibers. Collagen is a polymer held together by hydrogen bonds, and it is these cross-links that attribute to the collagen strength. Thermal energy causes a denaturing of the collagen, and the heat-stable intramolecular cross-links are preserved.[2] Skin tightening occurs because of a physical shortening of the collagen fibers with preservation of intramolecular hydrogen bonds, possibly increasing the elastic properties of the skin.[3,4] With increased delivery of thermal energy (ie, increased tissue temperature) there is a greater degree of collagen denaturation and thus resultant tissue tightening. Thermal injury also induces local fibroblasts to produce new collagen as a part of the wound-healing response. Balancing appropriate thermal injury without causing tissue necrosis remains the greatest challenge as the demand for improved efficacy and reproducible treatments rises.

Changes within the collagen occur in a time- and temperature-dependent manner, meaning short exposures to high temperatures or prolonged exposure to lower temperatures create a degree of collagen shortening. Bozec and Odlyha[5] demonstrated that denaturing of collagen fibrils occurs at approximately 65°C, with initial collagen injury occurring around 58°C. Additional studies agree that disruption and denaturing of collagen occurs in the 60°C to 65°C range with a greater degree of denaturation occurring at higher temperatures.[2,3,6,7] It is this initial collagen insult along with the resulting neocollagenesis that triggers the healing response responsible for the observed thermal tightening. However, the burn literature suggests that extensive cell membrane breakdown begins to occur at temperatures greater than 45°C.[8]

Disclosure Statement: The authors have nothing to disclose.
[a] Private Practice, Sieber Plastic Surgery, 450 Sutter Street, #2630, San Francisco, CA 94108, USA; [b] Department of Plastic Surgery, Clinical Center for Cosmetic Laser Treatment, 1801 Inwood Road, Dallas, TX 75390-9132, USA
* Corresponding author.
E-mail address: Davidsiebermd@gmail.com

Clin Plastic Surg 45 (2018) 571–584
https://doi.org/10.1016/j.cps.2018.06.003

As with any device, the user must understand the parameters of the device not only to optimize outcomes, but also to reduce possible treatment-related complications. Understanding and manipulation of five key parameters allows the user to master the laser device at hand instead of being at the mercy of preset manufacturer protocols. These five parameters for laser devices are[9]

1. Wavelength: determined by the target chromophore and its location within the tissue
2. Power: the amount of energy delivered to the tissue target
3. Spot size: used in correlation with the power to determine the power density
4. Pulse width: the delivery or exposure time of selected energy delivered to the tissue target
5. Cooling: allows for maximal depth of injury without harming more superficial tissue

Only through a complete understanding of the interplay of these five parameters is the user able to adequately treat the target tissue with lasers without unnecessarily damaging collateral tissue in the process. With each subsequent treatment the patient's tissue is uniquely changed and thus presents differently for each subsequent treatment. This leads to a need for slight modifications to the treatment parameters with each procedure.

LASER AND LIGHT THERAPY

Noninvasive laser devices may be divided into two categories: nonablative and ablative. Both share a similar goal of skin surface changes. When evaluating patients for laser or light therapy, the correct device needs to be chosen to address the specific skin disorder being treated, the target chromophore, and have acceptable downtime (**Table 1**). The most commonly used nonablative, ablative, and light-based devices in our practice are the fractionated 10,600-nm CO_2 laser, 2940-nm erbium:yttrium-aluminum-garnet (Er:YAG) laser, full-field Er:YAG, 1064-nm neodymium-doped:yttrium-aluminum-garnet laser, 532-nm potassium titanyl phosphate (KTP) laser, and an IPL device.

When using laser and light therapy, there are three main target chromophores within tissue: (1) hemoglobin, (2) melanin, and (3) water. Hemoglobin has three peaks at 400 nm, 532 nm, and 577 to 600, with 577 nm being the most selective for this chromophore. Melanin is found in a wider spectrum between 400 and 1100 nm of light, with the ranges of 400 to 475 nm and 630 to 810 nm being the most selective. Ablative lasers rely on water molecules stored within the tissue target (**Figs. 1** and **2**).

In our hands for skin resurfacing, the full ablative 2940-nm Er:YAG laser has the most dramatic effect on skin resurfacing at the cost of increased down time. The Er:YAG laser has largely replaced the previous generation of CO_2 lasers credited to the Er:YAG's precise depth of ablation without the undesirable collateral tissue heating commonly seen with traditional CO_2 devices. Total ablative Er:YAG resurfacing has a much more significant recovery than any of the nonablative lasers. However, the Er:YAG is able to provide predictable results with visible end points. This is in part because of the Er:YAG's high absorption by water, which is 13 times greater than that of the CO_2 laser. Heating of this water with suprathreshold fluences leads to immediate cellular heating resulting in instant tissue vaporization. A high absorption by water allows for a more precise suprathreshold ablation, with less subthreshold collateral damage to the surrounding tissue. The main downside to the Er:YAG is the prolonged recovery, usually requiring 7 to 10 days for complete re-epithelialization as compared with nonablative modalities. Patients typically have prolonged redness for at least 2 to 3 months post-treatment and it may persist for up to 6 months. This may be shortened by use of IPL vascular treatments to reduce redness after a few weeks postresurfacing.

Fractionated lasers were developed with the hope of achieving an end result similar to the fully ablative CO_2 and Er:YAG lasers while allowing the patient a quicker recovery with less down time. Fractionated devices use extremely high fluences to deliver focused columns of energy into the tissue resulting in microthermal zones of injury. Areas surrounding these thermal zones only reach subablative temperatures, yet still undergo significant protein denaturation, tissue coagulation, and apoptosis.[10] The thermal injury sustained generally extends 200 to 300 μm, although it can go

Table 1
Choice of devices based on what is being treated and associated downtime

| | Downtime | |
	Hours	Weeks
Pigment	IPL	Erbium
Redness	IPL, YAG (1064), KTP (532)	
Wrinkles	Botox, fillers	TCA, Erbium, FCO₂
Acne	Fillers	Excision, Erbium, FCO₂
Laxity	Ultrasound, RF	Surgery

Abbreviations: KTP, potassium titanyl phosphate; YAG, yttrium-aluminum-garnet.

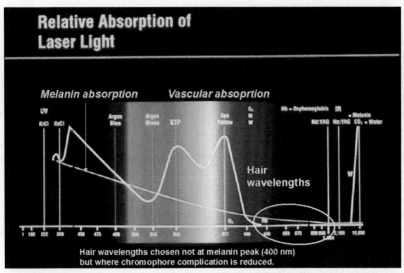

Fig. 1. Location of each device along the laser light spectrum and associated chromophores at each wavelength.

deeper, into the dermis, leading to the aforementioned cascade of heat-induced collagen shortening and neocollagenesis. By delivering a discontinuous, segmental injury to the tissue, reservoirs of healthy tissue remain to speed healing and to act as a source of keratinocyte migration.[11] Theoretically, these microthermal zones should produce sufficient injury so as to create a tissue response similar to the fully ablative CO_2 and Er:YAG lasers, yet this has not been the result experienced in our clinic.[12,13]

Doubling the frequency of a 1064-nm laser by way of a KTP crystal is what makes the higher-energy 532-nm KTP laser possible. Specific advantages of 532 nm over 1064 nm are that treatment energies for 532 nm are one order of magnitude less for the same chromophore (arteries or oxygenated hemoglobin), meaning when treating superficial telangiectasias located in the superficial dermis, less energy is needed to see a response. Whenever treating patients, the goal is

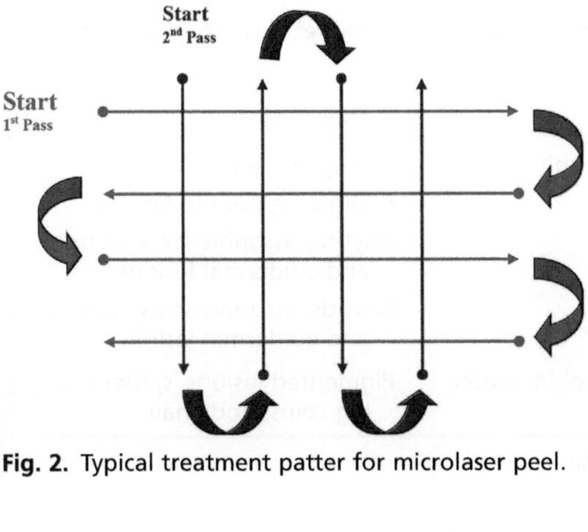

to use the minimum effective dose of energy at which a desired clinical end point is still evident. This prevents delivery of excess energy into target tissue and lessens the risk of subsequent adverse events.[14–16] A downside of the 532-nm laser is that it only has a superficial absorption length and is typically much less effective for vessels larger than 500 μm.[17] Additionally, use of the 532-nm laser in darker skin types must be approached cautiously, because melanin competes with hemoglobin at this wavelength.

The 1064 nm, however, is able to adequately treat deeper tissue and larger vessels, to a depth of 5 to 6 mm and a diameter up to 2 to 3 mm, all of this at the cost, however, of increased fluences because of decrease in absorption coefficient, resulting in more discomfort for the patient.

Although surgery remains the gold standard for facial rejuvenation, surgery alone is only able to address skin laxity and soft tissue deflation. Global facial rejuvenation must also address the skin surface. Years of sun exposure may result in static and dynamic rhytids, poor skin texture, and multiple dyschromias. Although initially there was some hesitancy to perform laser skin resurfacing at the same time as or as an adjunct to surgery, it has since been shown to be safe in select patients using moderate settings.[18–20] Despite its safety, many practitioners still prefer to wait 3 to 6 months after surgery before performing full-face laser skin resurfacing.

Intense Pulsed Light

IPL is our most commonly performed office procedure and has high patient satisfaction. Although commonly referred to as a laser, IPL is a flash lamp device, not a laser. This technology works

Fig. 2. Typical treatment patter for microlaser peel.

by generating a polychromatic light and most commonly has an output spectrum between 400 nm and 1400 nm within the electromagnetic spectrum. What differentiates IPL from a laser is that a laser most often emits a single wavelength, whereas IPL delivers an entire spectrum of light at the same time. IPL works by passing light through specific filters to block unwanted wavelengths, thus tailoring the emitted wavelengths for a desired chromophore. Although perception remains that because this is not a laser it is inherently a safer device, the opposite is true because it now emits up to 1000 different wavelengths and precise treatment of every chromophore is sometimes difficult to control. Simply, this is a device that scans for every chromophore because of the spectrum of light emitted and wavelength-limiting filters are used to regain some control. These filters are commonly "high pass filters," which block wavelengths lower than the number indicated on the filter while allowing longer wavelengths to pass through to tissue. Shorter wavelengths are absorbed in the more superficial targets and this allows targeting the deeper dermis without damaging upper skin structures. Pulsed light therapy may be used for correction of photoaging, treatment of pigment of vascular lesions, erythema, or acne.

Patient Selection for Laser and Light-Based Devices

The 532-nm KTP lasers are best suited for treatment of small veins, pigment, tattoos, and port wine stains, and for nonablative dermal remodeling.[21] Similar to the KTP laser, the 1064-nm neodymium-doped:yttrium-aluminum-garnet is commonly used for nonablative facial resurfacing, hair removal, treatment of acne, leg veins, pigmented lesions, and vascular anomalies.[22-30] Patients needing aggressive skin resurfacing for select pigments, skin texture, or rhytids are best treated

with Er:YAG.[31-35] IPL is the most versatile of the devices because of the broad range of wavelengths it produces. It may be used for treatment of telangiectasias, dyschromias, nonablative skin resurfacing, and hair reduction (**Table 2**).[24,36-39]

An excellent way to enhance facial rejuvenation is through placement of adipose or hyaluronic acid fillers with the addition of concomitant facial resurfacing.[40] Facial fat grafting is able to restore lost facial volume, and laser resurfacing addresses superficial and deep rhytids, improving facial contours and skin texture. We have performed upper lid surgery, facial fat grafting, and simultaneous laser resurfacing with excellent results. Laser resurfacing has also been shown to be safe and effective when performed at the same time as lower lid blepharoplasties.[41]

Technical Steps/Treatment Plan

Many patients undergoing more aggressive in-office procedures may require pretreatment with an anxiolytic agent in addition to an oral narcotic. We commonly use 0.25 to 0.50 mg alprazolam (Xanax) and oral hydrocodone containing such medications as acetaminophen/hydrocodone (Norco or Lortab). Pretreatment continues with application of a topical compound containing benzocaine, lidocaine, and tetracaine to all treatment areas. Although topical anesthesia is seemingly innocuous, care must be taken when treating large areas because of the potential risk for lidocaine toxicity.[42,43] Regional nerve blocks are sometimes required depending on the pain associated with the procedure and the pain threshold of the patient. Nerve blocks are typically placed using 0.25% to 1% lidocaine (Xylocaine) plain mixed with bicarbonate. Intraocular shield is often placed for corneal protection when the periorbita is being treated. Such procedures as aggressive fractionated CO_2 and erbium are

Table 2
Lasers and light-based devices with associated treatment wavelengths, target chromophores, and common uses

Laser	Wavelength (nm)	Chromophore	Common Uses
KTP	532	Melanin, hemoglobin	Telangiectasias
Nd:YAG	1064	Melanin	Benign pigmented lesions
Er:YAG	2940	Water	Rhytids, atrophic scars, dermal and epidermal lesions
CO_2	10,600	Water	Rhytids, atrophic scars, dermal and epidermal lesions
IPL device	400–1400	Melanin, hemoglobin, water	Pigmented lesions, spider veins, leg veins, body hair

Abbreviation: Ng:YAG, neodymium-doped:yttrium-aluminum-garnet.

challenging to manage in the office, so these patients are most comfortable under heavy sedation/anesthesia in a monitored setting.

Results

Patient example 1

The patient is a 54-year-old woman who presented to clinic desiring improvement of her acne scars, correction of excess upper eyelid skin, and overall improvement in the texture of skin. Risks and benefits of various procedures were explained to the patient and she elected to undergo in-office management of the aforementioned issues. She subsequently underwent bilateral upper eyelid blepharoplasty, placement of microionized fat to acne scars, and full-face fractionated erbium laser (Solta Medical, Hayward, CA). Her preoperative and postoperative results are shown in **Fig. 3**.

Patient example 2

This patient is a 56-year-old woman who presented to clinic complaining of a poorly defined jawline, excess skin on her upper eyelids, and poor facial skin texture with fine rhytids. A discussion was had with the patient regarding surgical versus nonsurgical options. She was not a good candidate for nonsurgical options because of the large amount of skin excess and lipodystrophy in her neck. The patient agreed to pursue upper lid blepharoplasty, neck lift, and full-face erbium resurfacing. Postoperatively the patient was treated with serial treatments of IPL. Six months after the initial procedure the patient had a treatment with erbium to her lower lids for increased skin tightening. Postoperative, the patient still thought there was persistent fullness in her right neck, so this was subsequently addressed with two treatments of Ultherapy (Ulthera Inc, Mesa, AZ) to even lipodystrophy of the neck. The patient's preoperative, postoperative after upper blepharoplasty, neck lift, full-face erbium, and after IPL and Ultherapy are presented in **Fig. 4**.

Patient example 3

This 43-year-old man presented to clinic complaining of unsatisfactory scarring from adolescent acne. The patient was counseled regarding his treatment options. He ultimately underwent micronized fat injections to the acne scars and 100-μm erbium laser peel in the same setting. He is seen in **Fig. 5** 4 months after treatment.

Postoperative Care

Light-based and nonablative therapy

Recovery is straightforward for these procedures. Patients may display redness for a few hours after the treatment. In patients with pigmentation, there may be accentuation of the pigmentation and ultimately a fine peel in some cases. Moisturizers and sun block are used appropriately. Multiple treatments are usually performed at 3- to 6-week intervals.

Fractionated CO_2 resurfacing

Patients experience pain and discomfort for 12 to 24 hours until re-epithelialization occurs. A light moisturizer is used three times a day to prevent excessive dryness of the skin. Once peeling occurs, patients may experience redness for 4 to 8 weeks post-treatment depending on how aggressive the treatment was. The patient is then transitioned back to their skin care regimen.

Full ablative erbium:yttrium-aluminum-garnet resurfacing

These patients experience considerable pain until epithelialization occurs somewhere between 2 and 4 days after treatment. Occlusive dressings significantly improve the patient experience and diminish the pain experienced. Dressings are changed at 48 hours so the skin can be assessed. Occlusion is associated with an increased risk for infection so close monitoring is essential. Once the dressing is removed, then a light moisturizer is used and continued through the peeling process, which lasts approximately 7 to 10 days. The patient is then transitioned back to their skin care routine.

Complications and Shortcomings

Complications for the 532-nm and 1064-nm devices include hypopigmentation, hyperpigmentation, and/or blistering, which all occur at or near the dermal/epidermal junction. Although seen infrequently, scaring is the most serious complication, occurring when a full-thickness wound is produced with any device. Postinflammatory hyperpigmentation (PIH) is the most commonly seen complication across all devices. PIH can sometimes be managed with a skin care regimen of tretinoin or retinol-containing products along with hydroquinone. Multiple treatments with a light TCA peel or IPL may also help improve the appearance of PIH. PIH often takes many months to resolve but most commonly does get better (**Fig. 6**). The main complication from CO_2 or Er:YAG is hypopigmentation caused by permanent destruction of melanocytes at the dermal/epidermal junction (**Fig. 7**). Another short-term issue that may arise with the use of ablative lasers is prolonged erythema, which may persist for 6 months post-treatment.

Although seemingly benign, IPL may create serious complications that are usually pigment

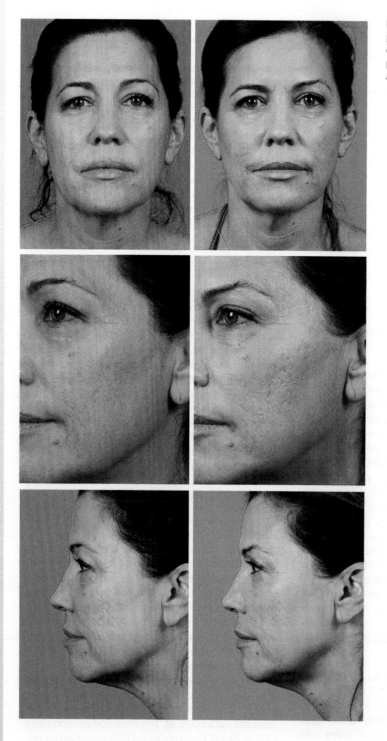

Fig. 3. A 54-year-old woman shown preoperative and 6 months postoperative after upper lid blepharoplasty, fat grafting to acne scars, and full-face fractionated CO_2 laser.

related and occur more commonly in patients with Fitzpatrick IV-IV skin. The most common adverse events include hyperpigmentation, hypopigmentation, and blistering, which can be a manifestation of skin type, target density, and device settings. When treating men, some may experience hair loss in their beard distribution from damage sustained by the hair follicle. Treatment of men later in the day creates more chromophore at the surface and may result in complications so caution should be used.

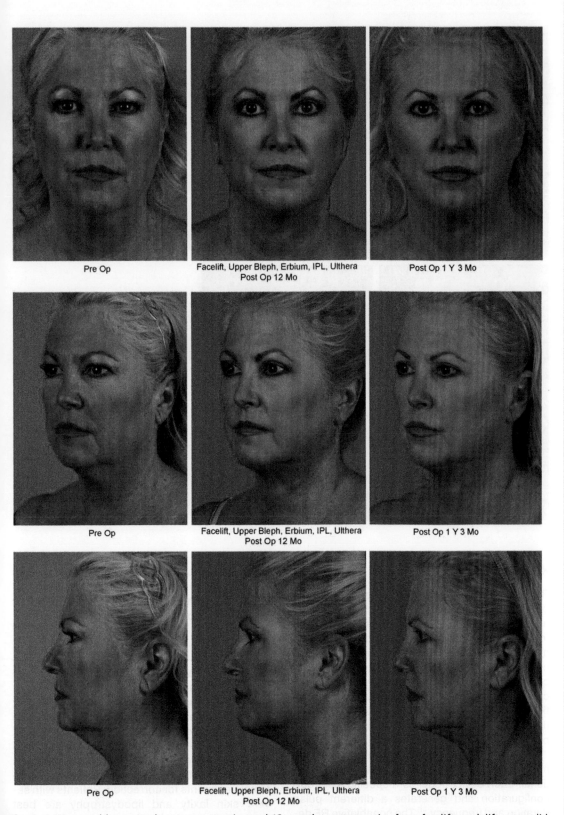

Pre Op | Facelift, Upper Bleph, Erbium, IPL, Ulthera Post Op 12 Mo | Post Op 1 Y 3 Mo

Pre Op | Facelift, Upper Bleph, Erbium, IPL, Ulthera Post Op 12 Mo | Post Op 1 Y 3 Mo

Pre Op | Facelift, Upper Bleph, Erbium, IPL, Ulthera Post Op 12 Mo | Post Op 1 Y 3 Mo

Fig. 4. A 56-year-old woman shown preoperative and 12 months postoperative from facelift, neck lift, upper lid blepharoplasty (*center photograph*), and post-procedure 15 months from full-face erbium, full-face IPL, and Ulthera to neck (*right photograph*).

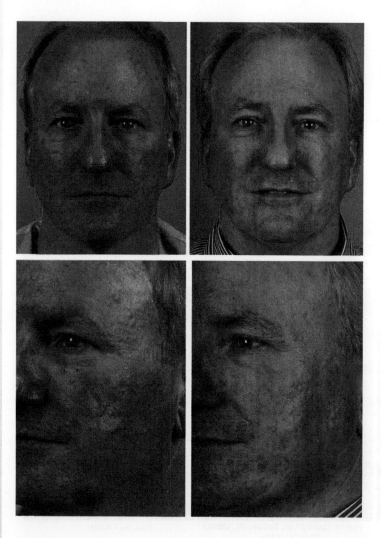

Fig. 5. This 43-year-old man complained of unsatisfactory scarring from adolescent acne. Photographs taken 4 months after micronized fat injections at the acne scars and 100-μm erbium laser peel.

RADIOFREQUENCY

RF devices use alternating electrical currents to polarize tissue within the electrical path using negatively and positively charged electrodes from which the electrical energy conducts. This alternating current causes oscillations in the target tissue ultimately generating heat. It is this heat that causes collagen break down and ultimately neo-collagenesis with subsequent collagen contraction. Because RF current is not scattered in tissue or absorbed by melanin, it is safe to use in patients of all Fitzpatrick skin types.[44]

Four types of RF devices area available: (1) monopolar, (2) bipolar, (3) multipolar, and (4) fractional. Each device requires a specific electrode configuration and generates a different pulse duration and frequency.[45] The nonablative RF devices used in medicine typically have an alternating current between 0.3 and 10 MHz.[46]

Varying the oscillations of energy delivered changes the target tissue depth, with lower frequencies having longer wavelengths and thus greater depth of penetration.

Patient Selection

RF devices are best used in patients with minimal to moderate skin laxity and lipodystrophy. As with any nonsurgical modality, the patient needs to understand that improvement in skin laxity and lipodystrophy especially in the neck may lead to other cosmetic deformities, such as exposure of platysmal bands or uneven correction of adiposity, which may require additional treatments for correction. Patients with severe skin laxity and lipodystrophy are best treated with surgical options.

Contraindications for use of RF include: pregnancy, any implanted electronic device, hip

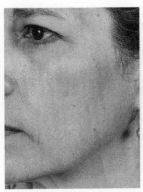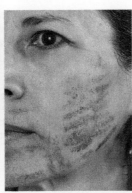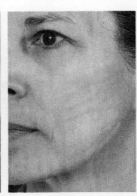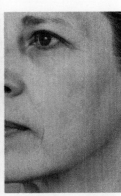

Fig. 6. This 48-year-old woman Fitzpatrick IV underwent her third IPL treatment. At that time, a suntan was not recognized and she subsequently developed localized PIH. This resolved with aggressive treatment after 6 months.

replacement, hip or femur surgery, any other metallic device that could be disrupted by RF energy, any active dermatologic or collagen vascular disorder, active or recent malignancy, any history of disease that may be exacerbated by heat, current use of isotretinoin, and history of blood coagulation disorders.[47]

Complications and Shortcomings

Possible complications related to RF therapy include: erythema, persistent pain, edema, ecchymosis, and burns. As with other nonsurgical devices used, there are about one-third of patients who have a noticeable positive response, another one-third with minimal change, and a final one-third who does not respond to therapy. Localized fat necrosis may occur in some patients. These typically are self-limiting and get better on their own. Temporary neuropraxia of the marginal mandibular nerve is seen and is most commonly transient. There are a few shortcomings of current RF and US devices. Often these devices decrease

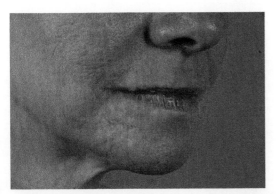

Fig. 7. This 54-year-old woman underwent fractionated CO_2 laser resurfacing 9 months prior. She presented with focal areas of hypopigmentation.

soft tissue excess to a greater extent than overlying skin laxity. This discrepancy can lead to unwanted contour deformities or exposure of underlying platysmal bands along with persistent skin excess.

ULTRASOUND

US technology is an acoustic energy-producing modality that is able to penetrate through tissues to a specific depth while leaving the neighboring tissue relatively unaffected.[48] As the US travels through the tissue it is coalesced into distinct areas called thermal coagulation points. These thermal coagulation points form because of a buildup of heat from friction between rapid vibrations of molecules caused by the ultrasonic waves.[49,50] This thermal insult leads down a similar path of collagen damage, collagen shrinkage, and finally neocollagenesis as part of the healing response. Studies have demonstrated clinical tightening and lifting of facial and neck skin.[51–53]

Patient Selection

Microfocused US therapy has Food and Drug Administration approval for lifting of the eyebrows, neck, and submental region. It is also beneficial in treatment of lines and wrinkles of the décolletage. Two-thirds of patients were satisfied with treatments, as were 60% of blinded reviewers. One shortcoming of this modality is that it has been found to be less efficacious in patients with body mass index greater than or equal to 30 kg/m^2.[54]

A common difficulty with neck rejuvenation is the disappointing longevity of the postoperative neck contours. Even though anterior plastysmaplasty often lasts for many years, the inherent characteristics of skin and soft tissue are not as durable leading to recurrent skin laxity. Microfocused US may be able to further tighten recurrent neck skin laxity without requiring additional operative procedures. For those patients unhappy with persistent or recurrent skin laxity, this modality provides a noninvasive alternative, which is well tolerated by many patients.

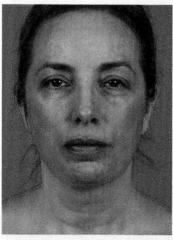 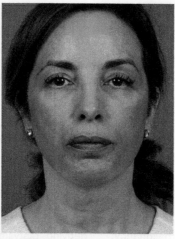

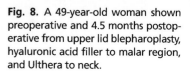

Fig. 8. A 49-year-old woman shown preoperative and 4.5 months postoperative from upper lid blepharoplasty, hyaluronic acid filler to malar region, and Ulthera to neck.

Pre Op   Upper Bleph, Hyaluronic Acid, & Ulthera   4½ Mo Post Op

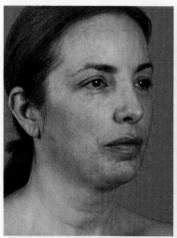 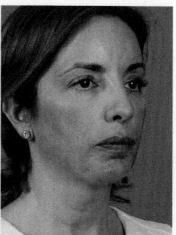

Pre Op   Upper Bleph, Hyaluronic Acid, & Ulthera   4½ Mo Post Op

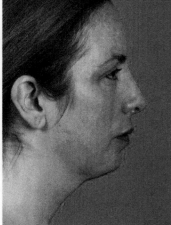 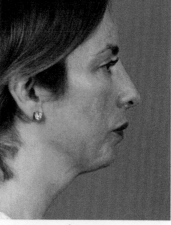

Pre Op   Upper Bleph, Hyaluronic Acid, & Ulthera   4½ Mo Post Op

Results

Patient example 4

This 49-year-old woman with a prior history of chin augmentation presented to the senior author's clinic complaining of excess upper eyelid skin, a prominent tear trough deformity, and she was unhappy with the excess skin and soft tissue along her jawline and neck. After explaining to the patient

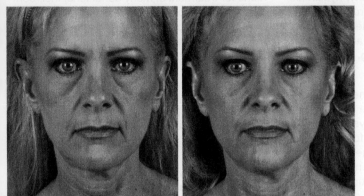

Fig. 9. A 55-year-old woman shown preoperative and 3 months postoperative from Ulthera to neck and hyaluronic acid filler to tear troughs.

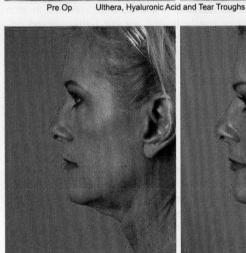 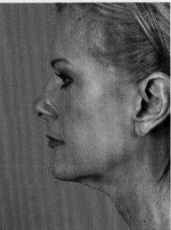

Pre Op   Ulthera, Hyaluronic Acid and Tear Troughs   3 Mo Post Op

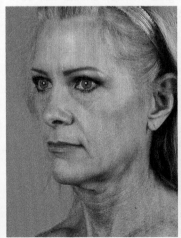 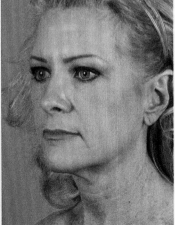

Pre Op   Ulthera, Hyaluronic Acid and Tear Troughs   3 Mo Post Op

the various approaches to address her concerns, she ultimately decided to pursue a treatment plan that could be performed locally in the office and with minimal downtime. She subsequently underwent bilateral upper lid blepharoplasty, hyaluronic acid to her tear troughs, and microfocused US with Ultherapy for treatment of her neck skin laxity and lipodystrophy. Her preoperative and postoperative results are demonstrated in **Fig. 8**.

Patient example 5

This patient is a 55-year-old woman who presented to clinic unhappy with the appearance of her excess neck skin and lipodystrophy. She also believed her tear trough deformities had gotten worse as she had aged. The patient had heard about Ultherapy for improvement of neck contours and came into clinic wanting to pursue this treatment option. She was a good candidate for Ultherapy and underwent treatment to her neck while also having hyaluronic acid placed to improve her tear trough deformities. Preoperative and postoperative results are seen in **Fig. 9**. The patient was ultimately not happy with the subtle improvement in her neck contours and went on to have a neck lift performed by the senior author.

Postoperative Care

Patients resume their normal skin regimen immediately after treatment.

Complications and Shortcomings

Complications related to US therapy include: procedural and post-procedural pain, ecchymosis, edema, dysesthesia, blisters, and erythema at treatment sites.

SKIN CARE

A well-balanced skin care regimen is crucial for optimizing surgical and nonsurgical results. All skin care regimens should include: sunblock, cleanser, tretinoin/exfoliant, antioxidant, and depigmenting agent when necessary. Much of the superficial skin resurfacing within epidermis can often be completed with a good skin care regimen and some patience.

COMBINING SURGICAL AND NONSURGICAL MODALITIES

Although surgery is still considered the gold standard for treatment of facial aging, there are a multitude of reasons patients seek out other nonsurgical options, usually related to cost, downtime, or some aversion to surgery. Surgery alone has its own limitations for what is achievable; this is especially true for central facial rejuvenation and treatment of sun-damaged skin. Although surgical and nonsurgical modalities are effective alone for treatment of many conditions, their combined synergy offers patients a more complete treatment plan to address their concerns.

First and foremost, providers must have a detailed understanding of all of the nonsurgical devices available. They need to understand the strengths and limitations of these devices because careless use may lead to irreversible damage to the patient. A safe approach with any new device is to start conservatively until a greater knowledge of the device is achieved.

Many patients who desire only a subtle change in appearance with minimal to no down time are ideal candidates for combined therapy. As with any therapy, a detailed discussion encompassing the patient's desires and the limitations of the treatments needs to be had in great detail. Those patients desiring a drastic improvement in skin laxity or lipodystrophy are still better served primarily with surgical options. However, these surgical results may still be optimized through use of the aforementioned modalities. There are multiple examples in the literature of combining rhytidectomy with laser or chemical facial resurfacing for complete facial rejuvenation.[18–20]

SUMMARY

Combing surgical and nonsurgical therapy allows the practitioner to optimize patient results. To maximize the benefits of each device, the provider must have a detailed understanding of the science behind them. Combined therapy is safe and is well tolerated by many patients in an office-based setting. Although surgery still remains the gold standard, nonsurgical therapy should still be a portion of all surgeon's practices.

REFERENCES

1. Statistics-American Society of Aesthetic Plastic Surgery. Available at: http://www.surgery.org/media/statistics2016. Accessed July 12, 2018.
2. Arnoczky SP, Aksan A. Thermal modification of connective tissues: basic science considerations and clinical implications. J Am Acad Orthop Surg 2000; 8:305–13.
3. Ross EV, Yashar SS, Naseef GS, et al. A pilot study of in vivo immediate tissue contraction with CO2 skin laser resurfacing in a live farm pig. Dermatol Surg 1999;25:851–6.
4. le Lous M, Flandin F, Herbage D, et al. Influence of collagen denaturation on the chemorheological

properties of skin, assessed by differential scanning calorimetry and hydrothermal isometric tension measurement. Biochim Biophys Acta 1982;717: 295–300.

5. Bozec L, Odlyha M. Thermal denaturation studies of collagen by microthermal analysis and atomic force microscopy. Biophys J 2011;101:228–36.

6. Lin SJ, Hsiao CY, Sun Y, et al. Monitoring the thermally induced structural transitions of collagen by use of second-harmonic generation microscopy. Opt Lett 2005;30:622–4.

7. Hsu TS, Kaminer MS. The use of nonablative radiofrequency technology to tighten the lower face and neck. Semin Cutan Med Surg 2003;22:115–23.

8. Despa F, Orgill DP, Neuwalder J, et al. The relative thermal stability of tissue macromolecules and cellular structure in burn injury. Burns 2005;31:568–77.

9. Farkas JP, Hoopman JE, Kenkel JM. Five parameters you must understand to master control of your laser/light-based devices. Aesthet Surg J 2013;33: 1059–64.

10. Geronemus RG. Fractional photothermolysis: current and future applications. Lasers Surg Med 2006;38:169–76.

11. Manstein D, Herron GS, Sink RK, et al. Fractional photothermolysis: a new concept for cutaneous remodeling using microscopic patterns of thermal injury. Lasers Surg Med 2004;34:426–38.

12. Farkas JP, Richardson JA, Burrus CF, et al. In vivo histopathologic comparison of the acute injury following treatment with five fractional ablative laser devices. Aesthet Surg J 2010;30:457–64.

13. Oni G, Robbins D, Bailey S, et al. An in vivo histopathological comparison of single and double pulsed modes of a fractionated CO(2) laser. Lasers Surg Med 2012;44:4–10.

14. Ozturk S, Hoopman J, Brown SA, et al. A useful algorithm for determining fluence and pulse width for vascular targets using 1,064 nm Nd:YAG laser in an animal model. Lasers Surg Med 2004;34: 420–5.

15. Major A, Brazzini B, Campolmi P, et al. Nd:YAG 1064 nm laser in the treatment of facial and leg telangiectasias. J Eur Acad Dermatol Venereol 2001;15:559–65.

16. Clark C, Cameron H, Moseley H, et al. Treatment of superficial cutaneous vascular lesions: experience with the KTP 532 nm laser. Lasers Med Sci 2004; 19:1–5.

17. Dudelzak J, Hussain M, Goldberg DJ. Vascular-specific laser wavelength for the treatment of facial telangiectasias. J Drugs Dermatol 2009;8:227–9.

18. Scheuer JF 3rd, Costa CR, Dauwe PB, et al. Laser resurfacing at the time of rhytidectomy. Plast Reconstr Surg 2015;136:27–38.

19. Weinstein C, Pozner J, Scheflan M, et al. Combined erbium:YAG laser resurfacing and face lifting. Plast Reconstr Surg 2001;107:593–4.

20. Hollmig ST, Struck SK, Hantash BM. Establishing the safety and efficacy of simultaneous face lift and intraoperative full face and neck fractional carbon dioxide resurfacing. Plast Reconstr Surg 2012;129: 737e–9e.

21. Ha RY, Byrd HS. Septal extension grafts revisited: 6-year experience in controlling nasal tip projection and shape. Plast Reconstr Surg 2003;112: 1929–35.

22. Cisneros JL, Rio R, Palou J. The Q-switched neodymium (Nd):YAG laser with quadruple frequency. Clinical histological evaluation of facial resurfacing using different wavelengths. Dermatol Surg 1998; 24:345–50.

23. Bencini PL, Luci A, Galimberti M, et al. Long-term epilation with long-pulsed neodimium:YAG laser. Dermatol Surg 1999;25:175–8.

24. Goldberg DJ. Laser- and light-based hair removal: an update. Expert Rev Med Devices 2007;4:253–60.

25. Tanzi EL, Alster TS. Long-pulsed 1064-nm Nd:YAG laser-assisted hair removal in all skin types. Dermatol Surg 2004;30:13–7.

26. Alster TS, Bryan H, Williams CM. Long-pulsed Nd: YAG laser-assisted hair removal in pigmented skin: a clinical and histological evaluation. Arch Dermatol 2001;137:885–9.

27. Bernstein EF, Kornbluth S, Brown DB, et al. Treatment of spider veins using a 10 millisecond pulse-duration frequency-doubled neodymium YAG laser. Dermatol Surg 1999;25:316–20.

28. Sadick NS. Laser treatment of leg veins. Skin Therapy Lett 2004;9:6–9.

29. Rogachefsky AS, Silapunt S, Goldberg DJ. Nd:YAG laser (1064 nm) irradiation for lower extremity telangiectases and small reticular veins: efficacy as measured by vessel color and size. Dermatol Surg 2002;28:220–3.

30. Eremia S, Li CY. Treatment of leg and face veins with a cryogen spray variable pulse width 1064-nm Nd: YAG laser: a prospective study of 47 patients. J Cosmet Laser Ther 2001;3:147–53.

31. Holcomb JD. Versatility of erbium YAG laser: from fractional skin rejuvenation to full-field skin resurfacing. Facial Plast Surg Clin North Am 2011;19: 261–73.

32. Alster TS, Lupton JR. Erbium:YAG cutaneous laser resurfacing. Dermatol Clin 2001;19:453–66.

33. Sapijaszko MJ, Zachary CB. Er:YAG laser skin resurfacing. Dermatol Clin 2002;20:87–96.

34. Jimenez G, Spencer JM. Erbium:YAG laser resurfacing of the hands, arms, and neck. Dermatol Surg 1999;25:831–4 [discussion: 834–5].

35. Hughes PS. Skin contraction following erbium:YAG laser resurfacing. Dermatol Surg 1998;24:109–11.

36. Angermeier MC. Treatment of facial vascular lesions with intense pulsed light. J Cutan Laser Ther 1999;1: 95–100.

37. Goldman MP, Weiss RA, Weiss MA. Intense pulsed light as a nonablative approach to photoaging. Dermatol Surg 2005;31:1179–87 [discussion: 1187].

38. Bitter PH. Noninvasive rejuvenation of photodamaged skin using serial, full-face intense pulsed light treatments. Dermatol Surg 2000;26:835–42 [discussion: 843].

39. Johnson F, Dovale M. Intense pulsed light treatment of hirsutism: case reports of skin phototypes V and VI. J Cutan Laser Ther 1999;1:233–7.

40. Ransom ER, Antunes MB, Bloom JD, et al. Concurrent structural fat grafting and carbon dioxide laser resurfacing for perioral and lower face rejuvenation. J Cosmet Laser Ther 2011;13:6–12.

41. Kim EM, Bucky LP. Power of the pinch: pinch lower lid blepharoplasty. Ann Plast Surg 2008;60:532–7.

42. Oni G, Brown S, Kenkel J. Comparison of five commonly-available, lidocaine-containing topical anesthetics and their effect on serum levels of lidocaine and its metabolite monoethylglycinexylidide (MEGX). Aesthet Surg J 2012;32:495–503.

43. Oni G, Brown S, Burrus C, et al. Effect of 4% topical lidocaine applied to the face on the serum levels of lidocaine and its metabolite, monoethylglycinexylidide. Aesthet Surg J 2010;30:853–8.

44. Sadick N. Tissue tightening technologies: fact or fiction. Aesthet Surg J 2008;28:180–8.

45. Weinkle AP, Sofen B, Emer J. Synergistic approaches to neck rejuvenation and lifting. J Drugs Dermatol 2015;14:1215–28.

46. Sadick NS, Makino Y. Selective electro-thermolysis in aesthetic medicine: a review. Lasers Surg Med 2004;34:91–7.

47. Belenky I, Margulis A, Elman M, et al. Exploring channeling optimized radiofrequency energy: a review of radiofrequency history and applications in esthetic fields. Adv Ther 2012;29:249–66.

48. Kennedy JE, Ter Haar GR, Cranston D. High intensity focused ultrasound: surgery of the future? Br J Radiol 2003;76:590–9.

49. White WM, Makin IR, Barthe PG, et al. Selective creation of thermal injury zones in the superficial musculoaponeurotic system using intense ultrasound therapy: a new target for noninvasive facial rejuvenation. Arch Facial Plast Surg 2007; 9:22–9.

50. Gliklich RE, White WM, Slayton MH, et al. Clinical pilot study of intense ultrasound therapy to deep dermal facial skin and subcutaneous tissues. Arch Facial Plast Surg 2007;9:88–95.

51. Fabi SG, Goldman MP. Retrospective evaluation of micro-focused ultrasound for lifting and tightening the face and neck. Dermatol Surg 2014;40:569–75.

52. Alam M, White LE, Martin N, et al. Ultrasound tightening of facial and neck skin: a rater-blinded prospective cohort study. J Am Acad Dermatol 2010; 62:262–9.

53. Kenkel J. Evaluation of the Ulthera system for achieving lift and tightening cheek tissue, improving jawline definition and submental skin laxity. Paper presented at: American Society for Laser Medicine and Surgery. Boston, MA.

54. Oni G, Hoxworth R, Teotia S, et al. Evaluation of a microfocused ultrasound system for improving skin laxity and tightening in the lower face. Aesthet Surg J 2014;34:1099–110.

Short Scar Neck Lift
Neck Lift Using a Submental Incision Only

Timothy Marten, MD*, Dino Elyassnia, MD

KEYWORDS

- Neck lift • Short scar neck lift • Submandibular gland reduction • Partial digastic myectomy
- Sub-platysmal lipectomy

KEY POINTS

- For a subset of patients, poor neck contour exists as a largely isolated problem and in many cases these patients can be treated with a short scar neck lift procedure in which no skin is removed.
- Typically, these patients include younger women with full, obtuse necks, and young and middle-aged men with poor neck contour.
- The procedure is performed through a submental incision without any removal of skin and relies on modification of deep-layer structures to improve neck contour.
- "Excess" skin is allowed to redistribute itself over the increased neck surface area created when deep-layer maneuvers are performed, neck contour is improved, and the cervicomental angle deepened.
- For properly selected patients, a short scar neck lift can produce a marked improvement in facial appearance.

INTRODUCTION

A well-contoured neck is paramount to a fit, healthy, decisive, and attractive appearance and improved neck contour is one of the most rewarding and gratifying changes a patient can make in his or her appearance. In many cases in which advanced aging is present elsewhere on the face, improving neck contour alone is a hollow victory and neck lift must be performed in conjunction with lifts of the face and jaw line and other areas if a harmonious, balanced and natural-appearing improvement is to be obtained. For a distinct subset of patients, however, poor neck contour exists as the predominant problem and an isolated neck lift procedure is artistically appropriate. In many cases, these patients can be treated with a short scar neck lift procedure in which skin need not be removed. Typically these patients include younger women with full, obtuse necks, and young and middle-aged men with poor neck contour. Often these patients report that their full obtuse necks have been present even in youth, and that their parents, siblings, and other relatives are all troubled by a similar appearance.

SHORT SCAR NECK LIFT: DEFINITION

Short scar neck lift is a term used to describe a neck lift performed through a submental incision only with no peri-auricular incisions, and one in which no skin is removed.

WHO ARE THE BEST CANDIDATES FOR SHORT SCAR NECK LIFT?

In general, men are the ideal candidates for short scar neck lift as male attractiveness is not as

Disclosure: The authors have nothing to disclose.
Marten Clinic of Plastic Surgery, 450 Sutter Street Suite 2222, San Francisco, CA 94108, USA
* Corresponding author.
E-mail address: tmarten@martenclinic.com

Clin Plastic Surg 45 (2018) 585–600
https://doi.org/10.1016/j.cps.2018.06.005

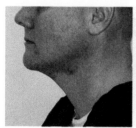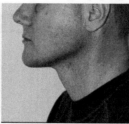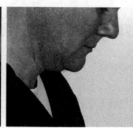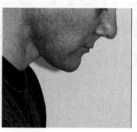

Fig. 1. Short scar neck lift in a young man with short hair. Before and after surgery views of a man who has had no prior surgery. Note lax skin, obtuse cervicosubmental contour, and "double-chin" appearance when the patient looks down in before views. A large submandibular gland can easily be seen in the lateral view and easily palpated on physical examination. His short hair ostensibly precludes traditional neck lift or facelift surgery. Same patient after short scar neck lift. The procedure included excision of excess subplatysmal fat, submandibular salivary gland reduction, superficial digastric myectomy, and anterior platysmaplasty. No incisions were made in the peri-auricular areas. Note well-defined jaw line and attractive, youthful-appearing neckline even when the patient looks down. The only scar is in the submental area. No skin was removed in the procedure. Surgical procedure performed by Timothy J. Marten, MD, FACS. (*Courtesy of* Timothy J. Marten, MD, FACS, Marten Clinic of Plastic Surgery, San Francisco, CA.)

closely tied to youth, and an appealing masculine appearance is not as dependent on the tight jaw line and inverted oval facial shape that typically defines the attractive female face. Indeed, a more bottom heavy, square facial shape, and a heavier jaw line are often regarded as essential to a masculine appearance, and as such a facelift in men can often be deferred until later in a man's life than is the case with women. Men also typically have thicker more elastic skin that better redistributes itself and contracts over the improved neck surface created in a short scar neck lift procedure. In many cases, a short scar neck lift is applicable to men well into their fifties or early sixties.

Carefully selected women can be very good candidates for a short scar neck lift procedure despite the considerations mentioned, but typically are in a younger age group, ranging from late teens to mid-thirties. As women enter their late thirties and beyond, a short scar neck lift is typically artistically less appropriate, as significant aging is usually present in the jowl and jaw line area by that time and simply targeting the under-jaw area creates disharmonious and unfeminine appearances. Skin type is also important, and better outcomes are typically obtained in darker-complected women of Mediterranean, Asian, and African ancestry, than in fair-skinned women of Northern European origin.

Another subset of patients who are usually excellent candidates for an isolated neck lift and short scar neck lift procedure are patients who have undergone previous well-performed facelifts but timidly performed neck lifts. These patients often will not benefit from additional skin excision, but problems of deep-layer origin in their necks have not been addressed and residual fullness due to deep-layer problems are still present. A

short scar neck lift can be transformative is such cases.

SHORT SCAR NECK LIFT: THE CONCEPT

Although submental liposuction alone will rarely produce optimal neck improvement for reasons discussed (see Timothy Marten and Dino Elyassnia's, "Neck Lift: Defining Anatomic Problems and Choosing Appropriate Treatment Strategies," in this issue), a neck lift performed through a submental incision without any removal of skin can create attractive cervical contour in many patients if proper modification of deep-layer structures contributing to cervicosubmental obtusity is made (**Figs. 1** and **2**).

This is because, unlike liposuction, a neck lift performed through a submental incision allows deep-layer problems and platysmal laxity typically present in most patients seeking neck improvement that comprise the overwhelming majority of their neck problems to be addressed.

SHORT SCAR NECK LIFT: WHAT ABOUT THE EXTRA SKIN?

A common question creating an obstacle to adopting the short scar neck lift strategy is "how can good neck contour be created without removing and tightening the skin?" and its corollary "what happens to the 'excess' skin if only the deeper layer treatment is made and no skin is excised?" The answer to these questions and this conundrum is twofold: first is the simple but often difficult to accept concept that in a properly performed neck lift, improved contour is created by modification of deep layers of the neck, *not* by tightening the skin. Skin is intended to be a

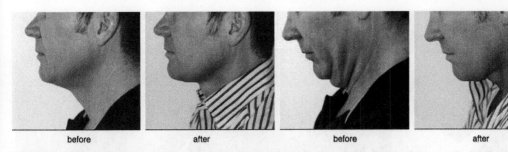

before | after | before | after

Fig. 2. Short scar neck lift in a man with a full neck. Before and after surgery views of a man who has had no prior surgery. Note lax skin, obtuse cervicosubmental contour, and "double-chin" appearance when the patient looks down in the before views. A large submandibular gland can be partially seen in the lateral view and is easily palpated. His young age and short haircut make him reluctant to submit to having peri-auricular scars. A marked amount of excess skin appears to be present. Same patient after short scar neck lift. The procedure included excision of excess subplatysmal fat, submandibular salivary gland reduction, superficial digastric myectomy, and anterior platysmaplasty. No incisions were made in the peri-auricular areas and no other procedures were performed. Note markedly improved cervicosubmental contour and attractive, youthful-appearing neckline even when the patient looks down. The only scar is in the submental area. No skin was removed in the procedure. This case demonstrates that the apparent skin redundancy is really a "pseudoexcess" and that "excess" skin redistributes itself over the deeper, geometrically larger and longer anterior neck surface created by treating deep neck problems. Surgical procedure performed by Dino Elyassnia, MD, FACS. (*Courtesy of* Dino Elyassnia, MD, FACS, Marten Clinic of Plastic Surgery, San Francisco, CA.)

covering layer and serve a covering function. It was meant to stretch and give as we move and express ourselves. It was not intended to be a structural supporting layer, or to hold up sagging muscle and fat or lift hypertrophied structures lying beneath it. The second part of the answer lies in the increase in neck surface area that occurs when deep-layer techniques are used and neck contour is improved. Improving neck contour by removing collections of subplatysmal fat, reducing the size of enlarged submandibular glands, and performing other deep-layer maneuvers as indicated, followed by appropriate treatment of lax platysma, will result in a deepened cervicomental angle, a longer, curvilinear distance from the mentum to the sternal notch, and a more concave and geometrically larger and longer anterior neck surface. When neck skin is re-draped and redistributed over the deeper, more concave surface created by reducing subplatysmal fat excess and submandibular gland reduction, "excess" skin is absorbed and none need be removed (**Fig. 3**). These simple but not intuitive or immediately obvious facts underlie the reason that skin excision need not be performed as part of a neck lift in many patients with good skin quality and mild to moderate skin excess to obtain a good result.

WHY NOT REMOVE SOME SKIN FROM THE SUBMENTAL INCISION?

Once the fact that increased neck surface area is produced by deepening the cervicomental angle by treatment of deep-layer subplatysmal neck problems is acknowledged, it becomes clear

why it is counterproductive to excise any skin from the submental incision, as this can create a "bowstring" effect and actually blunt the cervicomental angle (**Fig. 4**). Skin removal along this vector is not helpful in most patients. The submental skin incision is used for access to the neck only in a properly performed neck lift, and if skin excision is necessary, it is more practically, effectively, and logically removed from the postauricular area (extended neck lift or a facelift procedure, see Timothy Marten and Dino Elyassnia's, "Neck Lift: Defining Anatomic Problems and Choosing Appropriate Treatment Strategies," in this issue) along a more appropriately directed lateral vector.

It is also the case that when more than a modest amount of skin is removed as an ellipse about the submental incision that objectionable "dog-ears" will result at each end of the incision. If these are left in place, an attractive and natural submental contour will not be present. If dog-ears are removed by chasing them laterally, the submental incision ends up being unnecessarily long, with each end of the resulting scar extending objectionably up onto visible area on the jaw line.

IS IT NECESSARY TO MAKE A SUBPLATYSMAL DISSECTION AND TO REMOVE SUBPLATYSMAL FAT AND REDUCE THE SUBMANDIBULAR GLAND IN ALL PATIENTS?

The fundamental problem with our past efforts to rejuvenate the neck, be it with a noninvasive procedure, a short scar procedure, an extended neck lift, or neck lift performed with a facelift, and the core concept in the modern neck lift, is

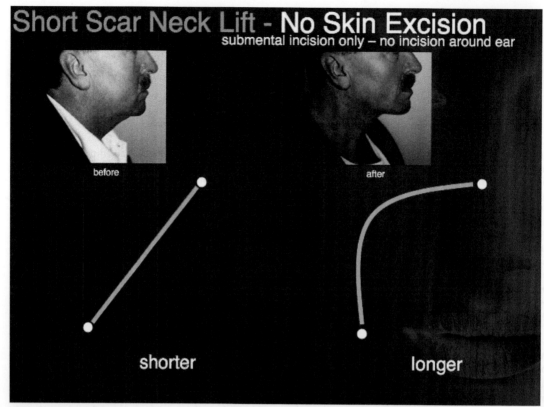

Fig. 3. Redistribution of "excess" skin in short scar neck lift. In the preoperative condition (*left*), subplatysmal full-ness (subplatysmal fat and large submandibular glands) has resulted in an oblique neck and the neck skin is distributed over a straight surface between the chin and the sternum. This straight line comprises the shortest distance between the 2 points and to the eye excess skin appears to be present. In the postoperative condition (*right*), subplatysmal fullness has been eliminated and a deeper, more concave, and geometrically larger and longer neck surface has been created. The skin is redistributed over a curved line that takes a longer path between the 2 points. Surgical procedure performed by Timothy J. Marten, MD, FACS. (*Courtesy of* Timothy J. Marten, MD, FACS, Marten Clinic of Plastic Surgery, San Francisco, CA.)

that poor neck contour is largely the result of excess and hypertrophy of structures in the sub-platysmal "deep neck" layer. As such, improved neck contour is and must be created by modifica-tion of the deep-layer anatomy and not by tightening skin or the platysma. Although the con-dition of the neck skin envelope and the platysma muscle contribute to poor neck contour, limiting our efforts to liposuction and other means of over-treatment of the subcutaneous layer and superfi-cial neck as we traditionally have, even when combined with platysma muscle and skin tight-ening, is conceptually flawed and has proven over time to be a practical failure. Simple logic, when the underlying origins of neck problems are recognized and acknowledged, tells us so.

It is fundamental to all branches of surgery that the underlying cause of a problem must be defined before appropriate treatment can be undertaken, and that any such treatment must address the anatomic problems present. Simply applying an arbitrary, formulaic, "cookie cutter" strategy to all patients without identifying the anatomic basis of their neck problems is not sound decision making and cannot be expected to predictably result in favorable outcomes. Treatment must be based on the anatomic problems present, and must address them in a logical way.

Regrettably, addressing deep neck problems has traditionally been viewed as something exotic performed as occasional treatment of problems that only uncommonly occur. The reality is that deep-layer problems are consistently seen in the aging neck and the young neck with poor contour once one learns to recognize them, and treating them forms the basis of the short scar neck lift and other forms of contemporary surgical neck treatment. Surgeons seeking consistent good results in the neck must learn to recognize and treat deep neck problems, and will need to apply needed treatment of them in many if not most cases.

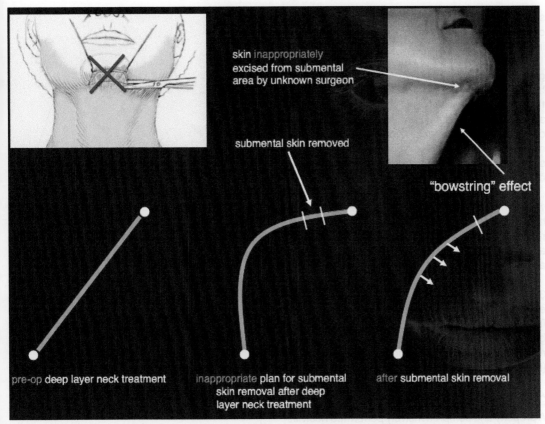

skin inappropriately
excised from submental
area by unknown surgeon

submental skin removed

"bowstring" effect

pre-op deep layer neck treatment

inappropriate plan for submental
skin removal after deep
layer neck treatment

after submental skin removal

Fig. 4. Improper excision of skin from the submental incision and "bowstring effect." Once it is recognized that increased neck surface area and deepening the cervicomental angle is created by treatment of subplatysmal neck problems, it becomes clear why it is counterproductive to excise any skin from the submental incision, as this can create a "bowstring" effect and actually blunt the cervicomental angle. This maneuver will also result in objectionable "dog-ears" at each end of the incision that spoil cervicosubmental contour. If skin excision is necessary, it is more practically, effectively, and logically removed from the postauricular area. (*Courtesy of* Marten Clinic of Plastic Surgery, San Francisco, CA.)

Because most neck problems are of subplatysmal origin, there are both advantages and disadvantages for surgeons who endeavor to improve the neck. The advantage is that in many cases a significant and often stunning improvement in neck appearance can be made using only a small incision under the chin, as set forth in this article. The disadvantage is that it means we must think differently from what we have and were taught, we must learn and do something new, and we must try a bit harder. Although the advantages are significant and far exceed the disadvantages, the disadvantages are nonetheless formidable and are difficult for many to overcome.

We feel the results shown in this article speak for themselves and should serve as evidence that the key to good outcomes in the neck rests in treating the deep neck problems, and that a subplatysmal dissection and excision and reduction of hypertrophied subplatysmal structures, including subplatysmal fat, the submandibular gland, and anterior

belly of the digastric muscles, are useful and effective maneuvers that form the foundation of thoughtful logical treatment of the cervicosubmental area.

WHY NOT PERFORM A SHORT SCAR NECK LIFT ON EVERYBODY?

There is a limit to the amount of neck skin that can be absorbed and managed by the short scar neck lift technique, however, and an isolated neck lift performed through a submental incision only is typically best for male patients and younger women with mild to moderate skin excess, good skin elasticity, and minimal or modest aging in the mid-face, cheek, jowl, and jawline.

SURGICAL TECHNIQUE
Planning the Submental Incision

Traditionally, the submental incision for neck lifting has been placed directly in and along the submental crease in a well-intended but ultimately counterproductive attempt to conceal the resulting scar (**Fig. 5**).

This incision plan should be avoided, as it will surgically reinforce the crease and accentuate a "double-chin" or "witch's chin" deformity. Exposure of the submental region will also be compromised, and difficulty will be encountered when suturing or dissecting low in the neck. A more posterior placement of this incision will avoid these problems, but still result in an inconspicuous and arguably better concealed scar (**Figs. 6** and **7**; see **Fig. 9**).

The submental incision should be placed well within the mandibular shadow and well posterior but parallel to the submental crease at a point lying roughly one-half the distance between the mentum and hyoid. This usually corresponds to a site situated 1.0 to 1.5 cm posterior to the crease (**Fig. 8**).

The incision should be approximately 3.0 to 3.5 cm in length, but may be made longer if neither end will be advanced up on a visible portion of the face when skin flaps are shifted. Healing will be best, and the scar will be best concealed, if it is made as a straight, and not as a curved line (**Figs. 9** and **10**).

Anesthesia

A properly and comprehensively performed neck lift is a time-consuming, technically demanding procedure, and can test the patience and composure

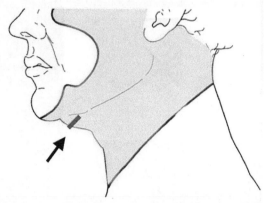

Fig. 6. Correct location for the submental incision. Placing the submental incision 1.0 to 1.5 cm *posterior* to the submental crease prevents accentuation of the "double chin" and witch's chin deformities and provides for easier dissection and suturing in the anterior neck (compare with **Fig. 10**). Note that this incision plan allows the submental crease to be undermined and submental retaining ligaments to be released, and the fat of the chin pad and submental neck to be blended to create a smooth transition between them (see **Fig. 12**). Yellow shaded area represents area of subcutaneous dissection. (*Courtesy of* Marten Clinic of Plastic Surgery, San Francisco, CA.)

of almost any surgeon. It is highly recommended that any surgeon new to these techniques enlist the services of an anesthesiologist or competent registered nurse anesthetist. This is particularly important when the procedure is to be performed on a patient who is apprehensive, or has a history of anesthetic difficulties, hypertension, sleep apnea, or other significant medical problems.

Most of our neck lifts are performed under deep sedation administered by an anesthesiologist using a laryngeal mask airway ("LMA") with a flexible shaft. The use of a laryngeal mask allows the patient to be heavily sedated without compromise of the airway, and the patient need not receive muscle relaxants and can be allowed to breath spontaneously. An LMA is also less likely to become dislodged during the procedure than an endotracheal tube, and will not trigger coughing and bucking when the patient emerges from the anesthetic. The *flexible* LMA is particularly useful in neck surgery. When this device is used and the breathing circuit is separately draped, the breathing circuit can be moved from side to side as needed during the procedure to obtain unobstructed access to the cervicosubmental region. Additional details on anesthesia for neck lift can be found (see Timothy Marten and Dino Elyassnia's, "Neck Lift: Defining Anatomic Problems and Choosing Appropriate Treatment Strategies," in this issue).

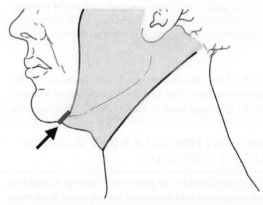

Fig. 5. Traditional, but *incorrect* plan for the submental incision. The incision should not be placed directly in the submental crease (*arrow*), as this will reinforce the submental retaining ligaments and accentuate the "double-chin" appearance. Note that the typical plan for skin undermining (*yellow area*) also promotes a double-chin appearance because the crease is not undermined, retaining ligaments are not released, and the fat of the chin and the submental neck cannot be readily blended to create a smooth transition between them. Yellow shaded area represents area of subcutaneous dissection. (*Courtesy of* Marten Clinic of Plastic Surgery, San Francisco, CA.)

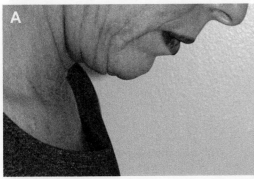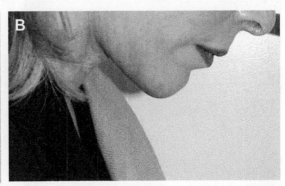

Fig. 7. Correction of the "double-chin" deformity. (*A*) Patient with "double chin" seen preoperatively. (*B*) Same patient seen after face and neck lift. The submental incision was made posterior to the submental crease (see **Fig. 6**) to allow undermining and release of the submental retaining ligaments and blending of chin and submental neck fat. Surgical procedure performed by Timothy J. Marten, MD, FACS. (*Courtesy of* Timothy J. Marten, MD, FACS, Marten Clinic of Plastic Surgery, San Francisco, CA.)

Preoperative Preparations

Patients undergoing short scar neck lift receive a full surgical scrub of the anterior scalp, face, ears,

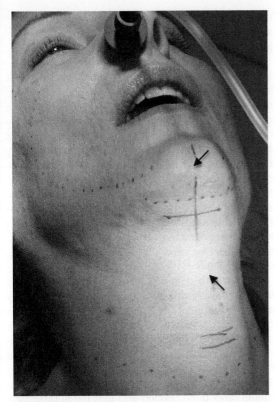

Fig. 8. Plan for the submental incision. The submental incision (*solid line*) should be placed posterior to the submental crease (*dotted line*), approximately one-half the distance between the mentum and hyoid (*arrows*). Usually this corresponds to a point approximately 1.0 to 1.5 cm posterior to the submental crease. (*Courtesy of* Marten Clinic of Plastic Surgery, San Francisco, CA.)

nose, neck, shoulders, and upper chest with full-strength (1:750) benzalkonium chloride (BAK or Zephran) solution after anesthesia is begun. The patient's head is then placed through the opening of a "split sheet" or a split adhesive–backed disposable transverse laparotomy sheet. A "turban" or "head drape" can be used, but if the patient has short hair it is typically simpler to prep the entire scalp. Additional details on preoperative preparation of the neck lift patient can be found (see Timothy Marten and Dino Elyassnia's, "Neck Lift: Defining Anatomic Problems and Choosing Appropriate Treatment Strategies," in this issue).

Administering Local Anesthesia

Local anesthetic is administered even if deep sedation or general anesthesia is used. This limits stimulation of the patient and the overall amount of narcotics and anesthetics needed. A significant and helpful hemostatic effect is also obtained when epinephrine-containing solutions are used.

Sensory nerve blocks and ring blocks around the area to be dissected are performed using 0.25% bupivacaine (Marcaine) with epinephrine 1:200,000. Skin marked for incision is then infiltrated with the same solution. Areas of subcutaneous dissection are generously infiltrated with 0.1% lidocaine (Xylocaine) with epinephrine 1:1,000,000 solution using a 1.6-mm multihole blunt-tipped infiltration cannula.

Skin Flap Elevation

The submental incision should be made 1.5 cm or more posterior to the submental crease approximately half way between the mentum and hyoid. Making the incision in this location helps conceal it in the shadow of the mandible, avoids surgical reinforcement of the crease and accentuation of

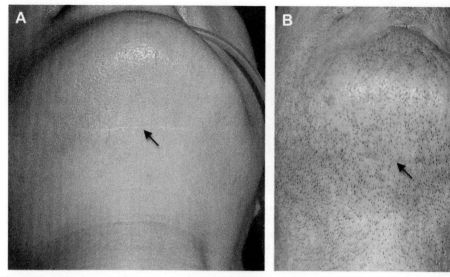

Fig. 9. Healed submental incisions. (*A, B*) Placement of the submental incision posterior to the submental crease will still result in an inconspicuous, well-concealed scar and simultaneously provide better access and exposure when working in the deep layers of the neck. *Black arrows* show location of healed submental scars. Surgical procedure performed by Timothy J. Marten, MD, FACS. (*Courtesy of* Timothy J. Marten, MD, FACS, Marten Clinic of Plastic Surgery, San Francisco, CA.)

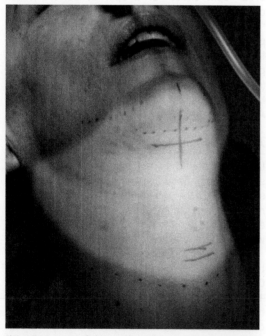

Fig. 10. Extent of skin undermining in short scar neck lift. Skin undermining is carried inferiorly below the level of the cricoid cartilage (*double solid lines*), laterally to the anterior border of the sternocleidomastoid muscle and superiorly beneath the submental crease (*dotted line*) and through the submental and mandibular retaining ligaments. Undermining and releasing the submental crease, and carrying the dissection retrograde up onto the chin allows the fat of the chin and submental area to be seamlessly blended. The solid line shown posterior to the submental crease is the site for the submental skin incision. (*Courtesy of* Marten Clinic of Plastic Surgery, San Francisco, CA.)

the "double-chin" and witch's chin deformities, and provides better exposure of the deep neck (see **Figs. 6** and **7**).

Once the submental incision has been made, the surgeon should stand at the head of the table during dissection of the submental region, while the assistant retracts the edges of the incision with a pair of 10-mm double-pronged skin hooks. Skin undermining should be made using a medium curved Metzenbaum scissors and the dissection should be made subcutaneously leaving most of the subcutaneous/preplatysmal fat on the platysma surface. This makes subcutaneous fat excision and sculpting easier later in the procedure if required. Preservation of a thicker layer of fat helps avoid a hard or overresected appearance in the cervicosubmental area, and objectionable overexposure of underlying neck anatomy postoperatively.

Skin undermining is carried inferiorly below the level of the cricoid cartilage and laterally to the anterior border of the sternocleidomastoid muscle. On completion of subcutaneous undermining of the anterior neck and submental regions, a retrograde dissection should be made subcutaneously up onto the inferior chin (see also **Figs. 5** and **9**). This will ensure the submental restraining ligaments have been divided and that the submental crease has been released and provides for subsequent blending of chin and submental fat after other neck maneuvers have been completed to obtain a seamless and optimally aesthetic transition for chin to submental region. Some bleeding is usually encountered from perforating vessels that accompany ligaments in this region during this maneuver, but this should not prevent one from carrying out this important step. Additional details on skin flap elevation can be found (see Timothy Marten and Dino Elyassnia's, "Neck Lift: Defining Anatomic Problems and Choosing Appropriate Treatment Strategies," in this issue).

Cervical Lipectomy

The key to obtaining good outcomes in neck lift lies in understanding the distribution of fat in the cervicosubmental region, and cervical fat can be seen to be present in 3 distinct anatomic layers: preplatysmal (subcutaneous), subplatysmal, and deep cervicosubmuscular ("interdigastric").

Although our traditional focus has mistakenly been on the preplatysmal layer (submental liposuction and related surgical and nonsurgical procedures targeting subcutaneous fat), most patients presenting with poor neck contour will instead be troubled by fat excess predominantly in the subplatysmal layer. Understanding and accepting this anatomic reality, and learning to appropriately treat subplatysmal fat, is essential to obtaining optimal outcomes.

Contrary to the traditionally taught technique, in all but the unusual case it is best to leave the subcutaneous fat layer untouched until all other maneuvers are completed and improvements obtained with them assessed. Only then should fat be removed from the subcutaneous layer.

The subplatysmal space is entered by incising the fascia between the medial platysma muscle borders using a Metzenbaum scissors or electrocautery. A combination of blunt and sharp scissors technique is used to isolate each muscle edge. The muscle edge is then grasped and retracted by the assistant using a 10-mm double-prong skin hook or an Allis forceps. The dissection is then carried laterally, over the anterior belly of the digastric muscle hugging the underside of the platysma. Subplatysmal fat should be left on the deep surface of the neck and not raised with the platysma flap. This will facilitate fat excision.

The plane tangent to the anterior bellies of the digastric muscles with the neck in neutral or slightly flexed position should be used as the landmark for subplatysmal fat removal. All fat present in the subplatysmal space lying *superficial* to this plane should be removed if optimal contour is to be obtained.

Fat situated deep to the plane tangent to anterior bellies of the digastric muscles and beneath the deep cervical fascia (deep cervical or "interdigastric" fat) should not be removed and the overwhelming temptation to "clean out" the deep submental space resisted. Platysmaplasty, invaginating platysma in a "corset" fashion, suturing the anterior bellies of the digastric muscles together, and other like maneuvers cannot compensate for overzealous excision of deep interdigastric fat and, in time, an objectionable submental depression will appear in the necks of patients so treated. Additional details on excision of subplatysmal fat can be found (see Timothy Marten and Dino Elyassnia's, "Neck Lift: Defining Anatomic Problems and Choosing Appropriate Treatment Strategies," in this issue).

Large Submandibular Glands

Prominent submandibular glands will be encountered as subplatysmal dissection is carried over the anterior belly of the ipsilateral digastric muscle. The prominent gland will appear as a smooth pink to tan-colored mass covered by a smooth capsule. Reduction is begun by incising the capsule overlying the gland inferomedially just lateral to the anterior belly of the digastric muscle insertion on the hyoid. The submandibular gland will be evident once exposed in this manner due to its distinctive lobulated appearance. Its inferior portion can be easily separated from adjacent tissue inside its capsule using a gentle blunt scissors-spreading technique. Although all vital structures are outside the glandular capsule, care should be taken when mobilizing the gland superior-laterally, as both the retromandibular vein and the marginal mandibular branch of the facial nerve are in proximity in that area.

An examination of the gland once mobilized inside its capsule will show it to be large, and not merely "ptotic," and this observation forms the basis of the recommendation that partial resection of the protruding portion be performed. Examination of the exposed gland will also clearly demonstrate that attempts to reposition it more superiorly by suture suspension, or by tightening overlying platysma muscle, will ultimately be ineffective.

Once adequately mobilized inside its capsule, the inferior portion of the gland is grasped, and pulled gently inferiorly and medially out of its fossa and away from adjacent structures. The redundant portion is subsequently excised incrementally under direct vision in a medial to lateral direction along the planned line of resection with coagulating current cautery. Excision of the excess part of the gland should be performed in such a manner that the portion protruding *inferior to the plane tangent to the ipsilateral anterior belly of the digastric muscle and the ipsilateral mandibular border* will be resected (see Timothy Marten and Dino Elyassnia's, "Neck Lift: Defining Anatomic Problems and Choosing Appropriate Treatment Strategies," in this issue). It is usually best that initial resection is conservative and that the gland is incrementally reduced thereafter as required.

Excision of the redundant and protruding portion of the submandibular gland should be performed using an extended flat-tipped cautery and a long, high-quality pair of atraumatic (DeBakey or similar) forceps. A flat-tipped, extended cautery is superior for controlling bleeding of an intraglandular vessel, should it be encountered, than is a needlepoint cautery tip. Additional details on reduction of the submandibular gland can be found (see Timothy Marten and Dino Elyassnia's, "Neck Lift: Defining Anatomic Problems and Choosing Appropriate Treatment Strategies," in this issue).

Partial Digastric Myectomy

After subplatysmal lipectomy and submandibular gland reduction have been performed, assessment should be made of the anterior bellies of the digastric muscles and whether partial digastric myectomy would produce further improvement in neck contour. In most cases, additional improvement in contour can be obtained by performing this simple procedure.

Typically, large digastric muscles will appear as a linear para-median fullness lying medial to the rounder and more laterally situated submandibular gland fullness (**Fig. 11**).

Superficial, subtotal anterior digastric myectomy is performed under direct vision, through the submental incision after the subplatysmal space has been opened and subplatysmal fat and protruding portions of the submandibular

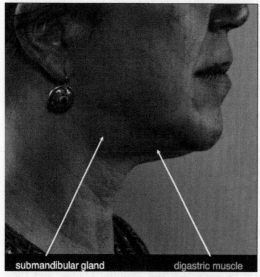

submandibular gland   digastric muscle

Fig. 11. External expression of large submandibular gland and digastric muscle. Large digastric muscles will appear as a linear para-median fullness lying medial to the rounder and more laterally situated submandibular gland fullness. (*Courtesy of* Marten Clinic of Plastic Surgery, San Francisco, CA.)

gland resected, if indicated. Tangential strip excision is performed by visually gauging the muscle redundancy, grasping the redundant portion with a DeBakey or similar forceps, and tangentially excising a strip of muscle longitudinally from the muscle belly with a Metzenbaum scissors or more commonly with electrocautery using coagulating current. Excision is begun near the muscle origin at the mentum and continuing to the muscle belly insertion at the lateral hyoid. The muscle is then reassessed and the action repeated until the protruding portion is fully removed and optimal contour has been established. Approximately 50% of the muscle is removed in the typical case, with the most muscle removed near the hyoid and the least near the chin (**Fig. 12**). Additional details on digastric muscle reduction can be found (see Timothy Marten and Dino Elyassnia's, "Neck Lift: Defining Anatomic Problems and Choosing Appropriate Treatment Strategies," in this issue).

Platysma Plasty

Anterior platysma*plasty* (see **Fig. 4** in the article by Timothy Marten and Dino Elyassnia, "Management of the Platysma in Neck Lift," in this issue) is performed as an integral part of short scar and other neck lift procedures. The purpose of platysmaplasty is to consolidate the neck, reduce irregularities due to horizontal platysmal laxity, and to enhance neck appearance when it is flexed and the patient is looking down. Platysmaplasty is performed by suturing the medial muscle borders of the platysma muscles together from mentum to thyroid cartilage (**Fig. 13** in the article by Timothy Marten and Dino Elyassnia, "Management of the Platysma in Neck Lift," in this issue). In short scar neck lifts, redundant muscle is uniformly present medially, as there is no superior and lateral advancement of the muscles that is seen when superficial musculoaponeurotic system flaps are raised when a facelift is performed. Excess muscle is gauged by pulling each to and across the midline and excess muscle along the medial border of each is excised before suturing is performed so that a smooth, edge-to-edge approximation of the medial muscle borders can be made without inversion, invagination, or imbrication (**Fig. 14** in Timothy Marten and Dino Elyassnia's, "Management of the Platysma in Neck Lift," in this issue). Experience has shown that this produces a better and more consistent outcome and reduces the likelihood that objectionable midline fullness or bands will result after healing and relaxation of tissues has occurred than when excess muscle is invaginated and a multilayer "plication" or "corset" is performed.

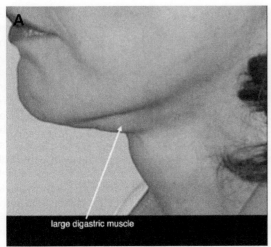
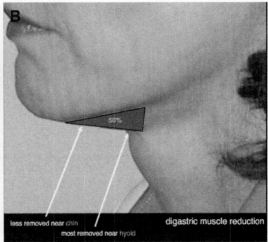

Fig. 12. Digastric muscle reduction strategy. (*A*) Typical appearance of a large anterior belly of the digastric muscle. (*B*) Digastric muscle fullness is treated in a manner that optimizes submental contour. Approximately 50% of the muscle is removed in the typical case with more muscle removed near the hyoid and less near the chin (*shaded gray area*). (*Courtesy of* Marten Clinic of Plastic Surgery, San Francisco, CA.)

Platysmaplasty is usually performed using multiple simple interrupted sutures of 3 to 0 polyglactin (Vicryl) (or suture of choice) on a medium to large tapered needle. The platysmaplasty repair should be snug but not tight. A tight "corset" and permanent sutures are not necessary, and a tight "corset" will not result in a sustained improvement in cervical contour if deep-layer problems are not addressed.

Optimal improvement generally cannot be obtained if repair is performed using a running suture, as some gathering and a "purse string" effect can occur. This will result in shortening along the line of repair and can cause bow-stringing and postoperative midline band formation. If the approximation is made using interrupted sutures, this problem is averted and the platysma is distributed over and into the concave surface created by deep-layer neck maneuvers. If partial suturing to the hyoid only is performed in the submental area, irregularities may result at the cervicomental angle. Additional details on platysmaplasty can be found (see the article by Timothy Marten and Dino Elyassnia, "Management of the Platysma in Neck Lift," in this issue).

Transverse Platysma Myotomy

Although anterior platysmaplasty will often result in an attractive neck at rest and on the operating table, objectionable-appearing "hard" dynamic platysma bands will often still be evident in conversation and during animation after surgery if additional steps are not taken to reduce longitudinal platysma muscle hyperfunction in patients troubled by this problem. Hard, dynamic platysma bands can usually be improved by performing *transverse platysma myotomy* (see **Figs. 6–8** in the article by Timothy Marten and Dino Elyassnia, "Management of the Platysma in Neck Lift," in this issue). If hard dynamic bands and longitudinal platysma hyperfunction are not present, platysma myotomy need not be performed.

Platysma myotomy, when indicated, should be performed after anterior platysma*plasty* has been completed, as the platysma muscle will be more uniformly distributed over the anterior neck and under slight tension. Myotomy should be performed low in the neck at the level of the *cricoid* cartilage and extended slightly superiorly as it is

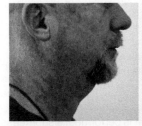
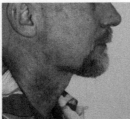
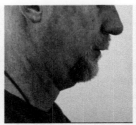
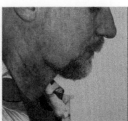

Fig. 13. Short scar neck lift in a man with a shaved head. Before and after surgery views of a man who has had no prior surgery. A chin implant has not been placed. Surgical procedure performed by Timothy J. Marten, MD, FACS. (*Courtesy of* Timothy J. Marten, MD, FACS, Marten Clinic of Plastic Surgery, San Francisco, CA.)

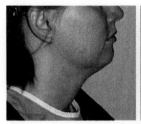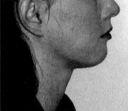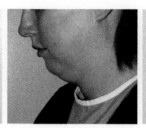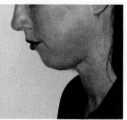

Fig. 14. Short scar neck lift in a young woman with a full neck. Before and after surgery views of a young woman who has had no prior surgery. A chin implant has not been placed. Surgical procedure performed by Timothy J. Marten, MD, FACS. (*Courtesy of* Timothy J. Marten, MD, FACS, Marten Clinic of Plastic Surgery, San Francisco, CA.)

extended laterally (Figs. 22A and 23A in the article by Timothy Marten and Dino Elyassnia, "Management of the Platysma in Neck Lift," in this issue). At this level, the muscle is thin and will bleed less, and the cut edges are less likely to be visible postoperatively, but muscle action will nonetheless be interrupted. In addition, a smooth transition across the cervicomental angle is maintained and lower lip dysfunction is avoided.

Anterior platysma myotomy is best begun just inferior to the inferior-most suture placed when platysmaplasty was performed (Fig. 23A in the article by Timothy Marten and Dino Elyassnia, "Management of the Platysma in Neck Lift," in this issue). The medial platysma border is identified over the cricothyroid area and grasped and lifted away from the deep cervical fascia with a long DeBakey-type forceps. Myotomy is then made by nibbling through the muscle in small increments with a Metzenbaum scissors (or alternatively using electrocautery). As the muscle is divided, it usually separates a centimeter or more, exposing the fascia beneath it. Myotomy is continued laterally and slightly superiorly according to the preoperative plan through as much of the area in which platysma hyperfunction is present as possible. In a short scar neck lift, a full-width myotomy (see **Fig 9**, Timothy Marten and Dino Elyassnia's, "Management of the Platysma in Neck Lift," in this issue) is usually not possible. Additional details on platysma myotomy can be found (see the article by Timothy Marten and Dino Elyassnia, "Management of the Platysma in Neck Lift," in this issue).

Drain Placement

Experience has shown that when subplatysmal fat excision and submandibular gland reduction is performed, it is prudent to place a 10-F round multiperforated Jackson-Pratt (or similar type) drain in both the subcutaneous and the subplatysmal space for at least several days after the procedure to reduce edema and induration in the submental area to reduce the chance of a fluid collection (lymphatic fluid leakage from the division of lymphatic vessels

during subplatysmal fat excision, and saliva leakage from the cut edge of the submandibular gland), and to speed the patient's overall recovery. It is additionally helpful if patients are placed on a "salivary rest" diet (see details that follow) for 10 to 14 days after surgery to reduce overall salivary output. In a male face, or in a large female face, 2 subcutaneous drains may be required to adequately drain the subcutaneous space. In short scar neck lift procedures, the subcutaneous undermining typically does not extend to the occiput, as it does when an extended neck lift or facelift is performed, and a 2.5-mm liposuction cannula can be used to tunnel from the post–auricular scalp to the subcutaneous space in the anterior neck and pull the drain tube retrograde into position. The drain can then be anchored to the occipital scalp with a 4 to 0 nylon suture (or other suture of choice). Additional details on drain placement can be found (see Timothy Marten and Dino Elyassnia's, "Neck Lift: Defining Anatomic Problems and Choosing Appropriate Treatment Strategies," in this issue).

Final Contouring of Cervicofacial Fat

Once correction of deep-layer neck problems has been made and platysmaplasty, has been performed, final contouring of subcutaneous fat should be performed. This can be done under direct vision using Metzenbaum scissors or a small suction cannula. Final fat sculpting should be continued until all contours are smooth and regular, but *it is essential that not all fat be removed if an attractive appearance is to be obtained*. In addition, if a "double chin" or "witch's chin" is present, an extended dissection of the peri-mental area and chin pad should be made and fat contributing to these problems sculpted and excised and the two regions seamlessly blended to ensure a smooth transition for the chin to the submental area (see **Figs. 6** and **7**).

Skin Closure

When a short scar neck lift is performed, a submental incision only will be present and this can be conveniently closed in 2 layers. Before closure, it is important to confirm that the wound edge thickness and amount of subcutaneous fat present on each side of the incision is similar. Typically, the wound edge of the cervical side will have a thinner edge and have less subcutaneous fat because of contact with instruments and retractors during the preceding steps in the procedure, and the mental, superior side will be thicker and have more fat. If a discrepancy is present, as it often will be, fat is carefully removed from the thicker superior side. The first layer of closure consists of several subcutaneous sutures of 5 to 0 Monocryl (or other suture of choice) to ensure that an equal amount of fat is present behind each edge of the closed wound and so that a depressed or irregular scar is avoided. Final approximation is then made with simple interrupted sutures of 6 to 0 nylon (or other suture of choice).

Dressings

No dressing is needed or applied, as closed suction drains effectively close down dead space. Unlike when an extended neck lift or facelift and neck lift are performed, a softly applied elastic neck band can be placed around the submental region and the top of the head if desired. The advantages and disadvantages of a dressing after neck surgery are discussed (see Timothy Marten and Dino Elyassnia's, "Neck Lift: Defining Anatomic Problems and Choosing Appropriate Treatment Strategies," in this issue).

POSTOPERATIVE CARE

Postoperative care of the patient with neck lift is discussed (see Timothy Marten and Dino Elyassnia's, "Neck Lift: Defining Anatomic Problems and Choosing Appropriate Treatment Strategies," in this issue).

After Surgery Diet

Patients undergoing neck lift that includes deep-layer subplatysmal maneuvers are placed on a "salivary rest" diet consisting of soft, wet easy-to-chew and swallow foods and are encouraged to avoid sweet, salty, sour, dry, citrus, chocolate, and difficult-to-chew foods for several weeks. It is particularly important to avoid the sorts of foods that stimulate salivation for 7 to 14 days if submandibular gland reduction has been performed if fluid collections and induration of neck tissues is to be avoided. Patients are asked to abstain from the intake of alcohol for 2 weeks after surgery.

Drain Removal

Drains are usually left in the neck until the patient's first clinic visit for suture removal 5 days after surgery. Typically, drain output often quickly falls on the first or second day after surgery during the time the patient is mostly supine and resting, but then typically picks up again when the patient begins to spend more time upright, starts to move his or her head about more, and begins to eat more. Leaving the neck drains in longer, for 5 to 7 days, will reduce the likelihood that collections will form and will speed the overall resolution of edema, ecchymosis, and induration in the neck area. Additional details on drain removal can be found (see Timothy Marten and Dino Elyassnia's, "Neck Lift: Defining Anatomic Problems and Choosing Appropriate Treatment Strategies," in this issue).

CASE EXAMPLES
Patient Example 1: Short Scar Neck Lift in a Man with a Shaved Head

Fig. 13 shows before and after surgery views of a man who has had no prior surgery. Note lax skin, obtuse cervicosubmental contour, and "double-chin" appearance when the patient looks down in the before views. A large submandibular gland is palpable but not visible due to a large collection of subplatysmal fat and lax platysma and skin. His shaved head ostensibly precludes traditional neck lift surgery.

Fig. 13 also shows the same patient after short scar neck lift. The procedure included excision of excess subplatysmal fat, submandibular salivary gland reduction, superficial digastric myectomy, and anterior platysmaplasty. No incisions were made in the peri-auricular areas and a chin implant has not been placed. Note well-defined jaw line and attractive, youthful-appearing neckline even when the patient looks down. He has a fit, athletic, and masculine appearance. The only scar is in the submental area. No skin was removed in the procedure.

Patient Example 2: Short Scar Neck Lift in a Young Woman with a Full Neck

Fig. 14 shows before and after surgery views of a young woman who has had no prior surgery. Note lax skin, obtuse cervicosubmental contour, and "double-chin" appearance when the patient looks down in the before view. A large submandibular gland is partially visible and palpable preoperatively but partially hidden due to a large collection of subplatysmal fat and lax platysma and skin.

Fig. 14 also shows the same patient after short scar neck lift. The procedure included excision of excess subplatysmal fat, submandibular salivary gland reduction, superficial digastric myectomy, and anterior platysmaplasty. No incisions were made in the peri-auricular areas and a chin implant has not been placed. Note improved jaw line and neckline even when the patient looks down. The only scar is in the submental area. No skin was removed in the procedure.

Patient Example 3: Short Scar Neck Lift in a Woman Who Had Undergone Previous LeForte 3 Advancement and Sliding Genioplasty

Fig. 15 shows before and after surgery views of a woman who has had previous LeForte 3 mandibular advancement and sliding genioplasty performed by an unknown surgeon. Note that despite these procedures, the patient has lax skin, obtuse cervicosubmental contour, and poor cervicosubmental contour. A large submandibular gland is palpable but not visible due to a large collection of subplatysmal fat and lax platysma and skin.

Fig. 15 also shows the same patient after short scar neck lift. The procedure included excision of excess subplatysmal fat, submandibular salivary gland reduction, superficial digastric myectomy, and anterior platysmaplasty. No incisions were made in the peri-auricular areas and no other procedures were performed. A chin implant has not been placed. Note well-defined jaw line and attractive, youthful-appearing neckline even when the patient looks down. The only scar is in the submental area. No skin was removed in the procedure.

Patient Example 4: Short Scar Neck Lift in a Young Man with a Full Neck

Fig. 16 shows before and after surgery views of a man, who has had no prior surgery. Note lax skin, obtuse cervicosubmental contour, and "double-chin" appearance when the patient looks down in the before views. A large submandibular gland is palpable but not visible due to a large collection of subplatysmal fat and lax platysma and skin. His young age and short haircut made him reluctant to submit to having peri-auricular scars.

Fig. 16 also shows the same patient after short scar neck lift. The procedure included excision of excess subplatysmal fat, submandibular salivary gland reduction, superficial digastric myectomy, and anterior platysmaplasty. No incisions were made in the peri-auricular areas and no other procedures were performed. A chin implant has not been placed. Note markedly improved cervicosubmental contour and attractive, youthful-appearing neckline even when the patient looks down. The only scar is in the submental area. No skin was removed in the procedure.

Patient Example 5: Short Scar Neck Lift in a Middle-Aged Man with a Full Neck

Fig. 17 shows before and after surgery views of a man who has had no prior surgery. Note lax skin, obtuse cervicosubmental contour, and "double-chin" appearance when the patient looks down in the before views. A large submandibular gland is palpable but not visible due to a large collection of subplatysmal fat and lax platysma and skin. It does not appear possible to improve his neck without removing skin.

Fig. 17 also shows the same patient after short scar neck lift. The procedure included excision of excess subplatysmal fat, submandibular salivary gland reduction, superficial digastric myectomy, and anterior platysmaplasty. No incisions were made in the peri-auricular areas and no other procedures were performed. A chin implant has not been placed. Note markedly improved cervicosubmental contour and attractive, youthful-appearing neckline even when the patient looks down. The only scar is in the submental area. No skin was removed in the procedure.

Patient Example 6: Short Scar Neck Lift in a Middle-Aged Man with a Full Neck

Fig. 18 shows before and after surgery views of a man who has had no prior surgery. Note lax skin,

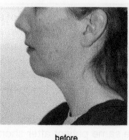 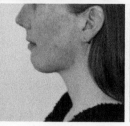 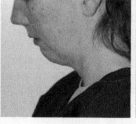 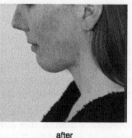

before   after   before   after

Fig. 15. Short scar neck lift in a woman who had undergone previous LeForte 3 advancement and sliding genioplasty. Before and after surgery views of a woman who has had previous LeForte 3 mandibular advancement and sliding genioplasty performed by an unknown surgeon. A chin implant has not been placed. The patient is shown 9 months following her procedure. Surgical procedure performed by Dino Elyassnia, MD, FACS. (*Courtesy of* Dino Elyassnia, MD, FACS, Marten Clinic of Plastic Surgery, San Francisco, CA.)

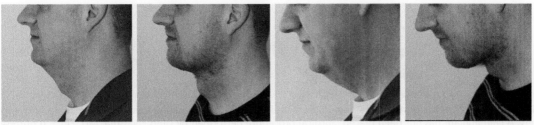

Fig. 16. Short scar neck lift in a young man with a full neck. Before and after surgery views of a man who has had no prior surgery. A chin implant has not been placed. Surgical procedure performed by Dino Elyassnia, MD, FACS. (*Courtesy of* Dino Elyassnia, MD, FACS, Marten Clinic of Plastic Surgery, San Francisco, CA.)

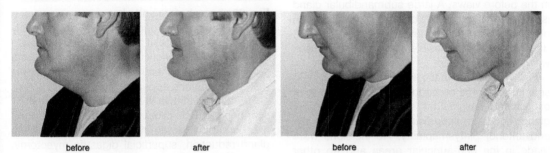

before   after   before   after

Fig. 17. Short scar neck lift in a middle-aged man with a full neck. Before and after surgery views of a man who has had no prior surgery. A chin implant has not been placed. Surgical procedure performed by Timothy J. Marten, MD, FACS. (*Courtesy of* Timothy J. Marten, MD, FACS, Marten Clinic of Plastic Surgery, San Francisco, CA).

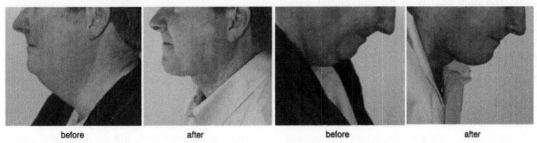

before   after   before   after

Fig. 18. Short scar neck lift in a middle-aged man with a full neck. Before and after surgery views of a man who has had no prior surgery. A chin implant has not been placed. Surgical procedure performed by Timothy J. Marten, MD, FACS. (*Courtesy of* Timothy J. Marten, MD, FACS, Marten Clinic of Plastic Surgery, San Francisco, CA.)

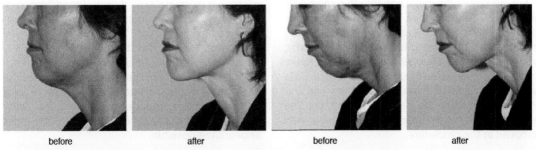

before   after   before   after

Fig. 19. Short scar neck lift in a middle-aged woman. Before and after surgery views of a woman who has had no prior surgery. A chin implant has not been placed. Surgical procedure performed by Timothy J. Marten, MD, FACS. (*Courtesy of* Timothy J. Marten, MD, FACS, Marten Clinic of Plastic Surgery, San Francisco, CA.)

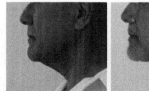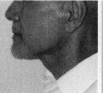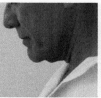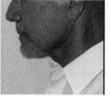

Fig. 20. Short scar neck lift in an older man. Before and after surgery views of a man who has had no prior surgery. A chin implant has not been placed. Surgical procedure performed by Dino Elyassnia, MD, FACS. (*Courtesy of* Dino Elyassnia, MD, FACS, Marten Clinic of Plastic Surgery, San Francisco, CA.)

obtuse cervicosubmental contour, and "double-chin" appearance when the patient looks down in the before views. A large submandibular gland is palpable but not visible due to a large collection of subplatysmal fat and lax platysma and skin. It does not appear possible to improve his neck without removing skin.

Fig. 18 also shows the same patient after short scar neck lift. The procedure included excision of excess subplatysmal fat, submandibular salivary gland reduction, superficial digastric myectomy, and anterior platysmaplasty. No incisions were made in the peri-auricular areas and no other procedures were performed. A chin implant has not been placed. Note markedly improved cervicosubmental contour and attractive, youthful-appearing neckline even when the patient looks down. The only scar is in the submental area. No skin was removed in the procedure.

Patient Example 7: Short Scar Neck Lift in a Middle-Aged Woman

Fig. 19 shows before and after surgery views of a woman who has had no prior surgery. She is arguably a candidate for a facelift procedure. Note lax skin, obtuse cervicosubmental contour, and "weak chin" appearance when the patient looks down. A large submandibular gland can be seen protruding in the lateral neck preoperatively. Note also paucity of subcutaneous fat. Liposuction would make the patient's appearance worse.

Fig. 19 shows the same patient after short scar neck lift. The procedure included excision of excess subplatysmal fat, submandibular salivary gland reduction, superficial digastric myectomy, and anterior platysmaplasty. No incisions were made in the peri-auricular areas and a chin implant has not been placed. Note improved jaw line and neckline even when the patient looks down. The only scar is in the submental area. No skin was removed in the procedure.

Patient Example 8: Short Scar Neck Lift in an Older Man

Fig. 20 shows before and after surgery views of a man who has had no prior surgery. He is arguably a candidate for a facelift procedure. Note lax, aged skin, obtuse cervicosubmental contour, and paucity of subcutaneous fat. Liposuction would make the patient's appearance worse.

Fig. 20 also shows the same patient after short scar neck lift. The procedure included excision of excess subplatysmal fat, submandibular salivary gland reduction, superficial digastric myectomy, and anterior platysmaplasty. No incisions were made in the peri-auricular areas and a chin implant has not been placed. Note improved jaw line and neckline even when the patient looks down. The only scar is in the submental area. No skin was removed in the procedure.

SUMMARY

For a distinct subset of patients, poor neck contour exists as a largely isolated problem, and in many cases these patients can be treated with a short scar neck lift procedure in which no skin is removed. Typically, these patients include younger women with full, obtuse necks and young and middle-aged men with poor neck contour. Although submental liposuction alone will rarely produce optimal neck improvement, a neck lift performed through a submental incision without any removal of skin can create attractive cervical contour in many patients if proper modification of deep-layer structures contributing to cervicosubmental obtusity is made. "Excess" skin is allowed to contract and redistribute itself over the increased neck surface area created when deep-layer techniques are used and neck contour is improved. For carefully selected patients, a short scar neck lift can produce some of the most satisfying and spectacular improvements in facial appearance possible.

Surgical and Nonsurgical Perioral/Lip Rejuvenation
Beyond Volume Restoration

Catherine Winslow, MD*

KEYWORDS

- Lip rejuvenation • SMAS • Perioral rejuvenation • Enhancement

KEY POINTS

- Rejuvenation of the perioral region is often overlooked, but contributes to successful holistic facial enhancement.
- Younger patients especially are seeking longer lasting options for volume enhancement in addition to rejuvenation.
- Comprehensive perioral rejuvenation requires proper assessment and skill at restoring youthful skin and lip proportions in addition to volumizing.

Addressing the neck and midface in lower facial rejuvenation is typically the highest priority for both patient and surgeon. Evaluation and treatment of the aging perioral complex on the other hand is seen as a secondary consideration, or often ignored completely. Especially relevant in the age of social media and the growing popularity of fillers, patients are with increasing frequency expecting rejuvenation of this area to be a part of global lower facial rejuvenation. It is thus crucial that facial plastic surgeons understand the anatomy, aging process, and treatment options for improving the aging perioral region, which is unaltered with rhytidectomy alone.

The perioral complex consists of the white upper and lower lip and mucosal surfaces of the lips, and is defined laterally by the melolabial folds coursing to the prejowl sulcus. Aging of the lower face and perioral region occurs globally, typically starting in the third to fourth decades. Loss of volume in the skeletal structure, midfacial fat pads, and subcutaneous fat lead to soft tissue descent.[1] The midface has both deeper and subcutaneous fat that serves to allow more tissue glide and

descent with age. The perioral region possesses skin with minimal subcutaneous fat and more aggressive muscular insertion into the skin. This accounts for not only the depth of the lateral fold owing to the midfacial descent, but also the obvious visibility of perioral rhytids.[2]

Aging of the nose–lip junction leads to tip ptosis and loss of rotation, contributing to the sagging appearance of the upper lip complex. Loss of maxillary bone and sometimes dentition contribute to less prominence of the lip. Diminishing collagen and elastin in the skin occur with age and are accentuated by ultraviolet exposure and nicotine use. Aging skin causes lengthening of the white lip, occurring in concert with shortening of the visible mucosal surface and flattening of the lip.[3] This feature is evident in a less conspicuous vermillion, cupid's bow, and philtral ridge definition and the introduction of "lipstick lines" or vertical rhytids emanating from the vermillion and extending in to the white upper lip. Overall, the lip changes from a 3-dimensional youthful protuberance to a 2-dimensional elongated and flattened structure.

Disclosure: The author has nothing to disclose.
Indiana University School of Medicine, 1130 West Michigan Street, Indianapolis, IN 46202, USA
* 2000 East 116th Street, Suite 200, Carmel, IN 46032.
E-mail address: Drwinslow@indyface.com

Clin Plastic Surg 45 (2018) 601–609
https://doi.org/10.1016/j.cps.2018.06.008
0094-1298/18/© 2018 Elsevier Inc. All rights reserved.

Surgical options to restore youth to the perioral complex involve 3 separate but complementary categories. First, volume restoration is critical to restoring 3-dimensional youth. Widely used injectable fillers are excellent for temporary improvements, but surgical permanent options exist that may be more attractive to patients. Second, changes in the length of the length of the white lip and relationship of white/pink show should be evaluated and addressed if necessary and appropriate. Finally, the intrinsic condition of the skin can be addressed to improve pigment and texture, elastin and collagen content, fine and coarse rhytids, and overall glow of youth.

VOLUME ENHANCEMENT

Injectable fillers are commonly used to improve lip volume and to sculpt and define the vermillion and philtral border as they flatten with age. They are also popular in youth, with younger patients desiring more volume than that they were naturally given. A recent study showed the ideal lip represented a 53.5% increase in volume over the natural lip of a youthful woman. Although culturally variable, an ideal upper:lower lip ration was noted as 1:2.[4] As a short-term alternative, fillers are an excellent option. However, they are painful to inject and currently no permanent injectable filler that is approved by the US Food and Drug Administration exists. Surgical options for long-term or permanent volume enhancement involve fat grafting or placement of an implant via a small incision in the mucosa. Most implants are fed through a small tunnel with curved tendon forceps. Because the mucosa is too thin to hide irregularities or asymmetries, the ideal implant is soft, symmetric, and integrates well with tissue. A few viable options exist, both in alloplastic and autologous form.

Alloplastic options include tissue and plastic implants. Tissue alloplasts such as cadaveric dermis have not shown permanence or consistent longevity and have been cost prohibitive for

short-term volumizing in the era of injectable fillers. Permanent plastic materials have been tried with variable success. Migration, infection, asymmetry, and palpability/visibility limit the use of such implants and complications typically require removal. Extended poly tetrafluroethylene (Gore-Tex) is an option popularized decades ago for its ease of placement and permanence (**Fig. 1**). One commercially available implant (Advanta) was packaged preloaded on a long thick needle for ease of insertion. Extended poly tetrafluroethylene has not been shown to be an ideal implant for the lips, however. Although tissue integration is excellent, the implant has a tendency toward shrinking and contracture that leads to an irregular and often asymmetric contour. The aggressive tissue integration makes the implant very difficult to remove without tearing and trauma to the mucosa. The material has largely been abandoned for the lips with the advent of injectable fillers and other more natural alternatives.

Another alloplastic option is a silicone implant. Currently, Surgisil Permalip implants are commercially available in different widths and lengths as a permanent alternative to injectables. A small incision is made in the mucosa and the implant is fed through a small tunnel with curved forceps. After ensuring midline placement, the incisions are closed with dissolvable sutures. The implant has the advantage of being able to be placed under local anesthesia and is easy to remove. Potential complications such as infection and significant asymmetry usually require implant removal. The cost is relatively low for patient and surgeon (cost to surgeon is approximately $300 per lip) and the implant is approved by the US Food and Drug Administration for lip enhancement. Perhaps the biggest detractor for this option is the palpability of the implant under the thin covering of the mucosal surface. Although the implant is soft, it still possesses the resilience of plastic. When the lip is rolled between the fingers, the implant is

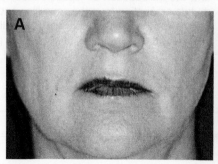 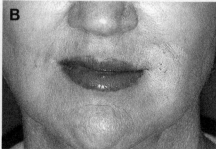

Fig. 1. Extended poly tetrafluoroethylene implant before (*A*) and after (*B*) placement with immediate volume improvements. This patient eventually requested removal owing to visibility with muscular contraction of lips.

palpable. In select patients with proper expectations, however, satisfaction is very high (**Fig. 2**).

Autogenous volume enhancement has the benefit of longevity over fillers while minimizing risks of alloplastic materials. Commonly used autogenous options include fat and fascia. Fat has been used for decades with variable results. A seemingly never ending debate over longevity and predictability has led to the continued search for different options. Fat requires a separate harvest site, but is easily injected in the lip. Complications such as prolonged swelling, asymmetry, and lumpiness are not uncommon. Contrary to other areas of the face, the permanence of fat in the lip seems less predictable, perhaps owing to the constant muscle contraction surrounding it.[5] Results typically last less than 1 year. Long-term objective results of persistence of volume are difficult to find, but with the advent of fillers lasting at least a year, surgical options must at least exceed the best results possible with fillers to have a distinct advantage for the increased risk.

As an alternative to fat, many surgeons have utilized the strips of the superficial musculoaponeurotic system (SMAS) harvested with SMAS facelifts as lip implants. The SMAS excision can be extended along the anterior border of the sternocleidomastoid muscle to increase the length of the strip harvested, especially if the strip is to be used for lip augmentation. After harvesting, the SMAS should be addressed to remove fat globules (typically by scraping with the side of a blade) and the ends tapered (**Fig. 3**). The SMAS is inserted through small incisions in the mucosa through which an isolated tunnel is created. The tunnel ideally is centered just below the vermillion to optimize the eversion and vermillion definition of the lip. The SMAS is passed with a curved tendon passer (**Fig. 4**) and the incisions are closed with a dissolvable suture after massaging the lip to ensure the tissue is fully stretched over the implant. The upper and lower lips should both be addressed to avoid disproportion in the lower face (**Fig. 5**).

Long-term outcomes with SMAS have been excellent. Studies have shown persistence of SMAS to and beyond 5 years with excellent patient satisfaction and very low complication rates.[6,7] Infection is very rare, and extrusion (**Fig. 6**) is treated fairly simply by excising the exposed SMAS and allowing the remainder to heal. Cost of harvest is nothing; the procedure takes approximately 10 minutes to perform at the time of a lift and thus adds little to operative time. Average self-reported patient cost for a lip implant is $2500 (RealSelf.com) and, thus, the return on investment for the procedure is excellent. The technique is simple and well worth the effort to learn as a means of improving the perioral region simultaneously with lower facial rejuvenation.

Take home points for volumizing the lips are as follows: volumizing the lips and changing the 2-dimensional aging lip to the 3-dimensional youthful lip is a crucial part of lower facial rejuvenation; plastic materials are commercially available, approved by the US Food and Drug Administration, and useful in select patients while possessing limitations. SMAS provides long-term/permanent lip volume in a natural fashion and can be added to a facelift to greatly improve patient satisfaction in a very cost-effective manner (**Fig. 7**).

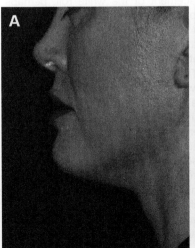
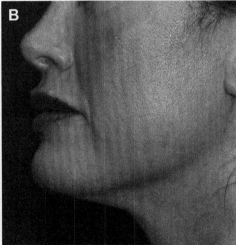

Fig. 2. Sillicone implant before (*A*) and after (*B*) placement with excellent volume improvements.

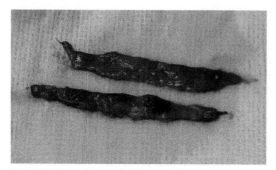

Fig. 3. Strips of superficial musculoaponeurotic system (SMAS) harvested from facelift, defatted, and tapered, ready for implantation.

ALTERATIONS IN LIP CONTOUR

In addition to volumetric changes, proportions of the lips alter with age. As noted, the lengthening of the white lip occurs on both the lower and upper lip in concert with loss of pink mucosal show height. Assessment of perioral aging should include an assessment of lip shape and vertical height of overall lip relative to the upper incisors as well as the proportion of white/pink lip as these all demonstrate changes with aging.[8] Volumizing can improve the amount of pink show somewhat, but does not alter the long white lip. Options for altering proportions of white/pink include subnasal lip lift and vermillion advancement. Mucosal V-Y advancement is occasionally performed as a "push" rather than "pull" to increase mucosal show without altering the lip height. A corner of the lip lift can create a vertical pull on the commissure and improve somewhat a deep marionette line. It is important to keep balance between the upper and lower lip and maintain the general proportion of mucosal show, which typically should be greater for the lower lip.

The subnasal lip lift is an excellent way to address a long upper lip when the inferior border

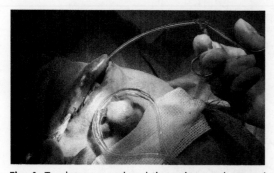

Fig. 4. Tendon passer placed through tunnel created in lip to pull the superficial musculoaponeurotic system through.

of the upper lip mucosa hangs below the upper incisor (**Fig. 8**). If the upper incisor is seen with the mouth slightly open, further shortening of the upper lip can lead to a "rabbit"-like foreshortened upper lip and should be avoided. The lift is performed with an incision that contours around the base of the nose with the incision hidden in the alar crease and contoured just inside the nasal sill. The white portion of the upper lip is measured and typically around one-third of the height is planned for excision with caliper measurements marking the planned excision. This usually corresponds with 5 to 10 mm of skin measured for removal.[9] The skin is excised and no undermining is required before layered closure. The procedure addresses the length of the central two-thirds of the lip, but does not address the lateral lip position and as a result the commissures may look inferiorly displaced relative to preoperative relationships. Additionally, it can affect the proportions between upper and lower lip mucosal show, and volumetric enhancement is not achieved with this procedure in isolation.

Vermillion advancement can be performed to both the upper and lower lips, and has the benefit of less "hard pull" of the upper lip because the mucosa is more effective unfurled. The incision is marked precisely at the vermillion margin and a skin excision is performed. The skin is meticulously closed. Absolute precision with suturing, preferably with a running subcuticular closure to avoid "railroad tracking" is required for acceptable results. The vermillion border is sacrificed with this procedure and great effort must be taken with closure to ensure a satisfactory cosmetic result. The technique is very useful when the patient has a preexisting deformity or scar of the vermillion that can be improved on (**Fig. 9**). Owing to the effacement of the white roll, perhaps the most important landmark of the lip, this procedure is not commonly performed other than in patients with preexisting imperfections or significant asymmetries of the vermillion.

The corner of the lip lift addresses the lateral downturn leading to a pronounced marionette line (**Fig. 10**). This procedure is useful in patients with a "droopy dog" inferior commissure displacement but does not address the central lip or volumetric status unless combined with another procedure such as SMAS placement. The lateral commissure itself is not altered with either vermillion advancement or subnasal lip lift and so this technique is useful in select patients with appropriate anatomy who are willing to trade permanent elevation of the commissure for a scar. The corner of lip lift uses a diamond-shaped excision centered on the commissure as the base. A line

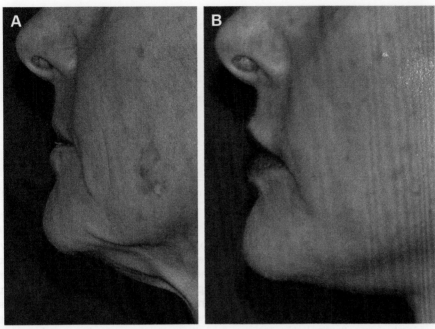

Fig. 5. Superficial musculoaponeurotic system implant, lift and 35% trichloroacetic acid peel before (*A*) and after (*B*). Note improvements both volumetrically and with skin tightening present at 1 year.

is drawn toward the tragus of 5 to 7 mm and then drawn an equidistance along the vermillion. Superiorly, an arc of skin is marked, measuring approximately 5 to 8 mm superior to the commissure. The skin is excised and the commissure is lifted with layered closure. An excellent improvement in lateral position is obtained, although volumetric losses in the marionette line are obviously unaltered. The procedure is quite useful in select patients, with the biggest downside being the rather

visible scar ("joker" line) extending from the lateral commissure. Despite meticulous closure, patients should be warned that the scar may continue to be visible and may require later resurfacing.

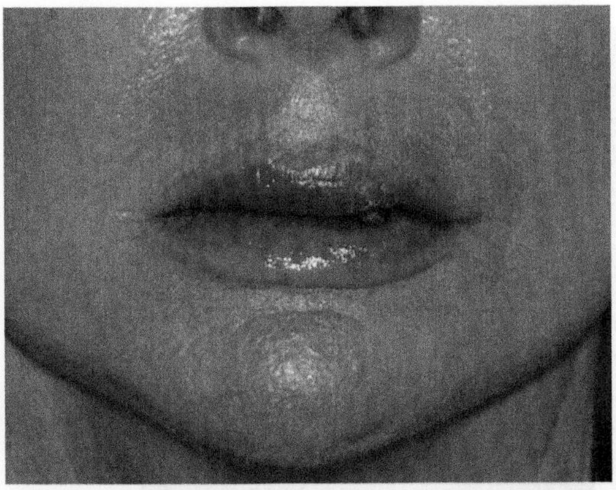

Mucosal show can be improved without altering lip height with a V-Y mucosal advancement. Typically 2 V-Y advancements are done side by side. As the flaps are meticulously closed intraorally, a small amount of increase in mucosal show is observed. The results are somewhat unpredictable, but the procedure can be done to the lower lip in conjunction with a subnasal lip lift to maintain upper/lower lip balance.

Take home points for surgical alteration of lip contour are as follows: not all patients are appropriate for lip lifts and anatomy; expected results and scars should be discussed thoroughly before proceeding; vermillion advancement more dramatically can improve the white/pink ratio at the expense of the critical definition of the white roll; and changing the lip contour in isolation will not alter signs of aging from volumetric or skin changes.

RHYTID IMPROVEMENT

Improving the lipstick lines and vertical rhytids of the white lip can be difficult. The causative factors, such as loss of collagen and elastin and continued muscular contraction, continue to worsen with age no matter the treatment rendered. The short-term

Fig. 6. Superficial musculoaponeurotic system (SMAS) extrusion, treated with antibiotics and excision of extruded portion. The remaining SMAS was firmly adhered and the lip healed with minimal asymmetry and no further sequelae.

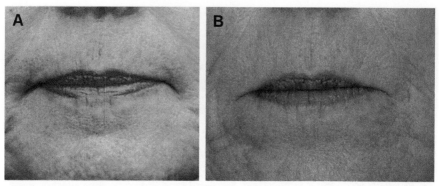

Fig. 7. Superficial musculoaponeurotic system before (A) and eight years after implant (B), still with notable volume improvements.

results seen can be frustrating to patient and physician alike. Muscular contractions from smoking or use of straws should be minimized, as should contributing factors to premature loss of elastin such as ultraviolet exposure and nicotine. Two short-term options that can improve the overall result of perioral rejuvenation include neuromodulators and injectable fillers. Neuromodulators can be used to significantly improve perioral rhytids on a short-term basis, but with a high level of patient satisfaction.[10] These options are useful for maintenance and complementing results of other perioral rejuvenation options.

Volume replacement will somewhat improve rhytids, especially at the vermillion, but optimally is combined with resurfacing. Resurfacing of the lip can more dramatically improve the appearance of perioral rhytids and is often performed with whole face resurfacing. Although the perioral complex can be resurfaced in isolation using the melolabial folds as landmarks, patients with moderate

to severe sun damage will still show lines of demarcation and thus would benefit from treatment to the face as one entity. Ablative resurfacing options in general include lasers, chemical peels, and dermabrasion. Ablative treatments remove the epithelium and require intact pilosebaceous units to provide epithelial cells for reepithelialization. These procedures have been shown to increase the amount of collagens I and III and improve the appearance of collagen and elastin fibers.[11]

Lasers are commonly used for skin resurfacing. Er:YAG lasers are ablative lasers that promote collagen remodeling while improving dyschromias and fine lines. The Er:YAG laser has shown less downtime with erythema and crusting but with less dramatic results for perioral rhytids than those seen with the CO_2 laser.[12] The CO_2 laser is a powerful ablative option that has become less attractive for most facial plastics surgeons after decades of observation showed high rates of

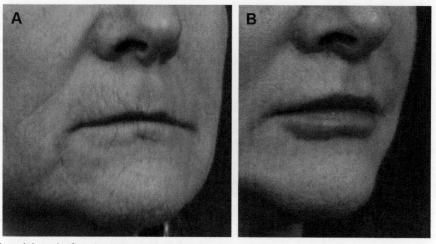

Fig. 8. Before (A) and after (B) sub nasal lip lift and superficial musculoaponeurotic system implantation. Combining procedures improves the overall lip enhancement.

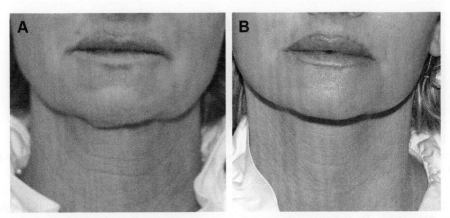

Fig. 9. Before (*A*) and after (*B*) vermillion advancement of upper and lower lips in patient with permanent makeup misadventure; white roll is effaced to effect greater mucosal show.

complications, thinning of the skin, and prolonged erythema and pain. Improvement to CO_2 systems such as the fraxelated approach treat approximately 30% of the surface area of the face and thus impart less risk, although at the expense of less effective results and the possible need for additional treatments.[13] Although the perioral region can safely undergo concurrent facelift with laser resurfacing, the literature is divided on the safety of simultaneous ablative laser full face resurfacing with rhytidectomy. With SMAS and sub-SMAS lifts, however, less subcutaneous dissection is performed, thus, increasing the safety of simultaneous treatments. Nevertheless, many surgeons prefer to wait 6 weeks to 6 months postoperatively before resurfacing. Intraoperative laser treatments require protective eyewear, special equipment, and safety precautions. The cost to surgeon and patient is moderate to high. Lasers are not indicated for patients with hepatitis or human immunodeficiency virus owing to the aerosolization of blood and skin.

Dermabrasion is a mechanical sanding of the skin to improve textural irregularities such as scars and deep rhytids (**Fig. 11**). It is performed with a rapidly spinning diamond fraise, although some surgeons use a sandpaper-type abrasion. Classic descriptions of this technique include ensuring the skin is pulled taut during the procedure. Cryogenic sprays were commonly used to minimize soft tissue movement. Bleeding petechial spots are first seen, indicating penetration through the epidermis. White fibrillar strands indicate the endpoint of reticular dermis. At the conclusion of the procedure, brisk bleeding is common; thus, the procedure is not advocated for patients with hematologic contagious conditions such as hepatitis or human immunodeficiency virus. Postprocedural pain is minimal and the area is kept moist with a semiocclusive dressing or petroleum layer. Healing is typically complete with reepithelialization by 5 to 7 days; however, erythema may persist for weeks. Results with dermabrasion are comparable in effacement of perioral rhytids to superpulsed CO_2 with less erythema and pain postoperatively.[14] It can be combined with laser resurfacing or chemical peels, with dermabrasion targeting specific areas, and with peels or lasers resurfacing the remaining face.[15] No lines of demarcation are seen when combining with full face trichloracetic acid performed first.

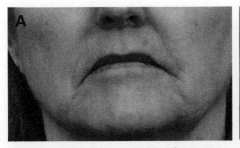
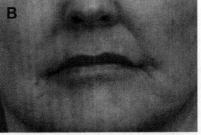

Fig. 10. Before (*A*) and after (*B*) corner of lip lift in patient with severe marionette line depression. The lateral scar is evident, although overall lip improvements are marked.

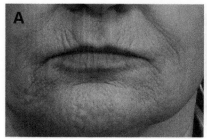
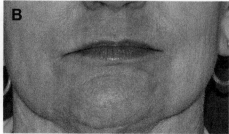

Fig. 11. Before (*A*) and three months post (*B*) perioral dermabrastion (with 35% trichloroacetic acid full face peel performed simultaneously) with some persistent erythema but significant improvement in rhytids.

Chemical peels are available at the superficial, medium, or deep levels. Superficial peels are not ablative and therefore are used for maintenance, not rejuvenation. Medium peels are ablative and extend into the papillary dermis. The most commonly used medium depth peel is 35% trichloracetic acid, often combined with Jessners' solution. This peel is easily applied to the entire face, and 20% trichloracetic acid can be taken onto the neck to avoid lines of demarcation. Medium depth peels are remarkably effective for fine lines and hyperpigmentation, but will not improve severe rhytids. For patients with less severe skin damage it is an excellent, low-cost addition to global facial rejuvenation, can be performed safely at the same time as surgery, and provides predictable improvements in collagen, elastin, and skin tone. Deep peels such as Baker-Gordon peels were formerly thought to be effective owing to phenol penetration into the reticular dermis. More recent research has shown resourcinol to be the main effective ingredient[16] and, thus, the paradigm has shifted toward a lower phenol concentration with the resourcinol concentration altered to the desired result. With any inclusion of phenol, the potential for cardiac, renal, and hepatic damage is unavoidable and thus these peels, although very effective for deep rhytids, are not commonly used.

Selection of treatment options for resurfacing is based on experience, comfort, patient preference, and cost. Newer technologies such as lasers and skin-tightening platforms require in initial financial investment and additional safety considerations. Older technologies such as dermabrasion and chemical peels require virtually no startup investment, but many surgeons lack proper training in these techniques. Technologies are often combined to improve results and minimize lines of demarcation and prolonged healing.

Take home points for lip resurfacing are as follows: addressing resurfacing of the perioral complex is often best done by resurfacing the entire face to minimize lines of demarcation; resurfacing

should be combined with other surgical and nonsurgical options for best cosmetic results of perioral aging; and older technologies such as chemical peels and dermabrasion are very effective and often much more cost effective than lasers and should not be neglected as a viable option for resurfacing.

SUMMARY

The perioral complex ages the lower face and reluctance to address this area leads to an incomplete rejuvenation of the lower face. Incorporating perioral rejuvenation into the plan for lower facial surgery can help to complete the youthful look sought by patients. Injectable fillers provide excellent but short-term benefits and additional options exist that offer the patient permanent improvements at a low cost. A thorough understanding and competence of different options to address volume restoration, lip proportion improvements, and aging skin are crucial to the facial plastic surgeon as tools to consistently obtain optimal results in the lower face, and improve overall satisfaction at a low cost.

REFERENCES

1. Sadick NS, Dorizas AS, Krueger N, et al. The facial adipose system: its role in facial aging and approaches to volume restoration. Dermatol Surg 2015;41(suppl 1):S333–9.
2. Karsan N, Ellis DA. The lip-cheek groove, a new analysis with treatment options. Arch Facial Plast Surg 2006;8:324–8.
3. Raschke GF, Rieger UM, Bader RD, et al. Perioral aging- an anthropometric appraisal. J Craniomaxillofac Surg 2014;42(5):a312–7.
4. Popenko NA, Tripathi PB, Devcic Z, et al. A quantitative approach to determining the ideal female lip aesthetic and its effect on facial attractiveness. JAMA Facial Plast Surg 2017;19(4):261–7.
5. Eremia S, Newman N. Long term follow up after autologous fat grafting: analysis of results from 116

patients followed at least 12 months after receiving the last of a minimum of two treatments. Dermatol Surg 2000;26(12):1150–8.

6. Leaf N, Firouz JS. Lip augmentation with superficial musculoaponeurotic system grafts: report of 103 cases. Plast Reconstr Surg 2002;109(1):319–26.

7. Richardson MA, Rousso DE, Replogle WH. Long term analysis of lip augmentation with superficial musculoaponeurotic system (SMAS) tissue transfer following biplanar extended SMAS rhytidectomy. JAMA Facial Plast Surg 2017;19(1):34–9.

8. Penna V, Stark GB, Voigt M, et al. Classification of the aging lips; a foundation for an integrated approach to perioral rejuvenation. Aesthetic Plast Surg 2015;39(1):1–7.

9. Waldman SR. The subnasal lift. Facial Plast Surg Clin North Am 2007;15(4):513–6.

10. Cohen JL, Dayan SH, Cox SE, et al. Onabotulinum-toxinA dose-ranging study for hyperdynamic perioral lines. Dermatol Surg 2012;38(9):1497–505.

11. El-Domyait MB, Attia SK, Saleh FY, et al. Trichloroacetic acid peeling versus dermabrasion: a histometric, immunohistochemical and ultrastructural comparison. Dermatol Surg 2004;30(2 Pt 1): 179–88.

12. Newman JB, Lord JL, Ash K, et al. Variable pulse erbium:YAG laser skin resurfacing of perioral rhytides and side-by-side comparison with carbon dioxide laser. Lasers Surg Med 2000;26(2):208–14.

13. Karsai S, Czarnecka A, Jünger M, et al. Ablative fractional lasers (CO2 and Er:YAG):a randomized controlled double blind split face trial of the treatment of periorbial rhytids. Lasers Surg Med 2010; 42(2):160–7.

14. Holmkvist KA, Rogers GS. Treatment of perioral rhytides: a comparison of dermabrasion and super-pulsed carbon dioxide laser. Arch Dermatol 2000; 136(6):725–31.

15. Roenigk HH. Dermbrasion: state of the art 2002. J Cosmet Dermatol 2002;1(2):72–87.

16. Hetter GP. An examination of the phenol-croton oil peel: part IV. Face peel results with different concentrations of phenol and croton oil. Plast Reconstr Surg 2000;105(3):1061–83.

Difficult Necks and Unresolved Problems in Neck Rejuvenation

Ryan M. Smith, MD[a], Ira D. Papel, MD[a,b],*

KEYWORDS

- Neck rejuvenation • Neck lift • Face lift • Aging face • Cosmetic surgery

KEY POINTS

- Aesthetic changes related to facial aging include excess skin laxity, volume loss, and contour irregularities and may impart an aged or unattractive facial appearance.
- Neck rejuvenation techniques aim to restore the features of facial beauty found in youth including a well-defined jaw contour, optimal cervicomental angle, smooth-appearing skin without laxity, and normally positioned soft tissue volume.
- Variations in anatomy, skin quality, and fat content make some cases inherently challenging and may limit the degree to which improvement can be made.
- Specific considerations and techniques may be used to address these problem areas and improve outcomes.
- Careful patient evaluation, counseling, and management of expectations is critical for patient satisfaction in difficult cases.

INTRODUCTION

The appearance of the neck has a profound impact on the overall youthfulness and attractiveness of the face. Changes of facial aging involve the skin, soft tissue, and underlying bone loss as this process progresses. Over time, excess skin laxity, volume loss, and contour irregularities combine to impart an aged and unattractive look. All facial rejuvenation procedures aim to restore the ideal features of facial beauty found in youth.

Facelift and necklift operations have grown in both societal acceptance and popularity since the 1970s.[1] A better anatomic understanding of the dynamics of facial aging coupled with improved techniques for superficial musculoaponeurotic system (SMAS) mobilization have established these procedures as powerful treatment options.[2,3] There are now a variety of sound techniques that can be performed safely and effectively.

However, the success of surgery does not solely depend on technique. Variations in anatomy, skin quality, and fat content make some cases inherently and particularly challenging. Additionally, psychological expectations vary based on the individual's perception of the problem and motivation for change. Patient satisfaction after surgery can be improved through careful communication of these inherent limitations and by setting realistic expectations. Only after rigorous patient evaluation and counseling can technical modifications of the surgical approach prove useful.

Disclosure Statement: The authors have nothing to disclose.

[a] Division of Facial Plastic and Reconstructive Surgery, Department of Otolaryngology–Head and Neck Surgery, Johns Hopkins School of Medicine, 601 North Caroline Street, 6th Floor, Baltimore, MD 21287, USA; [b] Facial Plastic Surgicenter, 1838 Greene Tree Road, Suite 370, Baltimore, MD 21208, USA

* Corresponding author. Facial Plastic Surgicenter, 1838 Greene Tree Road, Suite 370, Baltimore, MD 21208.

E-mail address: Ira.papel.md@gmail.com

Clin Plastic Surg 45 (2018) 611–622
https://doi.org/10.1016/j.cps.2018.06.009

The goal of this article is to examine the difficult neck. The most common difficult situations encountered during neck rejuvenation are presented and several unsolved problem areas discussed. Clinical examples as well as specific surgical approaches are included.

MOST COMMON DIFFICULT SITUATIONS
Anterior Hyoid and/or Retrognathia

The ideal neck displays a well-defined jaw and optimal cervicomental angle, which reflect a balance between underlying bony support and soft tissue projection. The variable anatomy of the hyoid bone and mandible may limit the ability to restore these features.

The hyoid bone is a horseshoe-shaped bone in the midline of the anterior neck typically found at or above the level of the fourth cervical vertebra. Unlike other bones, the hyoid is only loosely articulated with adjacent bony structures and mostly suspended by the suprahyoid and infrahyoid musculature.[4] In 1992, Guyuron[5] performed cephaloxerograms on 54 patients and reported a variable hyoid position in both the cranial–caudal and anteroposterior dimensions. This variation can influence the cervicomental angle as the suprahyoid muscles insert on the hyoid bone from their origin on the inferior mandible. Ideally, this angle should measure between 105° and 120°.[6]

A high and posterior hyoid position is most favorable, because the suprahyoid muscles course horizontally to create a sharp cervicomental angle. Conversely, a low and anterior position is associated with a vertical orientation and more obtuse angle. This configuration can lead to the appearance of a double chin or heavy neck.

The hyoid position is important to identify preoperatively, because it will influence the degree to which improvement can be made. The Dedo classification system was designed to categorize patients anatomically, with class VI representing a low hyoid position.[7] These patients must be counseled about the limitations of surgery and their expectations should be managed appropriately.

In addition to the hyoid, the position, size, and shape of the mandible can vary. Several methods for assessing chin projection have been described, using either the lower vermillion border or Frankfurt horizontal plane as landmarks.[8] In men, the chin should project to a point along a line tangential to the lower vermillion border. If the Frankfurt plane is used, projection should extend to a perpendicular line that is tangential to the nasion. In women, chin projection should be just posterior to these points. Retrognathia describes a poorly projected, or weak, chin and may be congenital or acquired with age owing to resorption. Micrognathia is a condition in which an underdeveloped chin is associated with dental malocclusion in Angle class II position. Microgenia is characterized by an ill-defined chin without associated occlusal abnormalities.[9] These conditions pose a challenge during neck lift surgery because the inherent structural deficiency of the chin cannot be overcome by improvement in the cervicomental angle alone. In these cases, the aesthetic goal of restoring definition of the jawline is difficult to achieve and the contour will likely remain blunted. Chin augmentation using alloplastic implants or orthognathic consultation in cases with associated malocclusion should be considered. Chin augmentation or advancement genioplasty can help mask the effects of an anterior hyoid position[10] (**Fig. 1**).

Thick/Heavy Skin

The skin is the most external tissue involved in the process of facial aging and, therefore, can betray the youthfulness of facial appearance even in the absence of other signs. Ultimately, the success of neck rejuvenation depends on the ability to correct excess tissue laxity, suspend the strength layers, and redrape the skin into a more youthful position. Definition of the jawline, cervicomental angle, sternocleidomastoid muscle, and trachea are the desired features associated with the aesthetic ideal.[11] This result requires skin that is able to conform, tighten, and contract. The

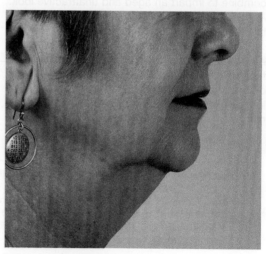

Fig. 1. Anterior hyoid position.

properties of thick skin make this process less likely to happen.

Subcutaneous fat superficial to the platysma may be associated with thick skin and contribute to the appearance of a double chin. Subplatysmal fat is located in a deeper plane and may contribute separately to the cosmetic deformity. Assessment of both the superficial and subplatysmal fat content is important to guide the surgical approach. Patients with thick skin may require more subcutaneous fat removal to allow favorable redraping of the skin, which can influence risk, recovery, and the likelihood for success[12] (**Fig. 2**).

Lax Skin Envelope/Solar Elastosis/Ehlers Danlos Syndrome

Skin-based techniques represent the earliest lifting attempts and have historically been favored owing to shorter operative time and less risk. An improved understanding of the relationship between the SMAS, facial retaining ligaments, and bony framework has led to the development of techniques with greater efficacy and longevity. Regardless of the method, eliminating skin laxity and allowing for smooth redraping of the soft tissue is desired. This process can be challenging in cases of excessive laxity.

Both endogenous and exogenous changes occur in the skin with aging. Endogenous changes include increased skin laxity, wrinkling, and dermal atrophy. This effect results from degradation and decreased mitogenic turnover of keratinocytes, fibroblasts, and melanocytes with a subsequent loss of collagen and elastin content. Exogenous changes accumulate during chronic sun exposure owing to the effects of ultraviolet light in a process called photoaging.[13] This process leads to deepening of wrinkles, leathery consistency, sallowness, pigmentation changes, telangiectasia, and the formation of solar lentigines and actinic keratoses.

Solar elastosis refers to the histopathologic degeneration of dermal elastic tissue owing to photoaging. Specific features include the accumulation of disorganized basophilic elastotic material between the papillary and reticular dermis. The degree of elastosis correlates with the cumulative ultraviolet exposure of the affected skin.[14] There are several pathologically distinct subtypes of solar elastosis that differ in terms of anatomic location and clinical severity. However, all lead to the appearance of yellow, thickened, and coarsely wrinkled skin.

Unlike solar elastosis, Ehlers Danlos syndrome is a genetic disorder of the connective tissue. Of the 13 different types of Ehlers Danlos syndrome that have been classified, type 1, or classical Ehlers Danlos syndrome, has the most severe skin involvement. Type 1 Ehlers Danlos syndrome is an autosomal-dominant condition caused by a

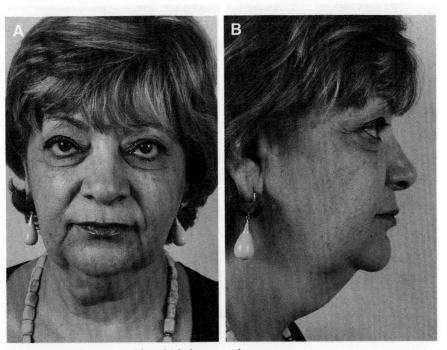

Fig. 2. (*A, B*) A 65-year-old woman with a thick, heavy neck.

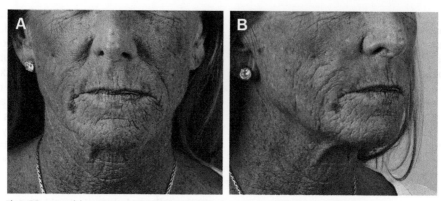

Fig. 3. (*A, B*) A 60-year-old woman with severe actinic damage with loss of elasticity.

mutation in the COL5A1 or COL5A2 genes, which affect type V collagen.[15] Histopathologically, this syndrome is seen as the presence of irregular and disorganized bundles of malformed collagen in the reticular dermis. Clinically, the condition is characterized by the presence of extremely elastic, smooth, and fragile skin that bruises easily and lacks subcutaneous fat.

Patients with excessive skin envelope laxity, as seen in solar elastosis and Ehlers Danlos syndrome, must be counseled carefully. The risks of bruising, bleeding, hematoma, skin flap necrosis, and scarring must be stated (**Figs. 3** and **4**).

Prominent Submandibular Gland

The submandibular glands are located within the submandibular triangle of the neck bound by the mandible, anterior and posterior bellies of the digastric muscle. The gland is composed of a deep and superficial lobe separated by the mylohyoid muscle. The submandibular duct exits the deep lobe to penetrate the floor of mouth.[16]

The location of the gland along the jawline can contribute to contour irregularity in the case of overly prominent glands. Congenital, developmental, inflammatory and postsurgical causes exist. When congenitally prominent, the glands are typically malpositioned; weak support of the

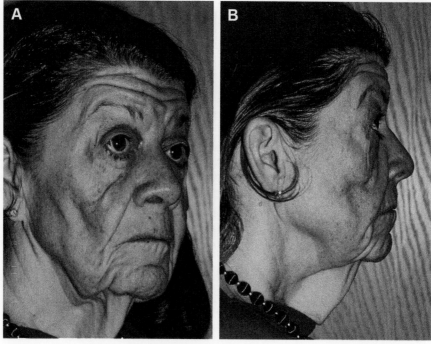

Fig. 4. (*A, B*) A 34-year-old woman with cutix laxa disease.

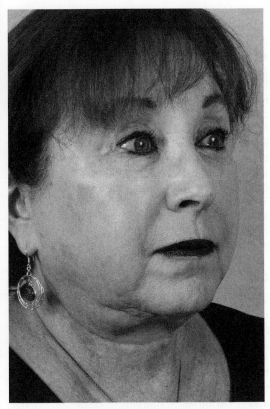

Fig. 5. Prominent submandibular gland in a woman seeking revision facelift surgery.

gland capsule allows them to occupy a more inferior, medial, and visible position. Developmental causes include age-acquired gland ptosis and tissue volume changes related to weight loss. In the case of ptosis, tissue laxity allows descent below the jawline. Chronic inflammation, gland hypertrophy, and sclerosis all have effects on gland size in this new position.[17]

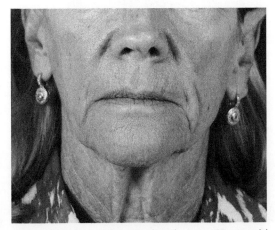

Fig. 6. Prominent platysma bands in a 66-year-old woman seeking facial surgery.

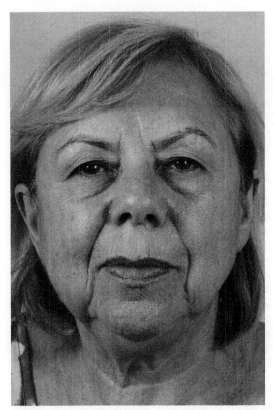

Fig. 7. Deep prejowl sulci in a 70-year-old woman interested in facelift surgery.

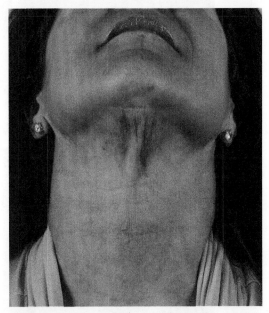

Fig. 8. Skin and subcutaneous fibrosis in a 45-year-old woman seeking revision 1 year after facelift surgery.

Prominent submandibular glands may contribute to the appearance of neck heaviness and contour irregularity in the primary neck lift candidate. Preoperative identification is crucial for appropriate surgical planning. The glands can usually be detected by palpation, even if surrounding tissue excess exists. Prominent glands may also become apparent after facelift if unnoticed or not properly addressed at the time of initial surgery (**Fig. 5**).

Persistent Platysmal Bands

The platysma muscle is a key structure defining the submental contour. With age, the platysma weakens resulting in laxity of the anterior muscular support of the neck. Anterior displacement of the muscle both at rest and with activity may produce unsightly vertical banding. This banding can be associated with the pattern of muscle decussation across the midline, which was found to be only partial in 75% of the population.[18] Without decussation, the muscle cannot serve as an effective sling and the dehiscence allows the medial edges to become prominent.

Persistent platysmal bands after prior treatment can be problematic and frustrating. This problem is seen after platysmaplasty to create a supportive muscular sling by suturing the medial muscle edges together. However, closure at the midline may allow more lateral platysma elements to prolapse medially and cause persistent banding. Even aggressive multilayered closures of the anterior platysma margins can result in persistent visible bands in some cases.[19] In 2016, Jacono and Malone[20] performed a cadaveric study showing significant limitation in rhytidectomy flap mobility with concomitant midline platysmaplasty. The authors suggest that this limitation on redraping can lead to recurrent neck ptosis itself. They present lateral distraction of the platysma as a technique that may avoid this issue in cases of mild to moderate platysmal banding[20] (**Fig. 6**).

Deep Prejowl Sulcus

Vertical descent of the facial soft tissue with aging creates areas of relative tissue excess and contour irregularity that can be seen as unsightly jowling along the mandible. The malar and buccal fat pads have minimal attachments to the underlying bone and become ptotic with age, especially as the platysma weakens and becomes inferiorly displaced. The

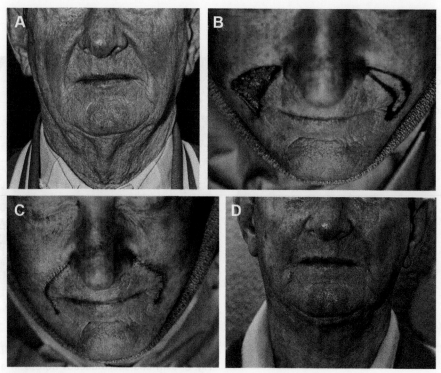

Fig. 9. (*A*) A 68-year-old man concerned with his deep nasolabial folds. (*B, C*) Excision technique. (*D*) Patient at 1 year postoperatively.

visual effect of jowling is amplified by the mandibular cutaneous retaining ligament, which originates on the periosteum and inserts into the dermis.[21] This ligament creates a demarcation between the immobile medial tissues and the lateral jowl along the prejowl sulcus.

A deep prejowl sulcus can be challenging to correct. Accurate preoperative assessment of facial volume changes is crucial for correct surgical decision making, and is best conducted systematically based on the subcutaneous fat compartments of the face. Establishing the correct vector for effacing the sulcus will guide incision planning and the degree of SMAS mobilization required. Ultimately, eliminating the shadow that draws attention to the jowls may require a

combination of lifting techniques and revolumization.[22] Mittelman's prejowl sulcus implant is an attempt to solve this issue.[23] The placement of filler material or fat grafting is also frequently employed (**Fig. 7**).

Revision Cases with No Superficial Musculoaponeurotic System/Platysmal Integrity

The importance of the SMAS layer in rejuvenation has been well-established, and represents one of the major advances in aesthetic facial surgery. The reliance on adequate mobilization and repositioned of the SMAS to effect lasting and significant improvement makes revision cases difficult. The integrity of the SMAS layer may be compromised by prior resection, dissection, suture

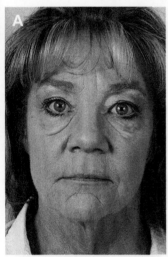
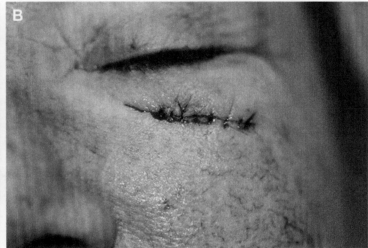
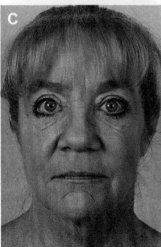

Fig. 10. (*A*) Large malar festoons. (*B*) Direct excision of the festoons. (*C*) Outcome at 6 months postoperatively.

suspension or scar formation, each of which can affect the viscoelastic properties of the tissue. The same is true of prior manipulation of the platysma.

In revision cases, details of the initial surgery may be unknown. Examination of surgical scars, palpation, and assessment of tissue laxity may provide some information. In most cases, this can only be assessed by direct observation after the incisions are made. Weakness, discontinuity, or absence of the SMAS or platysma may limit the success of revision surgery and these limitations should be explained to the patient. Alternative suspension techniques such

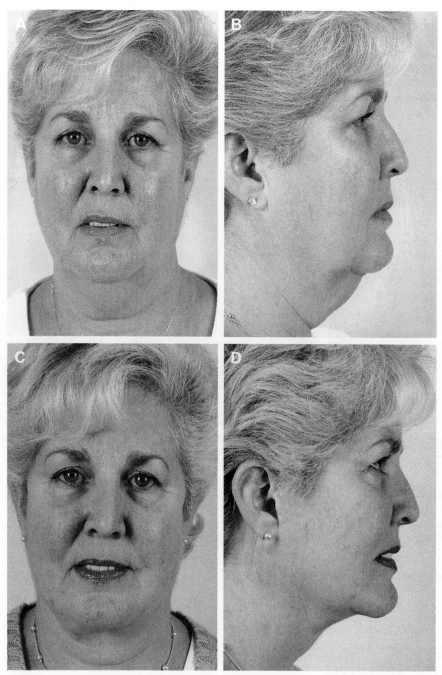

Fig. 11. A 60-year-old woman with a heavy neck. (*A, B*) Before facelift surgery. (*C, D*) Outcome at 1 year postoperatively.

as suture imbrication can be used to gain some elevation and repositioning of the deep tissues.[24]

Subcutaneous Fibrosis

A history of prior neck surgery may result in significant fibrosis of the skin envelope. This fibrosis can make elevation during revision surgery more technically difficult owing to distortion of the tissue planes and increased tissue rigidity. Although theoretically the skin flap in a revision case can be considered delayed, improved skin perfusion has not been shown. Complications of prior surgery, including seroma or hematoma, can increase the degree of subcutaneous fibrosis. Hematoma formation is the

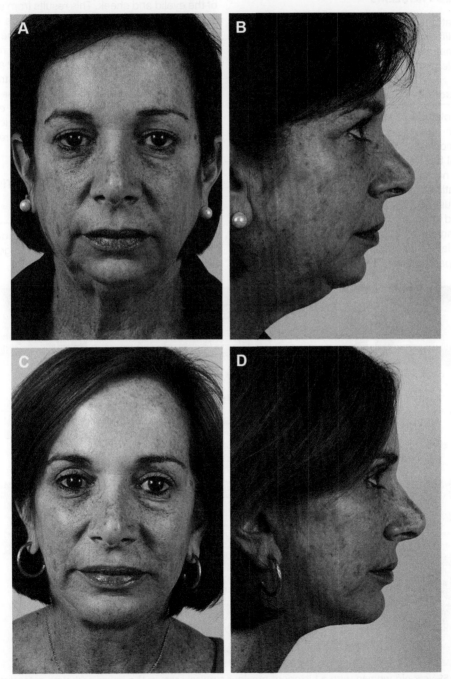

Fig. 12. A 62-year-old woman with retrognathia shown before (*A, B*) and 1 year after (*C, D*) facelift with mentoplasty.

most common postoperative complication with an incidence of up to 15%. Changes in the viscoelastic properties of fibrotic skin make it less distensible than healthy tissue, which may affect the ability to redrape the skin envelope and the degree of tension at incision sites (**Fig. 8**).

UNSOLVED PROBLEMS

Facial anatomy is diverse. This means that standard facelift procedures will not address the needs of some patients. In this section we discuss specific problem areas.

Deep Nasolabial Folds

Deep nasolabial folds, both in male and female patients, are challenging to meet patient expectations. Almost all aging face patients point to the nasolabial folds and ask if they will be eliminated. Because no facelift procedures can either eliminate or satisfactorily treat this area, patient expectations must be diminished through counseling or addressed through a series of increasingly aggressive techniques. The least invasive is using commercial fillers, such as hyaluronic acid or hydroxyapatite. These fillers will help to reduce

the shadow of the folds temporarily. Fat augmentation can also be helpful and of longer duration. Direct excision as shown in **Fig. 9** is the most aggressive, and usually results in good cosmetic outcomes.

Malar Edema/Festoons

Malar festoons (or malar bags) form at the junction of the eyelid and cheek. This results from a combination of factors, including soft tissue edema, laxity of the lower eyelid complex, the effects soft the orbital retaining ligament, and midfacial fat atrophy. Treatment varies in intensity and may involve facial skin energy devices (ultrasound, radiofrequency), resurfacing techniques (CO_2 laser, chemical peels), or direct surgical excision. Results are variable depending on unique patient characteristics. **Fig. 10** demonstrates direct excision of large malar festoons.

CLINICAL EXAMPLES WITH DESCRIPTION OF SURGERY REQUIRED
Heavy Neck

Fig. 11 presents preoperative and postoperative images of a patient who underwent surgery for a heavy neck.

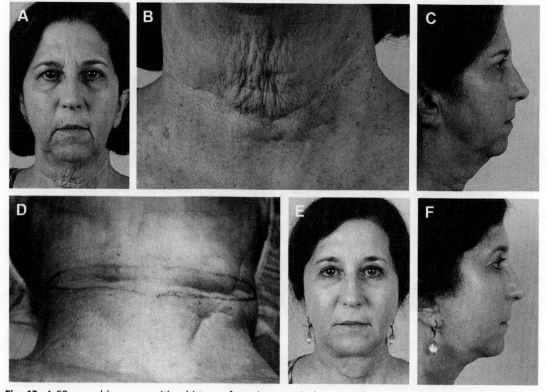

Fig. 13. A 58-year-old woman with a history of previous surgical scars in the lower neck with extensive fibrosis from radiation therapy. (*A–C*) Preoperative views. (*D*) Planned excision of damaged skin done 3 months after facelift surgery. (*E, F*) The 1-year postoperative result.

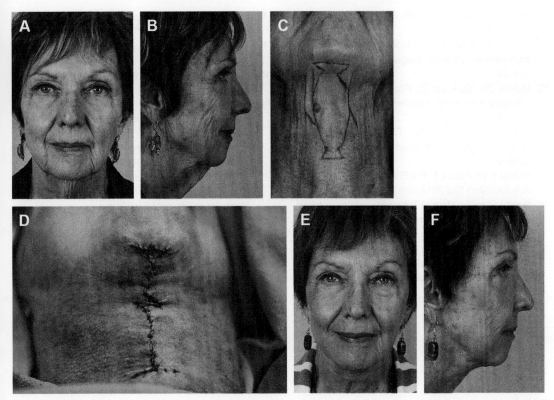

Fig. 14. (*A, B*) A 74-year-old woman with persistent platysma bands and lax tissue several years after facelift surgery. (*C, D*) Direct cervicoplasty excision incorporating a central Z-plasty. (*E, F*) The 1-year postoperative views.

Retrognathia

Fig. 12 presents preoperative and postoperative images of a patient who underwent surgery for retrognathia.

Previous Fibrosis in Submental Area

Fig. 13 presents preoperative and postoperative images of a patient who underwent surgery for previous fibrosis in the submental area.

Persistent Platysma Bands (Direct Excision)

Fig. 14 presents preoperative and postoperative images of a patient who underwent direct excision for persistent platysma bands.

REFERENCES

1. Rodriquez-Bruno K, Papel ID. Rhytidectomy: principles and practice emphasizing safety. Facial Plast Surg 2011;27(1):98–111.
2. Gonzalez-Ulloa M, Flores ES. Senility of the face – basic study to understand its causes and effects. Plast Reconstr Surg 1965;36:239–46.
3. Mitz V, Peyronie M. The superficial musculo-aponeurotic system (SMAS) in the parotid and cheek area. Plast Reconstr Surg 1976;58(1):80–8.
4. Shimizu Y, Kanetaka H, Kim YH, et al. Age-related morphological changes in the human hyoid bone. Cells Tissues Organs 2005;180:185–92.
5. Guyuron B. Problem neck, hyoid bone, and submental myotomy. Plast Reconstr Surg 1992;90(5):830–7.
6. Ellenbogen R, Karlin JV. Visual criteria for success in restoring the youthful neck. Plast Reconstr Surg 1980;66:826–37.
7. Dedo DD. "How I do it"—plastic surgery. Practical suggestions on facial plastic surgery. A preoperative classification of the neck for cervico-facial rhytidectomy. Laryngoscope 1980;90(11 Pt 1):1894–6.
8. Fedok FG, Chaikhoutdinov I, Garritano F. The difficult neck in facelifting. Facial Plast Surg 2014; 30(4):438–50.
9. Sykes JM. Orthognathic surgery. In: Papel I, editor. Facial plastic and reconstructive surgery. 4th edition. New York: Thieme; 2016. p. 910–30.
10. Frodel JL, Sykes JM. Chin augmentation/genioplasty: chin deformities in the aging patient. Facial Plast Surg 1996;12:279–83.
11. Liu TS, Owsley JQ. Long-term results of face lift surgery: patient photographs compared with patient

satisfaction ratings. Plast Reconstr Surg 2012;
129(1):253–62.

12. Espinosa J, Valencia DP. Management of the neck in thick-skinned patients. Facial Plast Surg 2013;29: 214–24.

13. Mokos ZB, Curkovic D, Kostovic K, et al. Facial changes in the mature patient. Clin Dermatol 2018; 36(2):152–8.

14. Calderone DC, Fenske NA. The clinical spectrum of actinic elastosis. J Am Acad Dermatol 1995;32(6): 1016–24.

15. Malfait F, De Paepe A. The Ehlers-Danlos syndrome. Adv Exp Med Biol 2014;802:129–43.

16. Bond L, Lee T, O'Daniel TG. Strategies for submandibular gland management in rhytidectomy. Clin Surg 2017;2(1446).

17. Mendelson BC, Tutino R. Submandibular gland reduction in aesthetic surgery of the neck: review of 112 consecutive cases. Plast Reconstr Surg 2015;136(3):463–71.

18. de Castro CC. The anatomy of the platysma muscle. Plast Reconstr Surg 1980;66(5):680–3.

19. Feldman JJ. Corset platysmaplasty. Clin Plast Surg 1992;19(2):369–82.

20. Jacono AA, Malone MH. The effect of corset platysmaplasty on degree of facelift flap elevation during concomitant deep plane facelift: a cadaveric study. JAMA Facial Plast Surg 2016;18(3): 183–7.

21. Furnas DW. The retaining ligaments of the cheek. Plast Reconstr Surg 1989;83:11–6.

22. Shire JR. The importance of the prejowl notch in face lifting: the prejowl implant. Facial Plast Surg Clin North Am 2008;16(1):87–97, vi.

23. Fedok FG, Mittelman H. Augmenting the prejowl: deciding between fat, fillers, and implants. Facial Plast Surg 2016;32(5):513–9.

24. Beaty MM. A progressive approach to neck rejuvenation. Facial Plast Surg Clin North Am 2014;22(2): 177–90.

The Avoidance and Management of Complications, and Revision Surgery of the Lower Face and Neck

Fred G. Fedok, MD

KEYWORDS

• Facelift • Rhytidectomy • Complications • Avoidance • Rejuvenation

KEY POINTS

- The preoperative assessment of the patient's medical history is important to assess the risk of complications.
- The preoperative discussion of risks and limitations is an important avenue to create favorable patient engagement.
- When complications occur, consultation with the medical literature and colleagues are valuable to formulate corrective action.
- Although many of the complications of rhytidectomy are not life-threatening, they will have a negative impact to the patients well-being and should be dealt with in the most responsible and humanistic manner.

INTRODUCTION

Patients are seeking various forms of facial rejuvenation at an increasing rate. It is anticipated that this trend will continue. It is this author's opinion that much of these individuals' desire to seek facial rejuvenation is an extension of the increase in life expectancy we have witnessed over the last 20 years.[1] The current adult population is not only living longer, but its members also want to be active longer. They want to work and play and enjoy life in a manner that they were able to decades earlier. To help accomplish that goal, they also want to look younger, rejuvenated, energetic, and vital.

The tools of facial rejuvenation have also expanded in the number and in the fundamental nature of interventions. It was just a few decades ago that practitioners were bound to a limited variety of surgical procedure options and a limited spectrum of skin peeling options and dermabrasion. Since the early 1990s, that toolbox has expanded to include a widening variety of energy devices, off-the-shelf fillers and neuromodulators, devices, cosmeceuticals, and biologically derived products. This increase has enabled a multidimensional approach to facial rejuvenation so that one is not limited to addressing only the vertical position of soft tissue, but also the volume of a given facial area, as well as the fundamental nature and the movement of the skin and other soft tissues. There has also been an expanding understanding of the underlying anatomy, the involution of suspensory elements, the changing volume elements, and other events that occur in facial structure with aging.

Disclosure: The author has nothing to disclose.
Facial Plastic and Reconstructive Surgery, Fedok Plastic Surgery, 113 East Fern Avenue, Foley, AL 36535, USA
E-mail address: drfredfedok@me.com

Clin Plastic Surg 45 (2018) 623–634
https://doi.org/10.1016/j.cps.2018.06.010

THE IMPORTANCE OF PREOPERATIVE ASSESSMENT IN THE AVOIDANCE OF COMPLICATIONS

Most adult patients are candidates for some form of facial rejuvenation. To be meaningful, the preoperative assessment should include a detailed interview to discern the patient's goals, their motivations, and realistic expectations of outcome of facial rejuvenation. This discussion should include the disclosure of potential shortcomings and complications.[2] Noting the patient's underlying features should reveal what aspects of their anatomy lend themselves to be rejuvenated, and what aspects of their anatomy will pose limitations in the final results.[3] For instance, the patient who presents with significant microgenia and/or an anterior and inferiorly positioned hyoid bone will present a challenge in the attempt to achieve a classical, ideal cervicomental angle and jawline[4–6] **(Fig. 1)**. The management of informed and realistic outcomes is an important determinate of the realization of favorable patient satisfaction. This foundation of communication provides the basis for the practitioner and patient to partner positively should any less favorable issues develop.

The exploration of the patient's underlying past medical history is important to gauge the risks of undergoing various procedures and methods of anesthesia. A basic evaluation should include questions about blood pressure, blood clotting, the use of anticoagulants, medications, vitamins and supplements, cigarette smoking, drug use, allergies, healing issues, and scarring. Medical issues that are important to explore in the preoperative evaluation include a history of past surgical issues, history of cardiac disease, lung disease, liver disease, diabetes, human immunodeficiency virus infection, hepatitis C virus infection, and other health issues that will impact the risks and results of any anesthesia and surgery. The deleterious impact of cigarette smoking and diabetes are well-known risks to favorable wound healing and the response to surgical trauma.[7–12]

The patient's overall health should also be assessed to gauge their candidacy for not only the particular surgical intervention, but also their underlying risk and candidacy for the anesthesia, anesthetic, and sedation methods to be used. These risk factors are largely in the pulmonary and cardiac spectrum of health issues. The disclosure of these health issues will guide the directing physician to advise the patient to have their procedure under local anesthesia and/or local anesthesia with some form of sedation or general anesthesia. Anesthetic complications are among the most concerning and most significant complications that can occur with facial rejuvenation procedures and include cardiac arrest, arrhythmia, pulmonary embolism, and death.[13]

The overall the risk of complications in facial rejuvenation procedures is derived from the cumulative impact of health issues, the type and biological aggressiveness of the procedure, the type of anesthesia and sedation, and the patient's anticipated outcome.[7,14] Also note that, if the patient has had previous interventions, including the placement of fillers or the use of energy devices, their biological response to these interventions will change and impact further rejuvenation interventions.

INTERVENTIONS USED FOR THE REJUVENATION OF THE LOWER FACE AND NECK
Aging of the Lower Face

The characteristics of aging of the lower face that compel patients to seek rejuvenation include laxity of the lower face and neck skin, the presence of platysma bands, the loss of an attractive jawline and cervicomental angle, changes in skin texture, wrinkling, and the aging of the perioral structures marked by a loss of volume, rhytids, and folds. The reasons for these observed aging changes in the lower face are multitudinous. Certainly, ultraviolet photodamage from sun exposure is a key factor in the loss of skin elasticity and other deleterious processes in the skin that contribute to laxity, rhytids, and texture changes.

Anatomically, the support of the lower facial soft tissues is borne principally by the mandible. In youth, there is a fullness and continuity of the inferior mandibular border that serves as the platform for the insertion of the lower facial musculature.

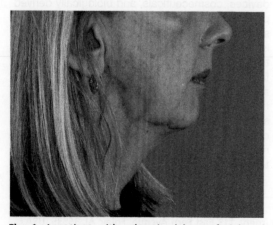

Fig. 1. A patient with suboptimal lower facial and neck anatomy for a facelift: microgenia and a relatively low and anteriorly positioned hyoid bone.

Age-associated changes occur in the skin, the subcutaneous tissues, and the bone. There is a loss of volume secondary to a loss of adipose tissue in the lower face and even a loss of structural bone. Atrophy of the mandibular bone occurs in a manner similar to what happens to other projecting regions of the facial skeleton like the chin and the orbital rims. The area of the anterior mandible immediately inferior to the mental foramen is one of the areas where the atrophic mandibular remodeling is pronounced. The resultant anatomic boney depression at that location is known as the anterior mandibular groove[15] (**Fig. 2**).

There are other age-related changes of the mandibular-associated structures, including atrophy of the superior and inferior mandibular fat compartments, and dehiscence of the mandibular septum. This contributes to a further descent of the regional soft tissue into the neck and further skin laxity. With aging, involutional changes occur that result in the disturbance of the smooth lower facial contours and cause the appearance of lumps, bulges, and depressions.

With the atrophy of the overlying fat compartments and the disruption of the normal muscular attachments, one notes changes in the lower central face, which include the deepening of the melomental folds and labiomandibular creases. The accompanying distortions result in anatomic characteristics which we identify as the appearance of jowls and a deepening prejowl sulcus[16] (**Fig. 3**).

The resultant involutional changes are further reflected into the lower face and the neck. In some patients, there is a further dehiscence of the platysma muscle attachments secondary to relaxation of posterior suspension elements.[17] This process results in visible platysma banding and laxity of the soft tissues.

As discussed elsewhere in this article, there are many factors that contribute to the aging in the lower face and neck. These involutional changes affect many different aspects of the local anatomy including the bone, soft tissue volume, muscle suspension, aberrant muscle activity, and finally changes in the skin itself. With these multiple facets of aging, it is logical that many different modalities of rejuvenation have been popularly developed.

These different modalities are directed at producing structural changes by augmentation of the bony structure, the replacement of volume, the modulation of muscle activity, the repositioning of anatomic structures, various facelift techniques to correct the position of the platysma muscles, and the elimination of laxity and textural changes of the skin.

Surgery continues to have a major role in the rejuvenation of the lower face and neck. Because much of the stigmata of aging involves laxity of the skin and changes in the positioning of muscles, only limited rejuvenation can be accomplished without the use of surgery. Various types and designs of facelifting methods are used and include short scar techniques, high superficial

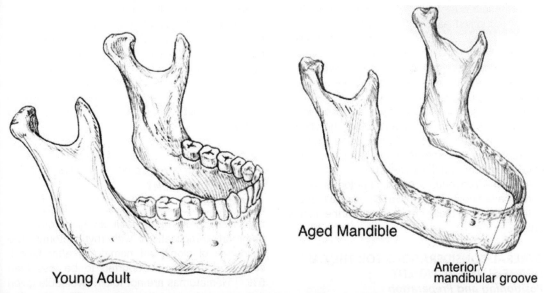

Young Adult

Aged Mandible

Anterior mandibular groove

Fig. 2. Bone wasting differences between the aged and youthful mandible. (*From* Fedok FG, Mittelman H. Augmenting the prejowl: deciding between fat, fillers, and implants. Facial Plast Surg 2016;32(5):513–9; with permission.)

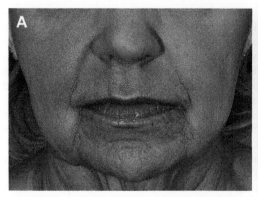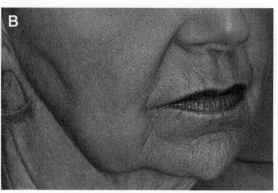

Fig. 3. (*A*) Frontal and (*B*) oblique clinical images of patient of patient with prominent marionette lines, jowls, prejowl sulcus, and submental crease. (*From* Fedok FG, Mittelman H. Augmenting the prejowl: deciding between fat, fillers, and implants. Facial Plast Surg 2016;32(5):513–9; with permission.)

musculoaponeurotic system (SMAS) techniques, deep plane techniques, and many other variations. Because the platysma is such a prominent feature of the aging neck, some form of platysmaplasty is frequently necessary to create corrections.[18] Volume deficiencies in the central midface and lower one-third of the face are a key aspect of facial aging. Fillers and fat transfer has been used to correct these deficiencies. Frequently, facelifting and fat transfer are used together.[19–21]

Energy-based tightening technology has had a limited impact in the correction of aging changes in the lower face and neck. Technologies have incorporated radiofrequency, ultrasonic, and microneedling technologies. Each has a spectrum of effectiveness and shortcomings.

Laser resurfacing continues to be a key component of successful facial rejuvenation. The CO_2 laser was the first laser technology that had broad adoption for significant resurfacing. Erbium laser and various fractional technologies as well as nonablative laser technologies have been used. Intense pulse light has a role for the rejuvenation of the facial and neck skin and décolleté.

The use of solid implants has waned in popularity since the introduction of injectable fillers. They, however, continue to have a key role in the focal augmentation of bone abnormalities and efficiencies in the chin, the cheeks and mandibular body.

All of the procedures and technologies noted herein have a host of benefits and possible complications. Some of these are reviewed further in this article.

GENERAL CONSIDERATIONS FOR THE CARE OF THE SURGICAL PATIENT
Positioning and Preparation

Lower facelift surgery, especially when paired with a combination of procedures, can be a lengthy and complicated procedure. Patients should be positioned appropriately to avoid pressure-related positioning complications.[22]

Use of Local Anesthetics

A relatively large volume of epinephrine containing local anesthetic is typically used to control bleeding during extensive facial flap elevation. To prevent toxicity, there should be strict attention paid to the volume and concentration of the solution used in reference to the patient's lean body mass.

Avoidance of Anesthetic Complications

The author has performed facelift procedures under local anesthesia or sedation, monitored anesthesia care, as well as general anesthesia. The choice of anesthetic method is usually best determined by a collaborative decision between the patient, surgeon, and the nurse anesthetist or anesthesiologist. Such discussion must include a consideration of the patient's underlying health, the length of procedure, the patient's general risks for anesthesia, and the procedure being performed.

PROBLEMS AFTER FACIAL REJUVENATION PROCEDURES: AVOIDANCE, EVALUATION, AND MANAGEMENT
Hematoma and Bruising

Significant bruising as well as hematoma are common complications with rhytidectomy. The incidence of significant hematoma after facelift surgery is frequently reported to be less than 5%.[11] Hematomas are not totally avoidable given the nature of surgical procedures. The minimization of risk starts with the preoperative assessment of whether the patient has adequate coagulation capabilities based on the physical examination, the history, and laboratory studies. Underlying hematologic abnormalities are relatively rare but should be looked for if the patient relates a suggestive history.

The use of medications that inhibit clotting such as warfarin and clopidogrel (Plavix), as well as others, is fairly common in the aging population. These medications should be stopped at the period of time as advised by the patient's managing physician(s) before any invasive procedure. The time frame of when the medication can be safety stopped, when it can be resumed, what bridges might be used, and other considerations are best determined through consultation with the physician who is managing the patient's anticoagulation medicine. It should be realized that the patient's underlying health issue that warrants the use of anticoagulants may in itself eliminate the patient's candidacy for the rejuvenation procedure. In addition, one should scan the patient's nonprescription medication and vitamin list to exclude those agents that will interfere with platelet function. These agents include various nonsteroidal pain medications and dietary supplements such as vitamin E, aspirin, nonsteroidal anti-inflammatory drugs, and similar agents. These medications and supplements are usually stopped at least 1 week before a surgical procedure if there is not a medical contraindication.

Avoidance, evaluation, and management of bleeding-related complications

Optimal preoperative screening and medication management is the beginning of avoidance of bleeding and hematoma issues. Intraoperative control of blood pressure and postoperative nausea and vomiting are relative easy preventive measures.[23,24] Decreasing the amount of narcotic use during anesthesia may aid in this control. The intraoperative control of bleeding and the postoperative use of drains and adequate dressings are the next step. Some practitioners have found the use of various tissue glues and fibrin products under the skin flaps to be helpful, although the evidence to support the practice is equivocal.[25–29] If the procedure is performed under general anesthesia, extubation and anesthesia emergence should be facilitated in the smoothest possible manner to avoid coughing and straining.

Finally, if a hematoma is suspected or recognized, it should be attended to and drained in a timely manner to prevent further skin compromise. A firm dressing and the use of a drain will minimize the chances of a recurrence.

Bruising and hematoma can even occur after less involved rejuvenation procedures. Bruising is common after the placement of implants and the injection of fillers and neuromodulators, as well as after fat transfer. The same general guidelines to assess the patient's candidacy for the particular procedure apply. There are several methods that are touted to lessen ,bruising such as the ingestion of arnica montana and fresh pineapple, the scientific support of these interventions is generally sparse.[30] It should be noted that males are reported to have a higher risk of complications, including hematoma, after aesthetic surgery.[31,32]

Motor Nerve Injuries

During facelifting, the facial nerve is noted to be at significantly higher risk in several anatomic areas. These areas include the frontal branch and the marginal mandibular branch of the facial nerve.[33] The patient should be assessed preoperatively to have their facial nerve function photodocumented and to note any asymmetries. Patients who have had a past medical history of Bell's palsy, and other nerve insults, even if they have very good recovery, may have a permanent underlying asymmetry.

The frontal branch of the facial nerve is usually at most risk during the temporal dissection for a brow lift. Most of these injuries are avoidable through careful dissection in the appropriate planes and avoiding certain danger zones, for instance where the facial nerve crosses the zygomatic arch. The nerve can have some variation in its course and as such may be injured even when the surgeon is following acceptable surgical methodology. It is reported that injuries to the facial nerve in this region are frequently due to traction injuries or cautery. Fortunately, most of these injuries will recover over time. The other area where the facial nerve seems to be at increased risk for injury is the marginal mandibular branch of the facial nerve. The nerve is particularly prone to injury where it crosses the mandibular border. This injury has been known to occur even with liposuction (**Fig. 4**).

Avoidance, evaluation, and management of motor nerve injuries

Again, the first step in the avoidance of an iatrogenic motor nerve injury starts with the initial evaluation of the patient and photodocumentation of the facial nerve function. It is fairly characteristic that after surgery patients will scrutinize their facial appearance and movement in front of a mirror more than they will have done before surgery. It is important that any asymmetries or after maladies be noted and documented beforehand.

The evaluation of a suspected nerve injury intraoperatively may start with the jump of the face noted with particular scissor snip during the

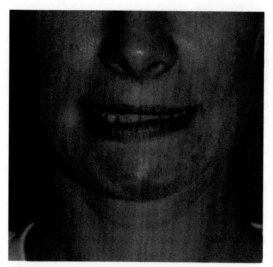

Fig. 4. Frontal clinical image of patient with left lower lip depressor weakness after minimal access cranial suspension lift and liposuction.

procedure. As with other recommendations made regarding traumatic nerve injuries, any facial nerve branch insult proximal to a vertical line tangent with the lateral canthus may be a candidate for acute nerve repair. These situations are rare and have never been encountered by the author. When a facial nerve injury is suspected postoperatively, the process is different. Facial nerve function may not fully recover the lidocaine-related neuropraxia for several hours after a procedure, so early assessment may be unreliable. If there is an isolated frontalis or lip depressor weakness noted, the patient should be informed and reassured that most of these injuries recover in a few months, especially if no direct nerve injury or aberrant dissection was suspected during the case.[34–36] The majority of isolated frontal and marginal mandibular nerve injuries recover over time. An exploration of the surgical site is usually not to warranted. Neuromodulators can be used to mask the asymmetry by weakening the noninvolved side. Recovery can take weeks to a year depending on the extent of injury and the capacity of the facial nerve to recover. Nerve stimulation has been advocated, but has mixed support of possible efficacy.

Injuries to a more proximal portion of facial nerve are exceedingly rare during rhytidectomy and should be evaluated differently. A proximal injury would be suspected if the entire side of the face is weak. The use of neurophysiologic electrical testing may be warranted if the entire side of the face is completely flaccid. If the patient shows significant denervation after a suspected proximal nerve injury, the nerve should be explored and

repaired if necessary. Once again, a severe injury such as this is exceedingly rare.

Sensory Nerve Injuries

The most common sensory nerve injured during facelift is the great auricular nerve. The nerve is most vulnerable in the postauricular area and the upper neck areas where there is a only a small amount of soft tissue between the skin dissection and the great auricular nerve as it courses over the upper portion of the sternocleidomastoid muscle.[37] If the nerve is injured, patients may complain of a burning pain. Because of proximity to the mental nerve, at least temporary numbness of the chin is possible with the dissection necessary to perform chin augmentation and genioplasty.

Avoidance, evaluation, management of sensory nerve injuries

Adhering to optimal planes of dissection and the cautious use of cautery are among the best methods to avoid sensory nerve injury. When injuries occur, unless one suspects that a nerve has been frankly transected, there will usually be an improvement over several months. If the patient has an intolerance to the dysesthesia, a trial with a low-dose tricyclic antidepressant or gabapentin may be used to minimize symptoms.[38]

Scarring and Other Skin Issues

Unfavorable scarring: widening or thickening of skin incision

All wounds heal with scarring. Unfavorable scarring occurs because of suboptimal incision design, planning, and execution. In facelifting, the avoidance of scarring has been one of the motivations for the adoption of short scar techniques. The avoidance of unfavorable scarring, however, does not necessarily dictate the use of the short scar techniques. Optimal incision placement and execution are more important. Incision design and placement should capitalize on various methods to minimize the scar's noticeability. Incisions can be placed in a trichophytic locations along hair-bearing areas. Incisions can be placed to take advantage of contour and color differences along facial structures. Finally, incisions that run counter to the relaxed tension lines and should be placed in a manner with minimal tension and tissue supported by deep sutures. In facelifting, these practices can be carried out to achieve barely noticeable scars (**Fig. 5**).

Epidermolysis

Epidermolysis can be mild or extensive. It is usually related to inadequate flap vascularity which can be affected by incision design, degree

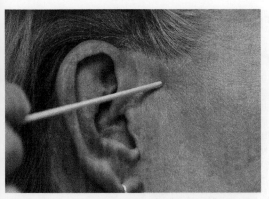

Fig. 5. Clinical postoperative image of patient after rhytidectomy showing well-planned and executed trichophytic, preauricular, and posttragal incisions.

of undermining, surgical disruption of the subdermal plexus, and wound tension.

Skin Loss and Necrosis

Severe epidermolysis and partial thickness and full-thickness loss of skin is relatively uncommon but not rare. This complication is by far among the most concerning that may occur after facelift surgery. These wound issues usually occur in the postauricular and preauricular areas. The underlying cause is vascular insufficiency of the skin flap. It can be due to underlying microvascular disease, pressure from hematoma, excessive tension on the wound, or flap design issues. A history of cigarette smoking, diabetes, and previous soft tissue insult increases a patient's risk of such an event.

Avoidance, evaluation, and management of scarring, skin loss, and necrosis

Unfavorable scarring can be minimized by optimal incision planning and execution, eliminating undue tension on the wound, by prudent skin incision, and the strategic placement of deep sutures. Intralesional steroids and the use of 595 nm laser therapy can be helpful in the management of thickened red scars.

The risk of significant epidermolysis and skin loss may be decreased with modification of incision design and flap length in the patient with a history of cigarette smoking. Some practitioners will not perform facelifts on patients who have had a past medical history of cigarette smoking, whereas others are comfortable in having them abstain from smoking for at least several weeks before the procedure. Nevertheless, those with a long history of smoking will have significant chronic microvascular disease, which leaves them at greater risk of healing problems. Diabetes and other causes of skin vascular insults will also present an increased risk of skin viability issues.[39]

When a portion of the skin shows evidence of compromise, some basic steps may be helpful. Releasing staples and sutures may reduce tension in the soft tissue to increase vascularity. The use of nitropaste is frequently cited as being useful, although there is little evidence to show that it really helps. Similarly, there may be a role for the use of hyperbaric oxygen in these circumstances. It is not without risk, so the pro and cons have to be weighed.[40–42] Except in unusual circumstances, these skin losses are usually managed conservatively while allowing the wound to heal by wound contracture and secondary intension. Only in extreme circumstances is it advisable to subject the patient to aggressive debridement and skin grafting. Surprisingly, the final cosmetic results can be quite good, but will take a long time to achieve (**Fig. 6**).

Sialocele

Sialocele is an uncommon complication of the lower facelift. This can occur with relatively nonaggressive forms of facelifting, but in all cases involves some insult of the parotid capsule or ductile system. In all except the most unusual cases this will resolve over time[43–45] (**Fig. 7**).

Avoidance, evaluation, and management of sialocele

Dissecting in a superficial plane will minimize the risk of sialocele. Given the current methods of SMAS flap and deep plane designs, it is surprising that sialocele does not occur more commonly. The evaluation is relative simple and based on physical examination. The presence of a sialocele can be confirmed with the aspiration of clear fluid. Fluid can be sent for amylase, but this step is usually not necessary. The use of drains, pressure dressings, and botulinum toxin facilitates resolution.

Aesthetic Complications

Although not as striking as some of the many technical complications, that is, hematoma, skin loss, and significant scarring, aesthetic shortcomings and complications can be equally if not more disappointing for the patient. Various shortcomings of procedures that are quite common include the persistence of the nasolabial folds, jowls, prejowl sulci, rhytids, and platysma bands. The persistence of jowls and the prejowl sulcus may be seen in isolation or along with a persistent nasolabial folds and other problems. Most surgeons who perform otherwise very successful facelifts encounter the problem of persistent platysma bands in some patients.

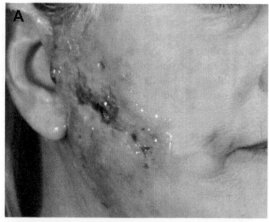
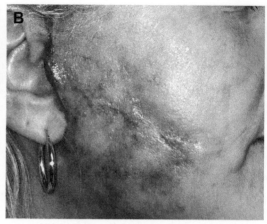
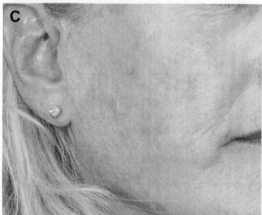

Fig. 6. Postoperative images of patient after rhytidectomy who had partial thickness skin loss and epidermolysis of right facial flap and was treated with conservative wound care measures and pulsed dye and fractionated CO_2 lasers: (*A*) 2 weeks after the procedure, (*B*) 5 weeks after the procedure, and (*C*) 11 months after the procedure.

Avoidance, evaluation, and management of aesthetic complications

The causes of a persistence of jowls, the marionette deformity and the prejowl sulcus include (1) a failure to adequately mobilize and reposition the midface and lower structures incorporated in the SMAS at the time of facelift and (2) a failure to adequately restore volume in the area of the

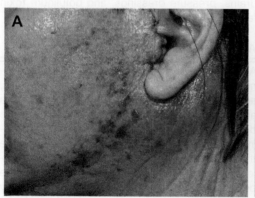
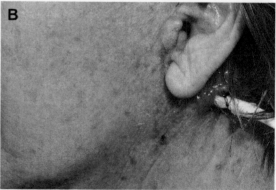

Fig. 7. Postoperative images of a patient after rhytidectomy who had evidence of sialocele. (*A*) Sialocele noted 8 days postoperatively by fullness below and behind ear lobe and confirmed with the aspiration of clear fluid consistent with saliva (skin erythema secondary to superficial laser resurfacing after facelift procedure). (*B*) Improvement 15 days after rhytidectomy with a drain in place and treatment with pressure dressing and botulinum toxin.

sulcus. This outcome can be prevented or remedied by incorporating SMAS management methods in the facelift, which adequately mobilizes this muscle–fascia complex during the initial procedure. High SMAS and deep plane methods and are viable options.[46–48]

The etiology of the prejowl sulcus was reviewed elsewhere in this article. Because of the deficiency of bone and adipose at this location, facelifting itself is usually inadequate to correct this. Hence, months after a very successful facelift and as edema resolves, one can find the reemergence of this age-related abnormality. To remedy the prejowl sulcus and to correct persistence afterward, the following recommendations are made. The void exhibited by the prejowl sulcus can be managed alone or at the time of a secondary lower facelift with the placement of volume, ideally fat transfer or with solid chin augmentation (**Fig. 8**).

If persistent platysma bands are noted postoperatively, some practitioners will attempt to lessen the noticeability with the injection of botulinum in the bands.[49–51] The best prevention is the optimal management of them during the first surgery. Methods to manage this include fairly standard anterior platysmaplasty techniques as well as adequate resuspension of the posterior portion of the platysma[52,53] (**Fig. 9**). Even with the best efforts, in some patients the will be a persistence of some portion of the bands.

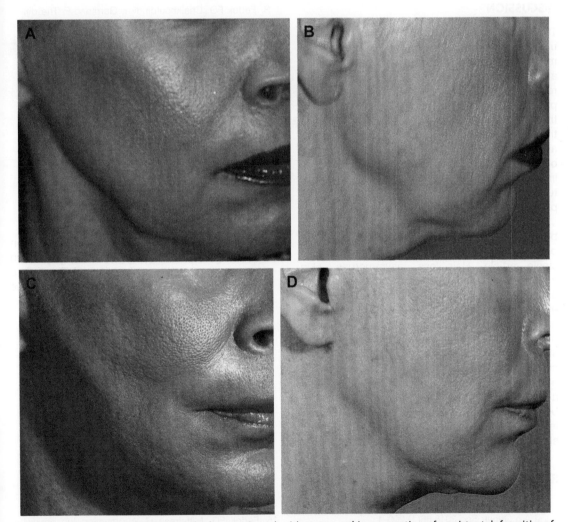

Fig. 8. A patient's lower face and neck after previous rhytidectomy seeking correction of persistent deformities of jowls, marionette lines, prejowl sulcus, and microgenia, (*A, B*) Preoperative appearance before secondary deep plane rhytidectomy, fat transfer to the lower face. and silastic chin augmentation. (*C, D*) At 12 months after secondary rhytidectomy including deep plane rhytidectomy, fat transfer to the lower face, and silastic chin augmentation.

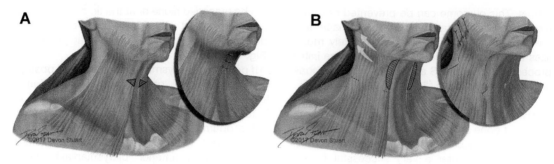

Fig. 9. Two methods to manage platysma bands. (*A*) Resection of triangle of muscle to allow midline advancement of more superior segment of anterior platysma muscle, and suturing anterior medial segment of platysma muscles together. (*B*) Partial division of the anterior and posterior borders of the platysma (*dotted line*) with resection of prominent platysma anterior bands (*shaded areas*) and posterior resuspension of platysma muscle to the sternocleidomastoid muscle.

DISCUSSION

Thorough rhytidectomy is a complicated procedure. As touched on in this article, there are a multitude of factors that need to be ascertained and managed as one engages the challenge of rejuvenating a patient's face. There are numerous patient factors and numerous technical factors that must be contended with. For each one of these factors that might be effective there is almost an equal number of things that can turn out suboptimally. These range from the most minimal concerns such as the spitting of deep sutures to significant cardiovascular and tissue problems.

Many of the more significant issues have been reviewed herein. Many issues have not been addressed because of the limitations in a single article. Hair loss, asymmetries, skin irregularities, and perioral limitations, for example, have not been addressed. As with every other aspect of surgery, shortcomings and complications typically decrease with experience of the surgeon. One should keep in mind should problems occur, formal or informal consultations with a trusted colleague may be helpful in elucidating plans for remedies. The adage, "First do no harm" should be remembered and behooves all of us to continually learn and sharpen our assessment and surgical skills.

REFERENCES

1. Clarfield AM. Healthy life expectancy is expanding. J Am Geriatr Soc 2018;66(1):200–1.
2. Kandinov A, Mutchnick S, Nangia V, et al. Analysis of factors associated with rhytidectomy malpractice litigation cases. JAMA Facial Plast Surg 2017;19(4):255–9.
3. Fedok FG, Chaikhoutdinov I, Garritano F. The difficult neck in facelifting. Facial Plast Surg 2014;30(4):438–50.
4. Ellenbogen R, Karlin JV. Visual criteria for success in restoring the youthful neck. Plast Reconstr Surg 1980;66(6):826–37.
5. Dayan SH, Arkins JP, Antonucci C, et al. Influence of the chin implant on cervicomental angle. Plast Reconstr Surg 2010;126(3):141e–3e.
6. Roy S, Buckingham E. The difficult neck in facelifting. Facial Plast Surg 2017;33(3):271–8.
7. Gupta V, Winocour J, Shi H, et al. Preoperative risk factors and complication rates in facelift: analysis of 11,300 patients. Aesthet Surg J 2016;36(1):1–13.
8. Bamba R, Gupta V, Shack RB, et al. Evaluation of diabetes mellitus as a risk factor for major complications in patients undergoing aesthetic surgery. Aesthet Surg J 2016;36(5):598–608.
9. Moyer JS, Baker SR. Complications of rhytidectomy. Facial Plast Surg Clin North Am 2005;13(3):469–78.
10. Salisbury CC, Kaye BL. Complications of rhytidectomy. Plast Surg Nurs 1998;18(2):71–7, 89.
11. Rees TD, Aston SJ. Complications of rhytidectomy. Clin Plast Surg 1978;5(1):109–19.
12. Baker TJ, Gordon HL. Complications of rhytidectomy. Plast Reconstr Surg 1967;40(1):31–9.
13. Abboushi N, Yezhelyev M, Symbas J, et al. Facelift complications and the risk of venous thromboembolism: a single center's experience. Aesthet Surg J 2012;32(4):413–20.
14. Marten E, Langevin CJ, Kaswan S, et al. The safety of rhytidectomy in the elderly. Plast Reconstr Surg 2011;127(6):2455–63.
15. Fedok FG, Mittelman H. Augmenting the prejowl: deciding between fat, fillers, and implants. Facial Plast Surg 2016;32(5):513–9.
16. Braz A, Humphrey S, Weinkle S, et al. Lower face: clinical anatomy and regional approaches with

injectable fillers. Plast Reconstr Surg 2015;136(5 Suppl):235S–57S.

17. Labbe D, Franco RG, Nicolas J. Platysma suspension and platysmaplasty during neck lift: anatomical study and analysis of 30 cases. Plast Reconstr Surg 2006;117(6):2001–7 [discussion: 2008–10].

18. Feldman JJ. Corset platysmaplasty. Clin Plast Surg 1992;19(2):369–82.

19. Chang CS, Kang GC. Achieving ideal lower face aesthetic contours: combination of tridimensional fat grafting to the chin with masseter botulinum toxin injection. Aesthet Surg J 2016;36(10):1093–100.

20. Glasgold M, Lam SM, Glasgold R. Autologous fat grafting for cosmetic enhancement of the perioral region. Facial Plast Surg Clin North Am 2007;15(4):461–70, vi.

21. Metzinger S, Parrish J, Guerra A, et al. Autologous fat grafting to the lower one-third of the face. Facial Plast Surg 2012;28(1):21–33.

22. Woodfin KO, Johnson C, Parker R, et al. Use of a novel memory aid to educate perioperative team members on proper patient positioning technique. AORN J 2018;107(3):325–32.

23. Beninger FG, Pritchard SJ. Clonidine in the management of blood pressure during rhytidectomy. Aesthet Surg J 1998;18(2):89–94.

24. Maricevich MA, Adair MJ, Maricevich RL, et al. Facelift complications related to median and peak blood pressure evaluation. Aesthetic Plast Surg 2014;38(4):641–7.

25. Berner RE, Morain WD, Noe JM. Postoperative hypertension as an etiological factor in hematoma after rhytidectomy. Prevention with chlorpromazine. Plast Reconstr Surg 1976;57(3):314–9.

26. Grover R, Jones BM, Waterhouse N. The prevention of haematoma following rhytidectomy: a review of 1078 consecutive facelifts. Br J Plast Surg 2001;54(6):481–6.

27. Jones BM, Grover R. Avoiding hematoma in cervicofacial rhytidectomy: a personal 8-year quest. Reviewing 910 patients. Plast Reconstr Surg 2004;113(1):381–7 [discussion: 388–90].

28. Kamer FM, Song AU. Hematoma formation in deep plane rhytidectomy. Arch Facial Plast Surg 2000;2(4):240–2.

29. Killion EA, Hyman CH, Hatef DA, et al. A systematic examination of the effect of tissue glues on rhytidectomy complications. Aesthet Surg J 2015;35(3):229–34.

30. Seeley BM, Denton AB, Ahn MS, et al. Effect of homeopathic Arnica Montana on bruising in face-lifts: results of a randomized, double-blind, placebo-controlled clinical trial. Arch Facial Plast Surg 2006;8(1):54–9.

31. Smith JW, Nelson R, Weaver K. Rhytidectomy in male patients. Aesthetic Plast Surg 1983;7(1):41–5.

32. Baker DC, Aston SJ, Guy CL, et al. The male rhytidectomy. Plast Reconstr Surg 1977;60(4):514–22.

33. Baker DC, Conley J. Avoiding facial nerve injuries in rhytidectomy. Anatomical variations and pitfalls. Plast Reconstr Surg 1979;64(6):781–95.

34. Pitanguy I, Ceravolo MP, Degand M. Nerve injuries during rhytidectomy. Considerations after 3,203 cases. Aesthetic Plast Surg 1980;4(1):257–65.

35. Castanares S. Facial nerve paralyses coincident with, or subsequent to, rhytidectomy. Plast Reconstr Surg 1974;54(6):637–43.

36. Lydiatt DD. Medical malpractice and facial nerve paralysis. Arch Otolaryngol Head Neck Surg 2003;129(1):50–3.

37. Lefkowitz T, Hazani R, Chowdhry S, et al. Anatomical landmarks to avoid injury to the great auricular nerve during rhytidectomy. Aesthet Surg J 2013;33(1):19–23.

38. Lewin ML, Tsur H. Injuries of the great auricular nerve in rhytidectomy. Aesthetic Plast Surg 1976;1(1):409–17.

39. Braddock SW. Cutaneous necrosis after rhytidectomy. Plast Reconstr Surg 1984;73(6):998.

40. Francis A, Baynosa RC. Hyperbaric oxygen therapy for the compromised graft or flap. Adv Wound Care (New Rochelle) 2017;6(1):23–32.

41. Mermans JF, Tuinder S, von Meyenfeldt MF, et al. Hyperbaric oxygen treatment for skin flap necrosis after a mastectomy: a case study. Undersea Hyperb Med 2012;39(3):719–23.

42. Vishwanath G. Hyperbaric oxygen therapy in free flap surgery: is it meaningful? Med J Armed Forces India 2011;67(3):253–6.

43. Lawson GA 3rd, Kreymerman P, Nahai F. An unusual complication following rhytidectomy: iatrogenic parotid injury resulting in parotid fistula/sialocele. Aesthet Surg J 2012;32(7):814–21.

44. Barron R, Margulis A, Icekson M, et al. Iatrogenic parotid sialocele following rhytidectomy: diagnosis and treatment. Plast Reconstr Surg 2001;108(6):1782–4 [discussion: 1785–6].

45. Feingold RS. Parotid salivary gland fistula following rhytidectomy. Plast Reconstr Surg 1998;101(1):245.

46. Hamra ST. The deep-plane rhytidectomy. Plast Reconstr Surg 1990;86(1):53–61 [discussion: 62–3].

47. Jacono AA, Malone MH, Talei B. Three-dimensional analysis of long-term midface volume change after vertical vector deep-plane rhytidectomy. Aesthet Surg J 2015;35(5):491–503.

48. Sundine MJ, Kretsis V, Connell BF. Longevity of SMAS facial rejuvenation and support. Plast Reconstr Surg 2010;126(1):229–37.

49. Kane MA. Nonsurgical treatment of platysmal bands with injection of botulinum toxin A. Plast

Reconstr Surg 1999;103(2):656–63 [discussion: 664–5].

50. Kane MA. Nonsurgical treatment of platysma bands with injection of botulinum toxin a revisited. Plast Reconstr Surg 2003;112(5 Suppl): 125S–6S.

51. Matarasso A, Matarasso SL, Brandt FS, et al. Botulinum A exotoxin for the management of platysma bands. Plast Reconstr Surg 1999;103(2):645–52 [discussion: 653–5].

52. Fedok FG, Sedgh J. Managing the neck in the era of the short scar face-lift. Facial Plast Surg 2012;28(1): 60–75.

53. Rohrich RJ, Rios JL, Smith PD, et al. Neck rejuvenation revisited. Plast Reconstr Surg 2006;118(5): 1251–63.

Gender Reassignment
Feminization and Masculinization of the Neck

Christopher J. Salgado, MD[a,*], Ajani G. Nugent, MD[a],
Thomas Satterwaite, MD[b],
Katherine H. Carruthers, MD, MS[c], Natalie R. Joumblat, BS[a]

KEYWORDS

- Mandibular angle reduction • Genioplasty • Chondrolaryngoplasty • Maxillofacial prosthesis
- Rhytidectomy • Transgender

KEY POINTS

- Facial features are strongly correlated with one's gender and is particularly important for transgender patients who seek social integration and gender congruity.
- Facial procedures related the feminization and masculinization have long been recognized as crucial to this process.
- This article focuses on these procedures as they relate to the lower facial third and neck.

INTRODUCTION

Gender dysphoria, quite often referred to as gender identity disorder, as renamed by the American Psychiatric Association in the *Diagnostic and Statistical Manual of Mental Disorders* in 2013, is defined by an individual's persistent discomfort with their assigned sex. Individuals with gender identity disorder have a desire to live as members of the opposite sex and therefore often modify their primary and secondary sex characteristics. Their facial appearance is central to their ability to pursue and maintain social interactions as their desired gender. Although most individuals will ultimately undergo bottom surgery, very few members of society will bear witness to the patient's actual genital modifications. This is unlike their facial appearance, where the dysphoric patient has the challenge of integrating into society as

the desired gender, despite difficulty camouflaging the characteristics of their assigned gender.

SEXUAL DIMORPHISMS OF THE ANATOMY
Skin

Skin texture
The skin of the face and neck in female individuals overall looks smoother and softer, with a reduced appearance of pores.[1,2] In comparison, male skin is significantly rougher,[3] with more pronounced pores and evidence of facial hair.[1]

Skin thickness
Throughout the body, male individuals have thicker skin than female individuals.[4] When looking at each layer of the skin, typically the dermis is thicker in male individuals and the epidermis is thicker in female individuals.[4] These

Disclosure Statement: The authors have nothing to disclose.
[a] Division of Plastic, Reconstructive, Aesthetic and Transgender Surgery, Department of Surgery, LGBTQ Center for Wellness, Gender and Sexual Health, University of Miami Hospital, Jackson Memorial Hospital, 1120 Northwest 14th Street, Miami, FL 33136, USA; [b] Brownstein & Crane Surgical Services, 575 Sir Francis Drake Boulevard, Suite 1, Greenbrae, CA 94904, USA; [c] Department of Surgery, Division of Plastic Surgery, West Virginia University, 1 Medical Center Drive, Morgantown, WV 26505, USA
* Corresponding author.
E-mail address: csalgado2@med.miami.edu

Clin Plastic Surg 45 (2018) 635–645
https://doi.org/10.1016/j.cps.2018.06.006

gender-related differences correlate to the effect that sex hormones have on specific layers of the skin.[4] Epidermal growth is influenced by estrogen, as demonstrated by postmenopausal women experiencing a thinning of their epidermis.[4] However, when looking at the face specifically, Whitton and Everall[5] found male individuals to have thicker epidermis than female individuals, measuring at 55 μm versus 40 μm, respectively.

Rhytids

Rhytids of the face and neck are considered by society to be a more masculine feature.[1] Generally, women tend to have fewer rhytids on the face and neck due to thicker subcutaneous tissue and smaller facial muscles that cause less contraction of the skin and subsequent expression lines.[1] When looking at gender-related differences in rhytids, Tsukahara and colleagues[3] found men to have significantly more inferolateral oral commissure lines in those 21 to 28 years old. However, when looking at the 65-year to 75-year range, postmenopausal women, with decreased circulating estrogen and thinning skin, were found to have significantly higher scores compared with men.[3]

Wound healing

Female skin tends to have superior wound healing and reduced scar formation compared with male skin.[4] This gender discrepancy is also influenced by the differing levels of circulating sex hormones. Estrogen enhances the signal transduction of cytokines that reduce harmful inflammation and promotes protein balance, thus accelerating cutaneous wound healing.[4]

Subcutaneous fat distribution

Overall, female individuals have a thicker subcutaneous fat than male individuals, which serves to obscure the muscular form and produce contours associated with femininity.[1,4] Cervical subcutaneous tissue is significantly more in female individuals.[6,7] Based on compartments described, Bredella[8] found that female individuals have more adipose tissue in the subcutaneous compartment, whereas the male distribution is primarily in the 2 intermuscular compartments (posterior and periverbetral).[9]

Musculature

Masseter

The masseter muscle is sexually dimorphic. The bulkier male masseter yields a more pronounced lower mandibular border and gonial angle, which is regarded by society as a more masculine feature.[2,10–15]

Cervical

Zheng and colleagues[16] and Rankin and colleagues[17] used MRI and ultrasound, respectively, to evaluate the gender-related differences in neck muscle volume. Male individuals were found to have their muscle volume occupy 7% more of the total neck volume compared with female individuals (male: 32%, female: 25%).[16,18] When looking at individual neck muscles as a percentage of total neck muscle volume, the sternocleidomastoid and longus capitis muscles were significantly larger in female individuals, whereas the obliquus capitis inferior muscle was significantly larger in male individuals.[16] However, when normalized for body mass, there was no significant size difference between genders.[17]

Submandibular Salivary Gland

Submandibular salivary glands, part of the mandibular subcutaneous soft tissue structures, can largely influence the contour of the jawline.[1] Scott[18] demonstrated sexual dimorphism in gland size, and Inoue and colleagues[19] supported this finding, where the bilateral summed volume in male individuals was found to be 34.1 cm³ and in female individuals to be 24.2 cm³.

Bony and Cartilaginous Architecture

The craniofacial skeleton establishes the architectural gender differences of the face.[20]

Mandible

Visual characteristics of the mandible can be used to determine gender with a high level of certainty.[21] A wider and sharper jaw is regarded as an indicator of masculinity.[1,22,23] The male mandible is 20% larger.[1,23] These features include a thicker external oblique ridge,[1,22] broader and longer ascending ramus,[1,21] larger condyle,[1] more pronounced mandibular flare,[1,11,23] more acute gonial angle,[1,11] and a larger bigonial diameter[21] (**Fig. 1**). In contrast, the female mandible is smaller, with a more obtuse gonial angle and less

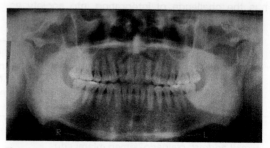

Fig. 1. Preoperative Panorex demonstrating wide bigonal distance before angle reduction.

mandibular flare, resulting in a softer and more narrow contour.[23] The mentum in male individuals is broader and longer with more projection, overall producing a larger silhouette that is associated with masculinity.[1,2,11,23] The female mentum, in contrast, is more narrow with less projection, yielding a more round chin that equates to a feminine contour.[2,11,24–26]

Thyroid

The prominent thyroid cartilage in male individuals, also knowns as an "Adam's apple" or "pomus adamus," is a defining masculine secondary sexual characteristic.[11,22,27] Before puberty, there is no significant gender difference in laryngeal size. During puberty, the male larynx enlarges significantly, resulting in more projection in the anterior midline.[27] The male thyroid cartilage is more acute (90°), with a relatively thinner thyroid gland resulting in a bulkier appearance to the neck.[1,11,22,27] The female thyroid cartilage tends to be obtuse (120°), with a larger thyroid gland, subsequently creating a slender neck silhouette.[1,11,22,27]

Neck

A feminine neck is classically described as long and slender, whereas the masculine counterpart is described as short and stout. Anthropometric parameters of the neck demonstrated that the female neck is 18% more slender than the male neck (length/circumference).[28]

NONINVASIVE METHODS

Nonsurgical techniques for sculpting the lower face and neck are an established and safe alternative to invasive procedures.[29,13] Both facial feminization and masculinization are highly amenable to the use of injectables and can be an appealing option, particularly for patients in the process of gender reassignment. In recent years, there has been an increasing interest in noninvasive treatments within the transgender population.[30] This may be, in part, due to cost considerations, as injectables are generally more affordable than surgical options while still holding the potential to offer patients dramatic, though in most cases temporary, results. Additionally, injectables may be a good choice for transitioning patients who want to delay surgery until their therapy with exogenous hormones has reached its maximum effect.

Although the use of injectable neurotoxins and fillers is generally considered a quick and safe procedure, a thorough examination is still essential. When examining the lower face and neck, the patient should always be seated fully upright, as soft tissue is dynamic and may shift slightly depending on the positioning. Key points to consider during preoperative planning include position and prominence of the mandibular angle, length of the mandibular body, thickness of the skin and subcutaneous tissue, dimensions of the chin, and the degree of the cervicomental angle.[31,32] For both men and women, a gender-appropriate jawline with adequate chin projection is considered a standard of beauty.

Neurotoxin for Masseter Hypertrophy

Masseter hypertrophy in particular can result in a square-appearing face.[28] The goal of noninvasive procedures is to reduce this muscular hypertrophy to create a slim and smooth facial contour without the inherent risks of surgery.[33]

Neurotoxin is a broad term that describes a wide range of commercially available products that provide a temporary neuromuscular blockade resulting in local muscular atrophy. The efficacy of neurotoxin in reducing masseter volume is well documented and has been evidenced on ultrasound, computed tomography, and photographic images.[34–36]

After defining the muscle borders, a line should be marked from oral commissure to the tragus, with injections only given inferiorly to avoid overhallowing at the zygoma.[10] Injections should be focused over the area of maximum muscle bulge when the patient clenches the jaw.[32,37] The needle is inserted perpendicularly to the skin and advanced until bone is reached.[38] Two to 3 injection sites are typically evenly distributed across this area with the equivalent of 4 to 8 units of onabotulinumtoxinA injected at each point.[32,37,38] Historical studies have shown that 20 units of neurotoxin is the minimal effective dose for clinically significant masseter reduction, with the maximum reported dose being a total of 40 units per masseter.[32] However, smaller frequent doses have been shown to produce a better overall effect than large infrequent doses.[5] Patients are instructed to massage the area over the next 48 hours to distribute the toxin throughout the muscle.[38]

A clinically visible reduction in muscle mass is typically seen by 1 month after the initial injection, with maximum results observed at 3 months.[37] A total reduction of 22% to 30% of the muscular volume has been reported.[33,34] Effects typically persist for 6 to 9 months, after which time patients will need retreatment to maintain the desired state of reduction.[28,33] Two to 3 maintenance treatments per year is reasonable in the first year; however, increasing effects may be seen with each subsequent injection.[10,33] It has even been suggested that long-term injections may lead to a reduction in the mandibular angle from the decreased stress placed on the bone.[5]

Contraindications to any neurotoxin injection include medication hypersensitivity, soft tissue inflammation, diseases of the neuromuscular system, and coagulopathy.[38] Complications are typically minor and include dizziness, headache, or injection site pain. The risk of more serious complications increases as the dose of the neurotoxin increases.[37] Rare but serious complications include weakness with mastication, deep hematomas, hallowing of the infrazygomatic region, and asymmetric smile.[37]

Neurotoxin for Platysma Hypertrophy

Although less commonly used than other noninvasive treatments of the lower face and neck, injection of the platysma with a neurotoxin can be a very effective tool for feminization through softening of the jaw line and elongating the appearance of the neck.[39,40]

When administering the injections, the patient should contract the platysma to allow the physician to hold the muscle between the thumb and index finger.[39] The needle should be inserted to allow for intradermal injections of 2 to 4 equivalent units of onabotulinumtoxinA per injection site spaced every 2 cm running laterally.[39,41] The neck usually requires larger doses than other parts of the lower face and the specific amount should be correlated with the degree of muscular hypertrophy.[12,42] However, deep, high-volume injections must be avoided, as this may lead to dysphagia or life-threatening respiratory compromise.[3] The recommended dose for platysmal injections is a total dose of 15 to 40 units per side, but up to 100 units has been reported without apparent complications.[32,40,42] Asking patients to actively contract the muscle has been shown to increase the local uptake and prevent distant absorption.[42]

Neurotoxin for Mentalis Hypertrophy

Hypertrophy of the mentalis muscle can lead to the appearance of a thicker, more masculine chin, and although infrequently performed, injections into the mentalis can be accomplished with a single midline injection at the origin of both muscle bellies, approximately 1 cm above the inferior most point of the chin and no closer than 1.5 cm from the lower lip.[32] Using this technique, it is important to maintain the injection in the midline, as lateral deviation in either direction could lead to injury to the mental nerve or paralysis of the depressor labii inferioris muscle, causing smile asymmetry.[32]

An alternative technique also exists, in which an injection is placed into each individual muscle belly, approximately 2 mm above the inferior boarder of the mandible and 5 mm to the left or right of the midline.[40] Using either technique, an equivalent total dose of 4 to 8 units of onabotulinumtoxinA should be delivered.[32,40]

Soft Tissue Fillers for Mandibular Contouring

Soft tissue fillers are one of the most common noninvasive procedures performed and are a good option for facial sculpting and 3-dimensional contouring, particularly in patients desiring facial masculinization.[29,43] Artfully placed fillers at the mandibular body and angle can create a significantly defined jawline and masculine contour.[32] In general, fillers are considered safe and relatively simple to inject under topical or local anesthesia.[29,43] In the hands of skilled practitioners, results are predictable and adjustable, while consistently providing a natural aesthetic.[29]

Both permanent and nonpermanent fillers are currently available on the market.[29] Temporary fillers approved by the Food and Drug Administration (FDA) include collagen, hyaluronic acid, calcium hydroxylapatite, and poly-L-lactic acid, to name a few.[44] Although the application of certain commercial products in the lower face and neck is considered to be off-labeled in nature, they have a long track record of use in these areas with good safety and efficacy.[29] Currently, there is no need for pretesting for allergies, and there is a low incidence of nodule formation. In the case of hyaluronic acid, the results are reversible with hyaluronidase.[29] In contrast, there is a far more limited market for permanent fillers. At the time of this publication, polymethyl methacrylate is the only FDA-approved permanent filler, although there have been concerns about the product's displacement over time.[44] Silicone injections should never be performed in the face, or any part of the body.

Both preprocedure marking and filler injections should be performed with the patient upright in an effort to prevent overfilling, which can lead to a witches chin deformity.[45] Typically, fillers are placed at 2 or 3 sites at the chin apex and at 2 or 3 sites on each side of the mandibular body.[32] The physician begins by grasping the skin above the mandible and injecting a temporary filler into the subcuticular space using a linear retrograde technique.[32] For permanent fillers, a deep tunneling supraperiosteal technique directed toward the midline is used with a slow injection, as this area is prone to deep hematomas.[32,46]

Several passes of the cannula at each injection site may be needed with small-volume boluses administered and subsequently massaged to prevent nodule formation.[31] It is important to constantly reassess for facial symmetry before and after each injection.[32] Dosing is specific to the product used and physicians should refer to individual manufacturer recommendations to decide the appropriate amount for optimal chin augmentation and mandibular contouring.[46]

Patients should also be counseled about possible complications. Allergic reactions to hyaluronic acid are rare but can occur, as can embolization of facial vessels, leading to local ischemic injury or blindness. Embolization can be temporized, in part, with injections of hyaluronidase, and it is generally recommended that physicians maintain a supply of hyaluronidase in their office for such occasions. More common side effects include swelling and bruising at the injection site, and pain with mastication.[29,31,46] Most minor complications resolve spontaneously within 4 to 8 days but more serious complications can persist, specifically with the use of permanent fillers.[46] In some cases, overcorrection with a permanent filler can result in superficial irregularities that can be improved via needle aspiration, but more serious changes can also occur, even years after the injections were placed.[46–49] Delayed presentation of large nodules or fluid-filled cysts have been reported, along with migration of the filler product from the site of the initial injection.[47] If there are concerns for these adverse changes, advanced imaging should be considered to allow for early detection, because surgical correction at the later stages can carry significant morbidity.[47]

In summary, neurotoxins to induce muscle paralysis are more commonly used for facial feminization and facial fillers along the jaw line are more commonly used for masculinization.

INVASIVE METHODS
Mandibular Contouring

As discussed previously, several anatomic components are responsible for mandibular gender characteristics, and although surgical alteration of the masseter has fallen out of favor, it is generally accepted that bony manipulation of the angle is a powerful maneuver to alter this aesthetic.[26]

The pogonion and menton are also aesthetically relevant regions of the lower facial third that can be altered to bring about features that are consistent with a patient's perceived gender (**Fig. 2**).

Before any bony manipulation, however, sound craniofacial principles of reviewing radiographs (Panorex/lateral cephalogram) or computed

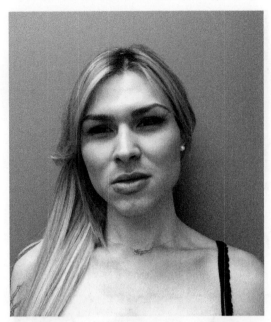

Fig. 2. Preoperative photograph demonstrating increased mandibular bi-gonal width, before mandibular reduction.

tomography images should be observed, in addition to evaluating for occlusal anomalies (see **Fig. 2**). Injury to the inferior alveolar nerve is not inconsequential, and thorough analysis of preoperative images will help reduce this risk.

Mandibular angle shave
Mandibular angle shave allows for narrowing of the coronal profile of the lower facial third and facilitates a smooth transition to the upper neck. It can be performed with local anesthesia, but nasotracheal intubation under general anesthesia allows for a more controlled operation. Hypotensive anesthesia and local anesthetic with vasoconstrictors will optimize visualization in the surgical field.[1] In addition, consideration should be given to intravenous steroids to aid with edema. A mucosal incision distal to the parotid duct, just lateral to the anterior ramus of the mandible, will allow direct surgical access. The buccinator muscle will be noted to originate from the oblique ridge of the mandible, posterior to which the pterygomasseteric sling will be identified. Care must be taken to avoid violation of buccinator, as release of the buccal fat pad will compromise visualization. A subperiosteal dissection is performed to elevate the masseter from the lateral and inferior surface of the mandible (**Fig. 3**). Reference should be made to the previously reviewed location of the inferior alveolar canal in relation to the mandibular border, to ensure safe but sufficient osteotomy of

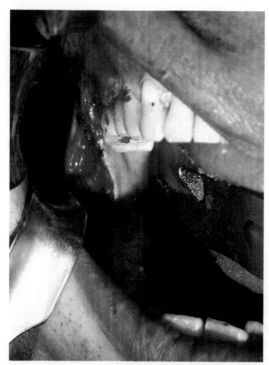

Fig. 3. Intraoperative photograph of exposure to right mandibular angle during mandibular angle reduction.

the angle. A reciprocating saw blade is positioned to perform an oblique osteotomy of the angle. It is important to not only shorten the vertical height of the mandibular angle, but to also narrow the bigonial distance with these cuts. If sharp edges remain, a burr is used to contour these down (**Fig. 4**). The incision should then be closed in layers, and the patient placed on a soft diet postoperatively (**Fig. 5**).

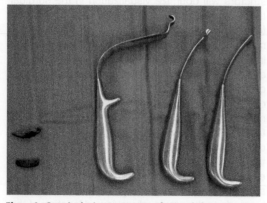

Fig. 4. Surgical instruments from bilateral split sagittal osteotomy tray used for angle reduction and osteotomized fragments of bone removed.

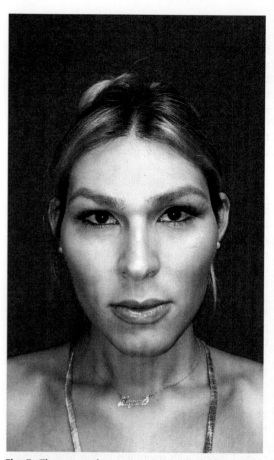

Fig. 5. Three months postoperative photograph after bilateral mandibular angle reduction.

Mandibular angle augmentation

Augmentation of the mandibular angle is a useful maneuver to provide more distinction and separation to the lower face and the neck. This can be achieved using alloplastic or autologous sources.

Alloplastic implants come from an array of sources; these include methylmethacrylate, silicone, titanium, and polyethylene to name a few. All of these materials have inherent properties that make them either favorable or unfavorable based on surgeon preference, the scope of which exceeds the purpose of this article. Regardless of the type of implant used, patient factors, including comorbidities, hygiene, and desired aesthetics should be considered. Although both an external or intraoral approach can be used to access the angle, an intraoral approach (similar to that described previously) is generally considered to be aesthetically superior, despite an increased risk for contamination. Another tenet to implant placement is ensuring that pocket dissection is just large enough to accommodate the prosthesis; failing to do so will increase the risk for postoperative malposition. The pocket created is usually placed medial to the masseter and lateral to the mandible, in a subperiosteal plane.

If surgeon preference or patient criteria preclude the use of alloplastic material, autologous calvarial bone grafts are a useful alternative. Although the soft tissue approach is generally the same, the plane of placement can be altered. Specifically, a ramus/angle-splitting osteotomy can be performed to create space within the cancellous bone for the graft. Autologous grafts have the advantage of decreased risk of infection, although potential resorption should be given consideration.

Genioplasty (Chin)

As mentioned previously, the relative width and protrusion of the chin has implications on perceived gender association. This can be manipulated via osteotomies or use of alloplastic implants. The size of the chin in relation to the face also should be noted. Generally, the chin is recognized as the portion of the lower face starting at the labiomental crease extending inferiorly to menton. In addition to being wider and having more projection, cis-males also usually have 2 points of light reflection, while cis-females have one.[27]

Osseous genioplasty
A mucosal incision is made in the gingivobuccal sulcus, preserving mucosa for closure (**Fig. 6**). The mentalis muscle is divided, while taking care to not traumatize the mental nerves. Depending on the desired movement of the mandible, a marking is made 5 mm inferior to the canine root and 6 mm below the mental nerve. A wedge can be removed to shorten the chin vertically, oblique osteotomies will facilitate creation of either a more or less pronounced chin depending on the trajectory, and horizontal osteotomies will increase or decrease the sagittal projection of the chin. The midline of the pogonion also can be divided vertically to allow for expansion and the creation of a wider-appearing chin. Fixation with titanium plates is used to maintain the new position. It is crucial to resuspend the mentalis muscle to prevent a "witch's chin" deformity.

Alloplast genioplasty
If a surgeon is not comfortable the aforementioned osteotomies, alloplastic material is a good alternative. Similar to mandibular angle augmentation, implants can be used to augment the chin. An intraoral approach is more favorable; however, a submental incision may be used alternatively.

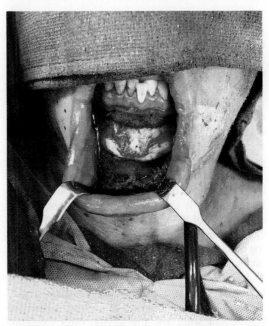

Fig. 6. Intraoperative photograph of prominent pogonion of cis-male mandible, as seen during intraoral approach for genioplasty.

The implant is tailored to the desired size, and secured to the menton with screws after a subperiosteal dissection is created.

Thyroid Cartilage

Surgical alteration of this structure is feasible and safe, but like other procedures, a strong command of the associated anatomy is paramount to success. Thyroid cartilage is crucial to the laryngeal function. It functions as the major domain for phonatory and respiratory tasks. The vocal cords insert on the inner surface of the thyroid cartilage, and are usually described as inserting at the midway point between the superior and inferior thyroid notch in male individuals. This insertion is displaced to the junction of the upper and middle third in female individuals. Disruption of vocal fold insertion at the anterior commissure can have devastating consequences, as it is not easily fixed, and can result in permanent and irreversible changes in pitch. This should be considered when performing chondrolaryngoplasty.

Chondrolaryngoplasty
This involves contouring the superior and anterior margins of the cartilage to decrease the stigmata of a cis-male neck. The incision can be placed directly over the thyroid cartilage if there is a prominent horizontal rhytid, however a submental incision is generally more pleasing.[27]

After the incision is made, the midline raphe of the strap muscles is divided vertically to allow for lateral retraction and exposure of the thyroid cartilage. Care should be taken to maintain midline dissection, as the internal and external laryngeal nerves enter the larynx laterally, and violation can result in laryngeal sensory loss or cricothyroid dysfunction with associated changes in pitch. Once the thyroid cartilage is identified, the perichondrium is incised and elevated anteriorly and posteriorly. This is carried out to approximately 1 cm below the superior margin or no more than half the distance between the superior and inferior borders. This is important to prevent inadvertent disinsertion of the vocal folds with cartilage excision. Instruments are then used to carefully excise the cartilage, which can be challenging if calcification is present. In our experience, we have found that Rongeurs work well; however, mechanical burrs, knives, and rasps may also be used. Extreme caution should be exercised to prevent inadvertent entry into the larynx. After excision, the strap muscles are re-approximated, and the skin closed in layers. We generally do not leave a drain; however, this is surgeon dependent (**Figs. 7** and **8**).

Thyroid cartilage masculinization
Augmentation of the thyroid cartilage in transmales was recently described by Deschamps-Braly and colleagues.[50] This technique has been reported to be useful to create a more prominent thyroid notch, which might be desired by some patients. The procedure uses costochondral cartilage, usually

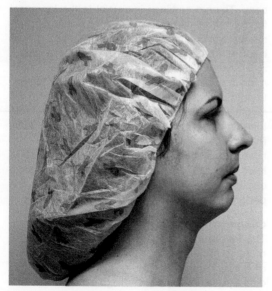

Fig. 7. Preoperative photograph before chondrolaryngoplasty.

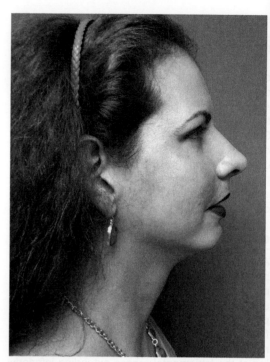

Fig. 8. Four months postoperative after chondrolaryngoplasty.

accessed through a prior mastectomy incision. The cartilage is then contoured with a #11 blade, secured to the existing thyroid cartilage with permanent sutures. The access to the thyroid cartilage is similar to that described previously. At the time of this publication, their group described a 6-month follow-up, with no notable resorption nor complications.

RHYTIDECTOMY

In general, male-to-female patients older than 35 should be advised that after mandible contouring, mandible angle reduction, and reduction genioplasty, there is a high chance that jowling may occur. In younger patients, this tissue will retract, but with an older patient population, there is a propensity for the tissue to remain lax. This will result in undesirable results, obscuring the results of the lower face bony contouring. This will be a pertinent issue particularly in older patients who have undergone a significant degree of bony reduction. If unsightly laxity exists postoperatively, then a face/neck lift should be performed to correct the iatrogenic jowling, typically at 6 to 12 months after the facial feminization (**Figs. 9** and **10**). It is advisable to stage the procedures. A facelift could be performed at the same time as the mandible contouring and genioplasty; however, this may result in unpredictable results.

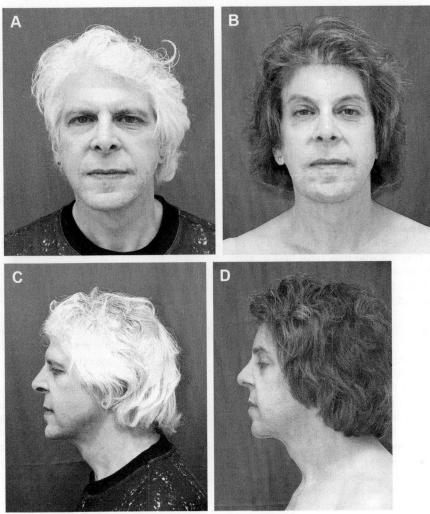

Fig. 9. (*A*) Anteroposterior (AP) view: pre-facial feminization surgery (FFS). (*B*) AP view: post-FFS. (*C*) Lateral view: pre-FFS. (*D*) Lateral view: post-FFS.

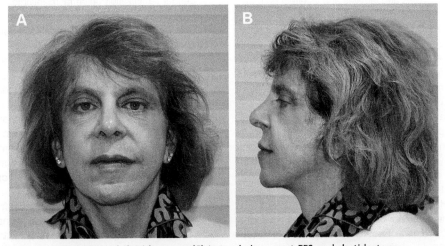

Fig. 10. (*A*) AP view: post-FFS and rhytidectomy. (*B*) Lateral view: post-FFS and rhytidectomy.

Components of the skin, subcutaneous fat, pre-platysmal fat, platysma, and subplatysmal fat should be carefully analyzed for each patient. Facial deflation should be assessed, and concomitant fat transfer can be considered. If the patient has not undergone permanent hair removal of the face, advise her to do this preoperatively, and to postpone any procedures 2 weeks before the operation. Patients are advised that they can resume hair removal at 6 weeks postoperatively. Incision placement should be discussed in detail with patients, and should be individualized based on how they wear their hair, and how much skin laxity they may have. In general, incisions at the hairline (both temporally and in occipital region) are preferred if a significant degree of skin excision is expected to prevent unsightly displacement of the hair. For patients who may have had a prior hairline advancement and open browlift, the temporal incision can be incorporated into this prior scar to prevent additional scars.

REFERENCES

1. Hage JJ, Becking AG, de Graaf FH, et al. Gender-confirming facial surgery: considerations on the masculinity and femininity of faces. Plast Reconstr Surg 1997;99(7):1799–807.
2. Shams MG, Motamedi MH. Case report: feminizing the male face. Eplasty 2009;9:e2.
3. Tsukahara K, Hotta M, Osanai O, et al. Gender-dependent differences in degree of facial wrinkles. Skin Res Technol 2013;19(1):e65–71.
4. Dao H Jr, Kazin RA. Gender differences in skin: a review of the literature. Gend Med 2007;4(4):308–28.
5. Whitton JT, Everall JD. The thickness of the epidermis. Br J Dermatol 1973;89(5):467–76.
6. Shigeta Y, Enciso R, Ogawa T, et al. Cervical CT derived neck fat tissue distribution differences in Japanese males and females and its effect on retroglossal and retropalatal airway volume. Oral Surg Oral Med Oral Pathol Oral Radiol Endod 2008;106(2):275–84.
7. Whittle AT, Marshall I, Mortimore IL, et al. Neck soft tissue and fat distribution: comparison between normal men and women by magnetic resonance imaging. Thorax 1999;54(4):323–8.
8. Bredella MA. Sex differences in body composition. Adv Exp Med Biol 2017;1043:9–27.
9. Janssen I, Heymsfield SB, Wang ZM, et al. Skeletal muscle mass and distribution in 468 men and women aged 18-88 yr. J Appl Physiol (1985) 2000;89(1):81–8.
10. Kim NH, Park RH, Park JB. Botulinum toxin type A for the treatment of hypertrophy of the masseter muscle. Plast Reconstr Surg 2010;125(6):1693–705.
11. Morrison SD, Vyas KS, Motakef S, et al. Facial feminization: systematic review of the literature. Plast Reconstr Surg 2016;137(6):1759–70.
12. de Almeida ART, Romiti A, Carruthers JDA. The facial platysma and its underappreciated role in lower face dynamics and contour. Dermatol Surg 2017;43(8):1042–9.
13. Kane MAC. Injectable and resurfacing techniques: botulinum toxin (BoNT-A). In: Rubin JP, editor. Plastic surgery: aesthetic surgery, vol. 2, 4th edition. New York: Elsevier Inc; 2018.
14. Guerrerosantos J. Managing platysma bands in the aging neck. Aesthet Surg J 2008;28(2):211–6.
15. Etcoff N. Survival of the prettiest: the science of beauty. New York: Anchor Books; 2000.
16. Zheng L, Siegmund G, Ozyigit G, et al. Sex-specific prediction of neck muscle volumes. J Biomech 2013;46(5):899–904.
17. Rankin G, Stokes M, Newham DJ. Size and shape of the posterior neck muscles measured by ultrasound imaging: normal values in males and females of different ages. Man Ther 2005;10(2):108–15.
18. Scott J. Age, sex and contralateral differences in the volumes of human submandibular salivary glands. Arch Oral Biol 1975;20(12):885–7.
19. Inoue H, Ono K, Masuda W, et al. Gender difference in unstimulated whole saliva flow rate and salivary gland sizes. Arch Oral Biol 2006;51(12):1055–60.
20. Plemons ED. Description of sex difference as prescription for sex change: on the origins of facial feminization surgery. Soc Stud Sci 2014;44(5):657–79.
21. Giles E. Sex determination by discriminant function analysis of the mandible. Am J Phys Anthropol 1964;22:129–35.
22. Altman K. Facial feminization surgery: current state of the art. Int J Oral Maxillofac Surg 2012;41(8):885–94.
23. Becking AG, Tuinzing DB, Hage JJ, et al. Transgender feminization of the facial skeleton. Clin Plast Surg 2007;34(3):557–64.
24. Spiegel JH. Facial determinants of female gender and feminizing forehead cranioplasty. Laryngoscope 2011;121(2):250–61.
25. Bruce V, Burton AM, Hanna E, et al. Sex discrimination: how do we tell the difference between male and female faces? Perception 1993;22(2):131–52.
26. Habal MB. Aesthetics of feminizing the male face by craniofacial contouring of the facial bones. Aesthetic Plast Surg 1990;14(2):143–50.
27. Wolfort FG, Dejerine ES, Ramos DJ, et al. Chondrolaryngoplasty for appearance. Plast Reconstr Surg 1990;86(3):464–9 [discussion: 470].
28. Vasavada AN, Danaraj J, Siegmund GP. Head and neck anthropometry, vertebral geometry and neck strength in height-matched men and women. J Biomech 2008;41(1):114–21.

29. Lee DH, Jin SP, Cho S, et al. RimabotulinumtoxinB versus OnabotulinumtoxinA in the treatment of masseter hypertrophy: a 24-week double-blind randomized split-face study. Dermatology 2013; 226(3):227–32.

30. Ballin AC, Brandt FS, Cazzaniga A. Dermal fillers: an update. Am J Clin Dermatol 2015;16(4):271–83.

31. Ginsberg BA, Calderon M, Seminara NM, et al. A potential role for the dermatologist in the physical transformation of transgender people: a survey of attitudes and practices within the transgender community. J Am Acad Dermatol 2016;74(2):303–8.

32. Moradi A, Watson J. Current concepts in filler injection. Facial Plast Surg Clin North Am 2015;23(4): 489–94.

33. de Maio M, Wu WTL, Goodman GJ, et al, Alliance for the Future of Aesthetics Consensus Committee. Facial assessment and injection guide for botulinum toxin and injectable hyaluronic acid fillers: focus on the lower face. Plast Reconstr Surg 2017;140(3): 393e–404e.

34. Wu WT. Botox facial slimming/facial sculpting: the role of botulinum toxin-A in the treatment of hypertrophic masseteric muscle and parotid enlargement to narrow the lower facial width. Facial Plast Surg Clin North Am 2010;18(1):133–40.

35. Klein FH, Brenner FM, Sato MS, et al. Lower facial remodeling with botulinum toxin type A for the treatment of masseter hypertrophy. An Bras Dermatol 2014;89(6):878–84.

36. Bae JH, Choi DY, Lee JG, et al. The risorius muscle: anatomic considerations with reference to botulinum neurotoxin injection for masseteric hypertrophy. Dermatol Surg 2014;40(12):1334–9.

37. Nguyen-Michel VH, Levy PP, Pallanca O, et al. Underperception of naps in older adults referred for a sleep assessment: an insomnia trait and a cognitive problem? J Am Geriatr Soc 2015;63(10): 2001–7.

38. Quezada-Gaon N, Wortsman X, Penaloza O, et al. Comparison of clinical marking and ultrasound-guided injection of Botulinum type A toxin into the masseter muscles for treating bruxism and its cosmetic effects. J Cosmet Dermatol 2016;15(3): 238–44.

39. Xie Y, Zhou J, Li H, et al. Classification of masseter hypertrophy for tailored botulinum toxin type A treatment. Plast Reconstr Surg 2014;134(2):209e–18e.

40. Andrade NN, Deshpande GS. Use of botulinum toxin (botox) in the management of masseter muscle hypertrophy: a simplified technique. Plast Reconstr Surg 2011;128(1):24e–6e.

41. Levy PM. Neurotoxins: current concepts in cosmetic use on the face and neck–jawline contouring/platysma bands/necklace lines. Plast Reconstr Surg 2015;136(5 Suppl):80S–3S.

42. Gart MS, Gutowski KA. Overview of botulinum toxins for aesthetic uses. Clin Plast Surg 2016;43(3): 459–71.

43. Matarasso A, Matarasso SL. Botulinum A exotoxin for the management of platysma bands. Plast Reconstr Surg 2003;112(5 Suppl):138S–40S.

44. Kane MA. Nonsurgical treatment of platysmal bands with injection of botulinum toxin A. Plast Reconstr Surg 1999;103(2):656–63 [discussion: 664–5].

45. Sykes JM, Fitzgerald R. Choosing the best procedure to augment the chin: is anything better than an implant? Facial Plast Surg 2016;32(5):507–12.

46. Chuang J, Barnes C, Wong BJF. Overview of facial plastic surgery and current developments. Surg J (N Y) 2016;2(1):e17–28.

47. Jansen DA, Graivier MH. Evaluation of a calcium hydroxylapatite-based implant (Radiesse) for facial soft-tissue augmentation. Plast Reconstr Surg 2006;118(3 Suppl):22S–30S [discussion: 31S–33S].

48. Belmontesi M, Grover R, Verpaele A. Transdermal injection of Restylane SubQ for aesthetic contouring of the cheeks, chin, and mandible. Aesthet Surg J 2006;26(1S):S28–34.

49. Liu HL, Cheung WY. Complications of polyacrylamide hydrogel (PAAG) injection in facial augmentation. J Plast Reconstr Aesthet Surg 2010;63(1): e9–12.

50. Deschamps-Braly JC, Sacher CL, Fick J, et al. First female to male confirmation surgery with description of new procedure for masculinization of the thyroid cartilage. Plast Reconstr Surg 2017;139(4):883e–7e.

Statement of Ownership, Management, and Circulation
(All Periodicals Publications Except Requester Publications)

UNITED STATES POSTAL SERVICE

1. Publication Title	2. Publication Number	3. Filing Date
CLINICS IN PLASTIC SURGERY	006 – 530	9/18/2018

4. Issue Frequency	5. Number of Issues Published Annually	6. Annual Subscription Price
JAN, APR, JUL, OCT	4	$525.00

7. Complete Mailing Address of Known Office of Publication *(Not printer) (Street, city, county, state, and ZIP+4®)*
ELSEVIER INC.
230 Park Avenue, Suite 800
New York, NY 10169

Contact Person
STEPHEN R. BUSHING

Telephone *(Include area code)*
215-239-3688

8. Complete Mailing Address of Headquarters or General Business Office of Publisher *(Not printer)*
ELSEVIER INC.
230 Park Avenue, Suite 800
New York, NY 10169

9. Full Names and Complete Mailing Addresses of Publisher, Editor, and Managing Editor *(Do not leave blank)*

Publisher *(Name and complete mailing address)*
TAYLOR E. BALL, ELSEVIER INC.
1600 JOHN F KENNEDY BLVD. SUITE 1800
PHILADELPHIA, PA 19103-2899

Editor *(Name and complete mailing address)*
JESSICA MCCOOL, ELSEVIER INC.
1600 JOHN F KENNEDY BLVD. SUITE 1800
PHILADELPHIA, PA 19103-2899

Managing Editor *(Name and complete mailing address)*
PATRICK MANLEY, ELSEVIER INC.
1600 JOHN F KENNEDY BLVD. SUITE 1800
PHILADELPHIA, PA 19103-2899

10. Owner *(Do not leave blank. If the publication is owned by a corporation, give the name and address of the corporation immediately followed by the names and addresses of all stockholders owning or holding 1 percent or more of the total amount of stock. If not owned by a corporation, give the names and addresses of the individual owners. If owned by a partnership or other unincorporated firm, give its name and address as well as those of each individual owner. If the publication is published by a nonprofit organization, give its name and address.)*

Full Name	Complete Mailing Address
WHOLLY OWNED SUBSIDIARY OF REED/ELSEVIER, US HOLDINGS	1600 JOHN F KENNEDY BLVD. SUITE 1800 PHILADELPHIA, PA 19103-2899

11. Known Bondholders, Mortgagees, and Other Security Holders Owning or Holding 1 Percent or More of Total Amount of Bonds, Mortgages, or Other Securities. If none, check box ▶ ☐ None

Full Name	Complete Mailing Address
N/A	

12. Tax Status *(For completion by nonprofit organizations authorized to mail at nonprofit rates) (Check one)*
The purpose, function, and nonprofit status of this organization and the exempt status for federal income tax purposes:
☒ Has Not Changed During Preceding 12 Months
☐ Has Changed During Preceding 12 Months *(Publisher must submit explanation of change with this statement)*

PS Form **3526**, July 2014 *(Page 1 of 4 (see instructions page 4))* PSN: 7530-01-000-9931 **PRIVACY NOTICE:** See our privacy policy on www.usps.com.

---

13. Publication Title	14. Issue Date for Circulation Data Below
CLINICS IN PLASTIC SURGERY	JULY 2018

15. Extent and Nature of Circulation		Average No. Copies Each Issue During Preceding 12 Months	No. Copies of Single Issue Published Nearest to Filing Date
a. Total Number of Copies *(Net press run)*		258	418
b. Paid Circulation *(By Mail and Outside the Mail)*	(1) Mailed Outside-County Paid Subscriptions Stated on PS Form 3541 (Include paid distribution above nominal rate, advertiser's proof copies, and exchange copies)	124	183
	(2) Mailed In-County Paid Subscriptions Stated on PS Form 3541 (Include paid distribution above nominal rate, advertiser's proof copies, and exchange copies)	0	0
	(3) Paid Distribution Outside the Mails Including Sales Through Dealers and Carriers, Street Vendors, Counter Sales, and Other Paid Distribution Outside USPS®	65	125
	(4) Paid Distribution by Other Classes of Mail Through the USPS (e.g., First-Class Mail®)	0	0
c. Total Paid Distribution *(Sum of 15b (1), (2), (3), and (4))*	▶	189	308
d. Free or Nominal Rate Distribution *(By Mail and Outside the Mail)*	(1) Free or Nominal Rate Outside-County Copies included on PS Form 3541	54	83
	(2) Free or Nominal Rate In-County Copies Included on PS Form 3541	0	0
	(3) Free or Nominal Rate Copies Mailed at Other Classes Through the USPS (e.g., First-Class Mail)	0	0
	(4) Free or Nominal Rate Distribution Outside the Mail (Carriers or other means)	54	83
e. Total Free or Nominal Rate Distribution *(Sum of 15d (1), (2), (3) and (4))*	▶	54	83
f. Total Distribution *(Sum of 15c and 15e)*	▶	243	391
g. Copies not Distributed *(See Instructions to Publishers #4 (page 3))*	▶	15	27
h. Total *(Sum of 15f and 15g)*	▶	258	418
i. Percent Paid *(15c divided by 15f times 100)*	▶	77.78%	78.77%

* If you are claiming electronic copies, go to line 16 on page 3. If you are not claiming electronic copies, skip to line 17 on page 3.

16. Electronic Copy Circulation		Average No. Copies Each Issue During Preceding 12 Months	No. Copies of Single Issue Published Nearest to Filing Date
a. Paid Electronic Copies	▶	0	0
b. Total Paid Print Copies (Line 15c) + Paid Electronic Copies (Line 16a)	▶	189	308
c. Total Print Distribution (Line 15f) + Paid Electronic Copies (Line 16a)	▶	243	391
d. Percent Paid (Both Print & Electronic Copies) (16b divided by 16c × 100)	▶	77.78%	78.77%

☒ I certify that 50% of all my distributed copies (electronic and print) are paid above a nominal price.

17. Publication of Statement of Ownership
☒ If the publication is a general publication, publication of this statement is required. Will be printed in the OCTOBER 2018 issue of this publication. ☐ Publication not required.

18. Signature and Title of Editor, Publisher, Business Manager, or Owner

STEPHEN R. BUSHING – INVENTORY DISTRIBUTION CONTROL MANAGER

Date 9/18/2018

I certify that all information furnished on this form is true and complete. I understand that anyone who furnishes false or misleading information on this form or who omits material or information requested on the form may be subject to criminal sanctions (including fines and imprisonment) and/or civil sanctions (including civil penalties).

PS Form **3526**, July 2014 *(Page 3 of 4)* **PRIVACY NOTICE:** See our privacy policy on www.usps.com.

Moving?

Make sure your subscription moves with you!

To notify us of your new address, find your **Clinics Account Number** (located on your mailing label above your name), and contact customer service at:

Email: journalscustomerservice-usa@elsevier.com

800-654-2452 (subscribers in the U.S. & Canada)
314-447-8871 (subscribers outside of the U.S. & Canada)

Fax number: 314-447-8029

Elsevier Health Sciences Division
Subscription Customer Service
3251 Riverport Lane
Maryland Heights, MO 63043

*To ensure uninterrupted delivery of your subscription, please notify us at least 4 weeks in advance of move.

Printed and bound by CPI Group (UK) Ltd, Croydon, CR0 4YY

08/05/2025

01864729-0003